Studies in Big Data

Volume 23

Series editor

Janusz Kacprzyk, Polish Academy of Sciences, Warsaw, Poland
e-mail: kacprzyk@ibspan.waw.pl

About this Series

The series "Studies in Big Data" (SBD) publishes new developments and advances in the various areas of Big Data-quickly and with a high quality. The intent is to cover the theory, research, development, and applications of Big Data, as embedded in the fields of engineering, computer science, physics, economics and life sciences. The books of the series refer to the analysis and understanding of large, complex, and/or distributed data sets generated from recent digital sources coming from sensors or other physical instruments as well as simulations, crowd sourcing, social networks or other internet transactions, such as emails or video click streams and other. The series contains monographs, lecture notes and edited volumes in Big Data spanning the areas of computational intelligence incl. neural networks, evolutionary computation, soft computing, fuzzy systems, as well as artificial intelligence, data mining, modern statistics and Operations research, as well as self-organizing systems. Of particular value to both the contributors and the readership are the short publication timeframe and the world-wide distribution, which enable both wide and rapid dissemination of research output.

More information about this series at http://www.springer.com/series/11970

Chintan Bhatt · Nilanjan Dey
Amira S. Ashour
Editors

Internet of Things and Big Data Technologies for Next Generation Healthcare

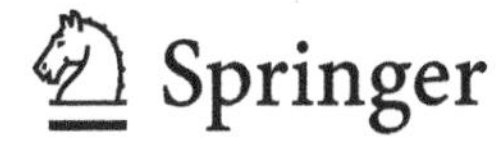

Editors
Chintan Bhatt
U & P U Patel Department of Computer Engineering
Charotar University of Science and Technology
Changa
India

Amira S. Ashour
Faculty of Engineering
Tanta University
Tanta
Egypt

Nilanjan Dey
Department of Information Technology
Techno India College of Technology
Kolkata
India

ISSN 2197-6503 ISSN 2197-6511 (electronic)
Studies in Big Data
ISBN 978-3-319-84228-8 ISBN 978-3-319-49736-5 (eBook)
DOI 10.1007/978-3-319-49736-5

Printed on acid-free paper

This Springer imprint is published by Springer Nature
The registered company is Springer International Publishing AG
The registered company address is: Gewerbestrasse 11, 6330 Cham, Switzerland

Preface

Internet of things (IoT) devices and services will guide healthcare toward new generation of proficient services while saving time and lives with high accuracy. Continuous progress in remote healthcare domain leads to the invention of wireless devices. Nowadays, a comprehensive view of the patient's overall health can be obtained through prototypes of the next generation emergency rooms. IoT technology facilitates the intercommunication and can alert the hospital staff based on the patient's vitals. It transforms the healthcare industry to more efficient, low cost and better patient care systems generation. Concurrently, the current era is filled with milestone improvements in the healthcare technology that has resulted in big data world. Big data is characterized by volume, variety, velocity and veracity. Big data and IoT are topical emerging technologies that attract focus from several researchers and engineers to develop the next generation of smarter connected devices/products. In addition, embedded medical devices are spreading to provide accessible information anywhere in the world. Healthcare organizations use the continuous engineering potential to design powerful future. They are intimately connected with enormous Internet-connected things/devices that generate massive amounts of data. Superior healthcare outcome is the foremost objective shared by hospitals, clinics and health organizations around the world. Healthcare combined with IoT drives the innovation of medical services along with cost reduction, accuracy improvement, and wide spread of the healthcare services to more population. Recently, healthcare stakeholders directed their attention toward big data analysis to support the healthcare sector instead of developing only automated medical systems, and digitizing medical records. Big data has the potential to assist healthcare organizations to equip providers with the necessary tools for better healthcare. The IoT healthcare devices acquire medical information in the form of signals and/or images. These acquired big data from the IoT requires analysis for accurate diagnosis. This provides the healthcare organizations with the required detailed data to achieve effective population health management. An unprecedented level of real-time data can be obtained by intelligent systems. Meanwhile, big data runs on open-source technologies with inconsistent security schemes. Thus, healthcare organizations have to ensure superior big data security.

This book consists of 15 chapters, including an intensive introduction about the IoT in healthcare with challenging topics followed by five chapters that reported various aspects in the IoT domain. These chapters addressed the 5th generation of IoT communication technology based medical body area network along with the nanotechnology in the IoT. In addition, the energy efficient network architecture for IoT health care applications including the major factors that affect energy efficiency to improve energy efficiency in IoT network is introduced. A novel strategic framework and computationally intelligent model to measure possible vulnerabilities for security context in e-health with the long term benefits in healthcare sector, medical emergencies, and e-health using robotics and IoT are reported. Furthermore, an overview regarding the importance of IoT in healthcare focusing on the proposed IoT solutions for smart services provided by an m-Health system is introduced. Moreover, the book contains another set of chapters that interested with the health care systems management for large amounts of data, which are driven by the patients' records and health/personal information. These chapters proposed Big Data based knowledge management system to develop the clinical decisions, and presented the storing/processing of big data using available tools, technologies and algorithms along with a case study in healthcare analytics. Thereafter, concepts of co-creation and co-production of knowledge in the field of global change and sustainable development linked to transdisciplinary and citizen's science was proposed along with introducing a case study of a preliminary early warning system based on a biometeorological model and a technological platform. Afterward, three chapters several health bioinformatics topics are introduced, prefering picture over the information/communication emerging technology enabling healthcare innovation through big data perspective, the HIaaS details in cloud along with cloud based architecture for hosting e-health services, and detailed illustration for wireless body area networks (WBAN) architectural analysis in healthcare domain. Big data in healthcare and risks involved in using social media for healthcare have been discussed to caution its usage as well as tumor segmentation has been implemented by extracting histogram and training support vector machine (SVM) for tumor detection. Finally, graphic processing units (GPU) and kinetic sensor devices for IoT computing environments in various application domains including mobile healthcare has been discussed. A novel training/testing process for building/testing a classification model for unusual human activities (UHA) using ensembles of neural networks running on NVIDIA GPUs is proposed.

This book concerns the IoT's big data analysis in healthcare domain supported by the research efforts. It addresses the difficulties and challenges that developing countries face in implementing IoT based healthcare systems and applications. This book aims to improve the understanding of the valuable role of the big data along with the IoT to improve the healthcare system in a specific context to the research community. It interests with measuring the progress and evaluates the newly developed systems' weaknesses. It includes comprehensive publications in the field of IoT and big data in healthcare. Trust, privacy, security issues, IoT and big data challenges, and related topics are addressed. This book provides interesting topics on recent IoT and big data devices. Moreover, it highlights the advanced improvement fields to guide the engineers developing different IoT devices as well as evaluating the different IoT techniques' performance. Additionally, the book explores the impact of such technologies on public, private, community, and hybrid scenarios in healthcare.

Essentially, this volume cannot be in this outstanding form without the promising group of authors' contributions to whom we offer our appreciation. Moreover, it was incredible to realize this quality without the impact of the anonymous referees who supported us during the revision and acceptance process of the submitted chapters. Our appreciation is extended to them for their diligence in reviewing the chapters. Special thanks are directed to our publisher, Springer, for the endless guidance and support.

We hope this book presents comprehensive concepts and outstanding research results to support further development of IoT and big data in the healthcare applications.

Changa, India — Chintan Bhatt
Kolkata, India — Nilanjan Dey
Tanta, Egypt — Amira S. Ashour

Contents

Part I
IoT Based Healthcare

Internet of Things Driven Connected Healthcare

Nilanjan Dey, Amira S. Ashour and Chintan Bhatt

Abstract The Internet of Things (IoT) is a physical device along with other items network that embedded with software, electronics, network connectivity, and sensors to collect objects in order to exchange data. The IoT impact in healthcare is still in its initial development phases. The IoT system has several layers that lead to implementation challenges where many engaged devices have sensors to collect data. Each has its manufacturer own exclusive protocols. These protocols using software environment associated with privacy and security raise new challenges in the IoT technology. This current chapter attempts to understand and review the IoT concept and healthcare applications to realize superior healthcare with affordable costs. The chapter included in brief the IoT functionality and its association with the sensing and wireless techniques to implement the required healthcare applications.

Keywords Internet of Things · Big data · IoT architecture · Sensor layer · Healthcare · Wide area network

---

N. Dey (✉)
Department of Information Technology, Techno India College of Technology,
Kolkata, India
e-mail: neelanjan.dey@gmail.com

A.S. Ashour
Department of Electronics and Electrical Communications Engineering,
Faculty of Engineering, Tanta University, Tanta, Egypt
e-mail: amirasashour@yahoo.com

C. Bhatt
U & P U Patel Department of Computer Engineering,
Charotar University of Science and Technology (CHARUSAT), Changa,
Gujarat, India
e-mail: chintanbhatt.ce@charusat.ac.in

C. Bhatt et al. (eds.), *Internet of Things and Big Data Technologies for Next Generation Healthcare*, Studies in Big Data 23,
DOI 10.1007/978-3-319-49736-5_1

1 Introduction

Information technologies and medicine convergence transforms healthcare to more advanced generations with accurate and efficient services. Such conjunction is developed through the Internet of Things (IoT) technology that has significant impact in medicine and healthcare applications. IoT consists of physical devices network along with embedded devices, sensors, software, and network connectivity to collect such system components for data exchange [1]. It can be defined as connecting objects/devices such as Internet TVs, smart phones, and sensors to the Internet in order to link the devices together in an intelligent way to enable new communication forms between devices, system components, and people [2]. The IoT integrates traditional domains including control systems and automation, embedded systems, wireless sensor networks for device to device (D2D) communication via the internet. The pre-requisite for implementing IoT systems is mainly the Radio Frequency Identification (RFID). Typically, it has business as well as private applications. From the perception of private users, e-learning, and healthcare are the foremost fields, while from perspective of the business users, logistics, automation, and industrial engineering are the significant domains [3].

The IoT is a platform that tolerates everything for information processing, data communication, and collaborative context analysis to serve individuals, businesses and organizations. In order to perform IoT such systems, a massive data amount having different content and formats has to be processed professionally, rapidly and intelligently using advanced techniques, algorithms, tools and models. This innovative paradigm is supported by the development of various technologies, such as the wireless communication, internet, cloud computing, machine learning algorithms and big data analysis [4]. Big data is considered to be another prototype to designate data processing to make sense from the data to the IoT users. It has five characteristics, namely velocity, volume, veracity, variety, and value [5]. Generally, equipped research communities with big data skills can offer additional opportunities, motivations, and innovation to their long-term strategies. Recently, the trend is to improve Big data in the IoT to provide "Everything as a Service". Thus, an innovative emerging services and analytics services can be the strategic solutions to organizations in order to adopt IoT and Big data.

Healthcare applications supported by the IoT, connected things anyplace, anytime, with anyone perfectly using any network and any service, which lead to smart health care. Embedded or worn on the body networked sensors gather rich information about the individuals' health [6]. Such information can produce a positive modification in the health care landscape. Data availability along with the new generations' intelligent processing procedures can (a) assist an evolution in medicine, (b) qualify personalization of management and treatment options, and (c) reduce the healthcare cost with improved outcomes.

2 Internet of Things Architecture

The architecture of IoT consists of several technologies suites to support the IoT. It demonstrates the integrated technologies related to each other to develop the IoT system modularity and scalability in different scenarios. The layers' functionality in the IoT system as reported in [7] depicted that the IoT architecture consists of several layers, namely:

- Sensor layer which is the lowest layer consisting of integrated smart objects along with the sensors. These sensors empower the interconnection of the real-world and the physical measurements for real-time information process. There are a variety of sensors where each is used with different purposes. The sensors can measure air quality, temperature, electricity and movement. In addition, sensors can have a memory to record a definite number of measurements [8–10].
  A sensor can measure a physical property for further conversion into understood able signal. Most sensors entail connectivity to the sensor gateways (aggregators) in the form of personal area network (PAN), such as Bluetooth, ZigBee, and Ultra-Wideband (UWB) or a local area network (LAN), and including WiFi and Ethernet connections. The wireless sensor networks (WSNs) represents sensors using low data rate connectivity and low power that form networks.
- Gateways and networks layer, where huge data volume is produced by tiny sensors, which requires a high performance and robust and wired/wireless network infrastructure. Such networks tied with different protocols to support machine-to-machine (M2M) networks and their applications. Recently, multiple networks with several access protocols and technologies are compulsory to integrate in a heterogeneous configuration [11–13].
  These networks can be public, private or hybrid models to support the communication requests for bandwidth, latency, or security. Converged network layer abstraction tolerates multiple hospitals and/or medical centers to share independently for their routed information without compromising their security, privacy and performance requirements. Each medical organization in the healthcare applications utilizes the network as if it is a private network.
- Management service layer includes information processing through security controls, analytics, and devices management. Various analytics methods are employed to extract applicable information from huge amount of raw data for processing in faster rate. Furthermore, data-in-motion analysis namely streaming analytics is obligatory to be executed in real time [14, 15]. Analytics reduces the network layer stress, and decreases the sensors' power requirements by less recurrent communication for faster responses to data established by the sensors. During data management, the information can be accessed, controlled and integrated. In addition, data filtering methods including data integration, data anonymisation, and data synchronization are applied for details hiding for the information. Data abstraction is applied to extract information to achieve greater agility and reprocess across domains. Finally, security should be performed across the whole IoT architecture dimensions. Security is applied to protect the

data travels across the whole system. Data integrity enables authentic and reliable decisions as it inhibits the IoT system unauthorized personnel or hacking. Researchers were interested to develop several security algorithms as depicted in [16–20]. Moreover, various authentication and encryption technologies for privacy and security using Message Authentication Code (MAC) and Rivest Shamir Adleman (RSA) guard the transaction data authenticity and confidentiality while transmission between networks. In addition, an authentication framework that used to support multiple authentication methods is the Extensible Authentication Protocol (EAP) [21].
For data privacy, technical implementations and policy approaches are engaged to ensure the removal of the data sensitive. The European Network and Information Security Agency (ENISA) proposed data privacy approach using data masking platform to guarantee data privacy. Using IoT-distributed systems that include embedded devices in public areas, threats produced from other networks attempts to spoof data access, thus IoT security has to be realized on a robust foundation at numerous interacting layers.

- Application layer includes the various applications of the IoT systems.

This IoT architecture is illustrated into layers using various technologies that can be classified into: (i) technologies concerned with network sharing, latency and capacity including software-defined radios and cognitive networks, (ii) technologies influences the microprocessor chips and devices, such as low power sensors and wireless sensor network, and (iii) services management to sustenance IoT applications such as in-memory and streaming analytics [22–24].

3 Internet of Things Based Healthcare

The IoT is a novel Internet revolution, where objects/devices are organized to realize intelligence system for enabling context related decisions. The information is accessible by other things, or components of complex services. This IoT system is associated with the cloud computing capabilities and the unlimited addressing capacity of the Internet transition towards IPv6. The communications and information rapid technology convergence occurs at technology innovation layers, namely the data, cloud, devices, and communication networks. The healthcare reliance on IoT is aggregating to develop access to care, to increase the care quality and to reduce the care cost [25].

The foremost IoT system must provide powerful, simple application access to IoT data and devices to aid designers for visualization dashboards, analytics applications, and healthcare-IoT applications. The major key abilities that leading platforms have to include:

- Easy device management: Easy device management empowers enhanced asset availability, minimized unintended outages, increased throughput, and reduced maintenance costs.

- Simple connectivity: A noble IoT platform makes it easy to perform device management functions and to connect devices. Scaled cloud-based services can be performed easily with applying analytics to achieve insight organizational transformation.
- Informative analytics: With massive IoT data volumes, analysis is necessary for superior decisions. Real-time analytics are essential to monitor the existing conditions and respond consequently.
- Intelligently transform: Information ingestion and store the IoT data to merge data and cloud in an integrating way. Data is consumed from platforms and diverse data sources, and then the indispensable values are extracted using valuable analytics.

Personalized healthcare is based on an individual's exclusive behavioral, biological, social characteristics. This leads to superior outcomes with making healthcare cost-effective. A supportable service focuses on the early disease detection, and homecare rather than the exclusive clinical one. IoT can handle the care personalization services and can preserve a digital identification for every individual. Various equipments are used in healthcare, to communicate and to make the omnipresent system-of-system. Thus, a categorization of the IoT based on personalized healthcare systems includes remote monitoring and clinical care [26], where:

- Remote monitoring allows the ready access to actual health monitoring through using dominant wireless solutions connected through the IoT to monitor the patients using the secured captured patient health data. Several complex algorithms and sensors are employed for data analysis, and then share this data via wireless connectivity to attain medical the professionals' health recommendations remotely.
- Clinical care employs noninvasive monitoring IoT systems for hospitalized. This clinical care system uses sensors for collecting physiological information that to be stored and analyzed using cloud. It delivers a continuous automated information flow, which improves the care quality with lower cost.

The general framework for the IoT's system consists of several architectures for health monitoring devices. The common features/uses of the IoT health monitoring are as follows:

- It gathers data from sensors using wireless sensor networks (WSNs)
- It supports user displays and interfaces
- It allows network connectivity to access infrastructure services
- It provides robustness, accuracy, reliability and durability.

The main components/requirements for the IoT system in healthcare applications are:

I. Wireless Sensor Networks (WSNs) connects a number of sensor and nodes in a network via wireless communication. This incorporates the network into a higher level system using a network gateway [27].

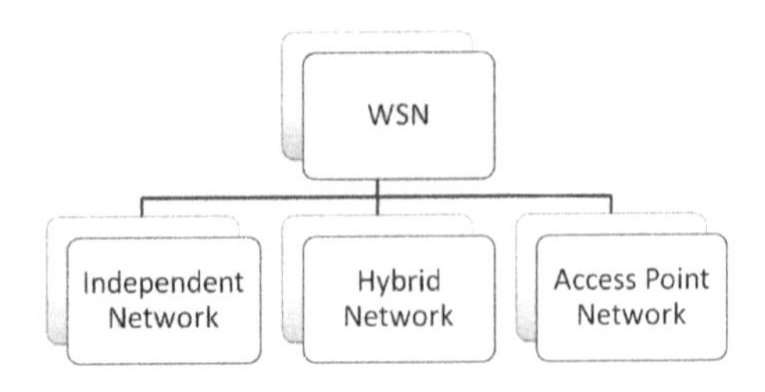

Fig. 1 Classification for the WSN

II. Ubiquitous Sensor Network (USN) is an extension of WSN combined with an IoT application system. It uses gateways which are information hubs that assemble sensor data, analyses data for further transmission to the cloud via wide area network (WAN). Physical data for the monitored parameters are measured using sensors. There are three approaches to connect the WSNs to the Internet as illustrated in Fig. 1.

Figure 1 depicted that the WSN has three approaches, namely independent network, hybrid network, and access point network [28–30].

III. User interface equirements includes the (i) interoperability which is realized by the device manufacturers, (ii) usability which is developed by empowering display devices to carry information using graphics user interfaces (GUIs), (iii) reliability represents the IoT adoption to provide correct information, (iv) mobility support by tolerating the association with the user even if the network scheme changes, and (v) extensibility and flexibility that allow changes in the devices to location mapping.

4 Internet of Things Applications in Healthcare

The evolution in the electronics, medical devices and computer science leads to remarkable technological progresses in the form of IoT realization. Since, multiple sensor nodes can connect the Internet from in-home monitoring devices to hospital-based imaging systems, thus healthcare industry devices offer enhanced care by systematizing the processes to facilitate the collaboration and securely for the transferred information. Intelligent systems provide physicians with easy and efficient access to health information to improve the patient experience [31]. Examples for several applications of the IoT for heathcare are addressed as follows.

- Heart rate monitoring, where the biometrics of each patient are independently monitored using specific threshold settings. Such monitoring system records the ECG Heart rate variability and reliability, respiration rate, activity level of the heart, body position. In addition, the vital signs such as the weight and blood pressure are remotely monitored using supplementary devices in conjunction. Generally, the heart rate monitoring system reports the rhythm to realize the cardiac role of impenetrable symptoms. Arrhythmia medication therapy is a further clinical applications the cardiac monitoring remotely at home or in the hospital [32].

- Aging Individuals monitoring through IoT ultrasound-based technology is employed in hospitals as a personalized home healthcare solution for locating and tracking the resident's activity. Emergency calls can be managed in a cost actual system for wide area communication interface. This system can be a waterproof worn sensor system that can be programmed to send a report including the position signal to the ultrasound receiver. The receiver in turn receives the signal through typical wireless WLAN connections to the homecare gateway. Generally, data analysis is performed by the gateway, afterward the significant data is broadcasted and the integrated wireless wide area network connection is employed to send out a help notification in the critical events [33–38].

5 Challenges and Future Perspectives

The Internet of Things changed our society anywhere and anytime. Over fast secure and reliable networks, personalized healthcare and monitoring. Recently, the standard web services is the most extensively adopted technology for the Internet. At the network edge, the wireless perceptible embedded healthcare systems requires functionalities which is challenging in the internet future. Ubiquitous networks and wireless sensor networks, where the sensors are controlled and connected by the embedded systems where services encapsulate the functionality and offer unified access to the system functionality. These components process information in several healthcare environments such as households, hospitals, and work as well as it lead to big data.

In future, innovative technologies and standards should address privacy and security features for network, users, data and applications. For network protocol security, the IPv6 (Internet Protocol Version 6) is the next generation protocol for the Internet. This protocol encompasses security control and addressing information to route packets through the Internet.

With IPv6, IPSec sustenance is integrated into the protocol connections and design that can be protected/secured when communicating with other IPv6 devices. The IPSec offers data integrity, data confidentiality and data authentication at the network layer. Thus, it offers several security services at the IP layer and above. Such security services include connectionless integrity, access control, protection, data authentication, encryption, and traffic flow confidentiality. Other IP-based security solutions are challenging to perform authenticated key exchanges over the IPSec protocol for payload secure delivery.

Generally, the most challenging issues includes settling on device capabilities, security, bridging the gaps between individuals,sensors fabrication and safety.

6 Conclusion

The Internet of things (IoT) is one of the most noteworthy technology trends. Innovations merging in the domains of communication and computing, leads to smart devices that applied in the IoT which not only user-machine interaction but also concerns with the approach in which the machines involve with each other. The IoT revolution in healthcare by this time is underway. As recent use cases are emerging, thus the IoT technology still addresses the urgent necessity for accessible and affordable care. Meanwhile, the building blocks of the IoT system for automated and machine-to-machine communication continue to be conventional. Service layer addition produces the complete IoT infrastructure. This revolution is characterized by connectivity solutions and end-to-end processing for IoT-driven healthcare. This chapter introduced the main concept and design of the IoT systems along with pointing out the most challenging problems.

References

1. Zanella, A., Bui, N., Castellani, A., Vangelista, L., Zorzi, M.: Internet of things for smart cities. IEEE Internet Things J. **1**(1), 22–32 (2014)
2. Kortuem, G., Kawsar, F., Fitton, D., Sundramoorthy, V.: Smart objects as building blocks for the internet of things (2011). Internet Comput. IEEE, **14**, 44–51 (2010)
3. Da Xu, L., He, W., Li, S.: Internet of things in industries: a survey. IEEE Trans. Industr. Inf. **10**(4), 2233–2243 (2014)
4. Sharma, S.: Expanded cloud plumes hiding big data ecosystem. Future Gener. Comput. Syst. **59**, 63–92 (2016)
5. Needham, J.: Disruptive Possibilities: How Big Data Changes Everything. O'Reilly Media, Inc (2013)
6. Bardram, J.E., Doryab, A., Jensen, R.M., Lange, P.M., Nielsen, K.L., Petersen, S.T.: Phase recognition during surgical procedures using embedded and body-worn sensors. In: IEEE International Conference on Pervasive Computing and Communications (PerCom), 45–53 March 2011
7. Evangelatos, N.O.: Efficient algorithms, architectures and implementations in internet of things and smart environments. Doctoral dissertation, University of Geneva (2015)
8. Haller, S., Karnouskos, S., Schroth, C.: The internet of things in an enterprise context. In: Future Internet Symposium. 14–28. Springer, Berlin September 2008
9. Miorandi, D., Sicari, S., De Pellegrini, F., Chlamtac, I.: Internet of things: vision, applications and research challenges. Ad. Hoc. Netw. **10**(7), 1497–1516 (2012)
10. Abdelwahab, S., Hamdaoui, B., Guizani, M., Rayes, A.: Enabling smart cloud services through remote sensing: an internet of everything enabler. IEEE Internet Things J. **1**(3), 276–288 (2014)
11. Jung, S., Ahn, J.Y., Hwang, D.J., Kim, S.: An optimization scheme for M2M-based patient monitoring in ubiquitous healthcare domain. Int. J. Distrib. Sens. Netw. (2012)
12. Elyengui, S., Bouhouchi, R., Ezzedine, T.: The enhancement of communication technologies and networks for smart grid applications. arXiv preprint arXiv:1403.0530 (2014)
13. Fuentes-Samaniego, R.A., Cavalli, A.R., Nolazco-Flores, J.A., Baliosian, J.: A survey on wireless sensors networks security based on a layered approach. In: International Conference on Wired/Wireless Internet Communication. 77–93. Springer International Publishing

14. Bossé, É., Solaiman, B.: Information fusion and analytics for big data and IoT. Artech House (2016)
15. Raj, P.: Big data analytics demystified. Handbook of research on cloud infrastructures for big data analytics, 38 (2014)
16. Dey, N., Biswas, S., Das, P., Das, A., Chaudhuri, S.S.: Feature analysis for the reversible watermarked electrooculography signal using low distortion prediction-error expansion. In: International Conference Communications, Devices and Intelligent Systems (Codis), pp. 624–627 (2012)
17. Dey, N., Maji, P., Das, P., Biswas, S., Das, A., Chaudhuri, S.: Embedding of blink frequency. In: Electrooculography Signal Using Difference Expansion Based Reversible Watermarking Technique. Buletinul Ştiinţific Al Universităţii "Politehnica" Din Timişoara, Seria Electronică Şi Telecomunicaţii Transactions on Electronics and Communications **57** (71) (2012)
18. Dey, N., Biswas, D., Roy, A., Das, A.: DWT-DCT-SVD based blind watermarking technique of gray image in electrooculogram signal. In: 12th International Conference on Intelligent Systems Design and Applications (ISDA), pp. 680–685 (2012)
19. Dey, N., Mukhopadhyay, S., Das, A., Chaudhuri, S.: Analysis of P-QRS-T components modified by blind watermarking technique within the electrocardiogram signal for authentication in wireless telecardiology using DWT. Int. J. Image, Graph. Sig. Process. **7**, 33–46 (2012)
20. Nandi, S., Roy, S., Dansana, J., Karaa, W.B., Ray, R., Chowdhury, S.R., Chakraborty, S., Dey, N.: Cellular automata based encrypted ECG-hash code generation: an application in inter human biometric authentication system. Int. J. Comput. Netw. Inf. Secur. **6**(11), 1 (2014)
21. Hurson, A.R., Ploskonka, J., Jiao, Y., Haridas, H.: Security issues and solutions in distributed heterogeneous mobile database systems. Adv. Comput. **61**, 107–198 (2004)
22. Akyildiz, I.F., Wang, X., Wang, W.: Wireless mesh networks: a survey. Comput. Netw. **47** (4), 445–487 (2005)
23. Chen, M., Gonzalez, S., Vasilakos, A., Cao, H., Leung, V.C.: Body area networks: a survey. Mobile Netw. Appl. **16**(2), 171–193 (2011)
24. Zhang, Y., Luo, J., Hu, H. (eds.): Wireless Mesh Networking: Architectures, Protocols and Standards. CRC Press (2006)
25. Frederix, I.: Internet of things and radio frequency identification in care taking, facts and privacy challenges. In: Wireless Communication, Vehicular Technology, Information Theory and aerospace and Electronic Systems Technology. In: IEEE 1st International Conference on Wireless VITAE, 319–323 May 2009
26. Simonov, M., Zich, R., Mazzitelli, F.: Personalized healthcare communication in internet of things. In: Proceedings of URSI GA08 (2008)
27. Pang, Z.: Technologies and architectures of the Internet-of-Things (IoT) for health and well-being, Doctoral Thesis, KTH—Royal Institute of Technology Stockholm, Sweden (2013)
28. Christin, D., Reinhardt, A., Mogre, P.S., Steinmetz, R.: Wireless sensor networks and the internet of things: selected challenges. In: Proceedings of the 8th GI/ITG KuVS Fachgespräch "Drahtlose Sensornetze" (FGSN), pp. 31–34, 2009
29. Alemdar, H., Ersoy, C.: Wireless sensor networks for healthcare: A Survey. Comput. Netw. **54**(15), 2688–2710 (2010)
30. Triantafyllidis, A., Koutkias, V., Chouvarda, I., Maglaveras, N.: An open and reconfigurable wireless sensor network for pervasive health monitoring. In: Second International Conference on Pervasive Computing Technologies for Healthcare, pp. 112–115 Jan 2008
31. Kumar, P., Lee, H.J.: Security issues in healthcare applications using wireless medical sensor networks: a survey. Sensors **12**(1), 55–91 (2011)
32. Bourge, R.C., Abraham, W.T., Adamson, P.B., Aaron, M.F., Aranda, J.M., Magalski, A., Jessup, M.L.: Randomized controlled trial of an implantable continuous hemodynamic monitor in patients with advanced heart failure: the COMPASS-HF study. J. Am. Coll. Cardiol. **51**(11), 1073–1079 (2008)

33. Dekker, A.L.A.J. US Patent No. 6,702,752. Washington, DC, US patent and trademark office (2004)
34. Ren, Y., Werner, R., Pazzi, N., Boukerche, A.: Monitoring patients via a secure and mobile healthcare system. IEEE Wirel. Commun. **17**(1), 59–65 (2010)
35. Jundanian, R.H.: US Patent No. 4,347,851. Washington, DC, US patent and trademark office (1982)
36. Unger, J.D.:US. Patent No. 5,458,123. Washington, DC, US patent and trademark office (1995)
37. Lubell, M., & Marks, S. US Patent 4,566,461. Washington, DC, US patent and trademark office (1986)
38. Trouva, E.: The mobile phone as a platform for assisting the independent living of aging people. Athens, June 2009

Internet of Things in HealthCare

Yesha Bhatt and Chintan Bhatt

Abstract The next era will be the connection between the physical things and internet. The things include goods, machine, appliances even we also become the part of it. The reason for integrating healthcare with Internet of Things features into medical devices improves the quality and effectiveness of service, bringing especially high value for elderly, patients with chronic conditions and those that require consistent supervision. Now research is going on-how to transform healthcare industry by increasing efficiency, lowering costs and put the focus back on better patient care. The Internet of Things will be a game changer for the healthcare industry. With an intelligent system and powerful algorithms, one can obtain an unprecedented level of real-time, life-critical data which is captured and analyzed to drive people in advance research, management and critical care. Taking care of patient's health at very low cost is an important factor. The main idea of applying IoT in healthcare is move out from traditional area to visit hospitals and thus waiting will come to an end. The concept here is that it can be able to sense, process and communicate with biomedical and physical parameters so that they can work on it. Many applications and devices have been designed for healthcare purpose and have been put for people to use. The view is to connect the doctors, patients and nurses via smart device and each entity can roam without any restrictions. The idea is 24 * 7 monitoring of patient.

Keywords HealthCare · Medical services · Remote monitoring · Sensing

Y. Bhatt (✉) · C. Bhatt
Computer Engineering, Charotar University of Science and Technology, Changa, Anand 388421, Gujarat, India
e-mail: 15pgce005@charusat.edu.in

C. Bhatt
e-mail: chintanbhatt.ce@charusat.ac.in

C. Bhatt et al. (eds.), *Internet of Things and Big Data Technologies for Next Generation Healthcare*, Studies in Big Data 23,
DOI 10.1007/978-3-319-49736-5_2

1 Brief to the Internet of Things

IoT [1, 2] known as Internet of Things can simply be described as connecting any device with Internet and we can switch it on and off and/or to each other. This includes home automation system, cell phone, wearable devices etc. Ubiquitous networking which is the next word comes in mind when we think of Internet of Things. Basically it is the technical term used for internet everywhere any time we need. For Internet of Things we can use the sensor; to sense the medium. For unique identity and sensing we can use RFID sensors. If we have any physical appliance for that then we can easily charge them. The Internet of Things will also provide us the real search engines. E.g. where are my car keys? What is the status of my order? Etc. With all these expectations The Internet of Things is still in its early stages.

We will understand with an example. Suppose in a mall we want a parking space. So far from the mall we want to know the empty parking space. For the transmission of the information of particular parking space, a constant messages should be transmitted for that the parking space should have a unique identity. It could be achieved with RFID sensor tags. RFID sensor tag can sense the data and it can constantly communicate the information about the place whether it is empty or not.

2 Introduction of Internet of Things in HealthCare

Internet of Things will be the phase changer of healthcare industry. From taking care of patient's health by taking care of comfort zone of both the parties at very low cost. Interconnected devices in the Internet provides more feasibility to the patients to connect them via specialist all over the world. In a single sentence we can say IoT as "It provides seamlessly healthcare system to the patients." The IoT in healthcare provides the observation of heartbeats, glucose level as well as the routine water level measurement of the body etc.

Mainly IoT in Healthcare focuses on:

- Critical treatments which have high risk of life.
- The routine medicine/check-up of the patient.
- Critical treatments by standard way and connect machine, people, data that can be deployed on machine or in the cloud.

The main idea of applying IoT in healthcare is move out from traditional area to visit hospitals and waiting will come to an end. The concept here is that it can be able to sense, process moreover communicate with biomedical and physical parameters so that they can work on it.

The view is to connect the doctors, patients via smart device and each entity can roam without any restrictions. The idea is constant monitoring of patient take some important information and upload it to doctor's side then he can suggest further steps to be followed. Here to upload the data patient can take the use of cloud services, the big data then the analysis of the data will do. The smart devices are the necessity of user's life. A user needs to access available wide area network with highly facilities applications which will solve the maximum problem of the user.

While designing something for health some criteria that need to be take care is

- IoT for healthcare should be in centre not the technology which is implemented.
- We think IoT as wireless sensor network (M2M) communication will happen. Here reliability is most important criteria for it.
- The flexibility that is provided should be mobile. One should be able to roam even after having it.

The communication protocol that is being design is the one of the important aspect while designing the device. But still it can be implemented using ZigBee network which uses Proactive and Reactive routing protocols.

Healthcare with IoT they are mainly based on the network connected devices that can directly communicate with each other to capture the data, process the data, through the secure service layer. Other useful healthcare devices can be independent living services, telehealth, wearable devices. Specifically in the field of telecare, remote monitoring of the users allow more self management of chronic disorders and cost reductions.

Figure 1 presents the planned architecture for HealthCare in Internet of things. With the help of figure we can say that basically it is made up of four layers. The first layer which is the Medical devices layer shows that it is made up of various device e.g. cylindrical magnetic resonance machine (MRI machine) which is with the help of Ethernet connected with the second layer which is M2M Multi-Service Gateway which consist of Remote Gateway Routers. The routers are responsible for uploading the data to central data repository. Third layer is M2M Integration Platform which is of central data repository which could be public/private cloud. The fourth layer of proposed architecture M2M Integration Platform which uses the data presented at the cloud for notifications regarding regular check-ups and reminder of medicines are sent as a notification to the patients, reports are generated. The cloud system might as well connected to the IT database for the live data purpose.

The future of Internet of Things mainstream will be based on efficient wireless protocols, cheap and low-power microprocessor, right standardization, support of communities etc. It is expected that by 2020 the number of connected devices will be around 50 billion and increased traffic from those devices will probably effect on the network. The medical care should provide the wearable devices, physician and associate system must facilitate the information and rigorously should protect the patient's privacy. To achieve this healthcare part in Internet of Things must be as flexible and rapidly scalable as they are highly secure [3].

The working of monitoring patients remotely when they are at their home known as telemonitoring system has one between operation that passes the sensed data to remote server which is responsible for critical event detection, analysis of collected

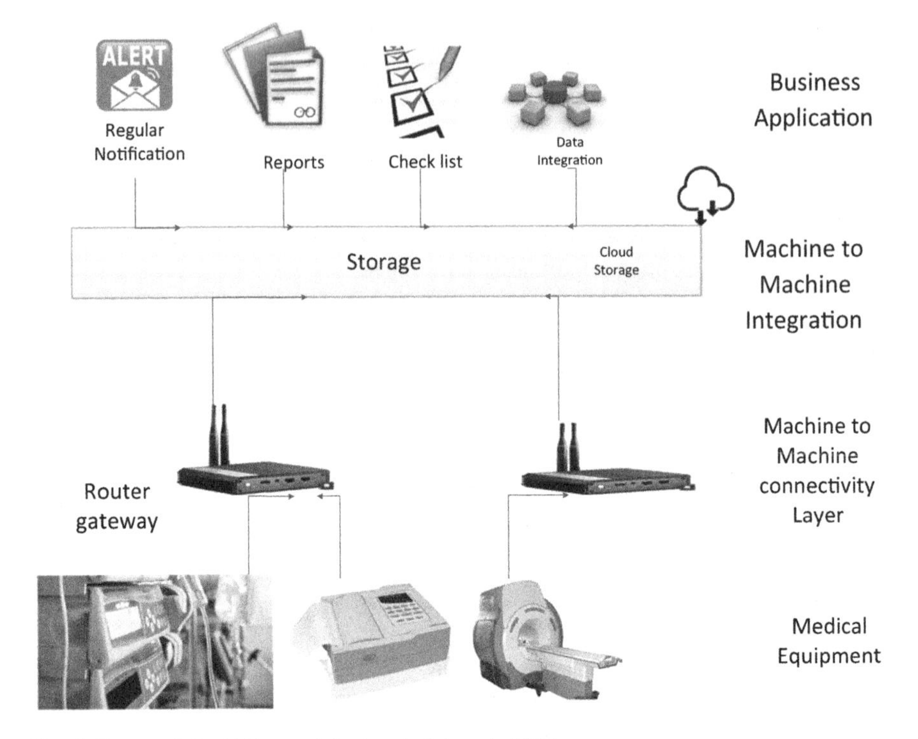

Fig. 1 Proposed HealthCare architecture in Internet of Things

data moreover for consolidation too. By this way associated with smart sensor which is responsible for smarter environment which pushes the information to medical teams to communicate, to technologies for citizen (especially for elders) to find best suitable condition to proceed with proper local treatments.

Few facilities that will be added when we talk about Internet of Things in HealthCare are:

- Flexible patient Monitoring

While most of the patient needs to move from very places, Internet of Things will allow patient to choose their comfort zone and then they can perform any treatment remotely without moving from their place.

- Improved Quality of Drug

One of the biggest problem for today's drug industry is to maintain and produce the drug. One solution for the drug management came into the picture is to tag each and every drug with one RFID tag which will enter inside the body and it will provide the medicine as well as it will also monitor the inside body structure. It will help to take advance step for any dieses like Cancer [4].

The HealthCare industry have vision to achieve some serious changes, mostly pushed by various innovations that mostly be around, which will solve a lot of problems which healthcare industry is facing at this point of time. The HealthCare technologies will support many features e.g. integration of real-time HealthCare data with tracking useful data of medical and non-medical streams as well as Electronic health records (EHRs).

Connected medical devices with the Internet is slowly becoming a part of the HealthCare system. Now we have to observe about the medical devices that how much they can integrate and store the information. There will be a combination and comparison of desirable services with new service categories as Internet of HealthCare Things progresses. IoT in Healthcare in next few years provides depth assessment of the global IoT healthcare market including growth drivers, vendor analysis, quantitative assessment, and value chain of the industry.

Target audience will be:

- Medical device Manufacturers and providers
- Internet of Things service and application developer
- Hospital, diagnostic center, clinics
- Wireless service providers
- Embedded system providers

2.1 Communication Between Devices

The 5th generation of communication technology for people and things (Internet of Everything) will be achiever network and trustworthy where both wireless and wired communications will be using the same infrastructure for communication. This future ubiquitous with ultra-high bandwidth communication infrastructure which will drive the future networked society.

Figure 2 shows that how the communication between devices in hospital. Various sensor network connected via Wi-Fi, 6LoWPAN and connected in various topology e.g. star, mesh observe the data broadcasted by the machine like cylindrical magnetic resonance machine (MRI machine). This data is related to patient and strictly prohibited to doctors only. Because this type of information should be provided to doctors only. The data broadcasted by the machine and the data observed by the sensor are stored inside a data repository via smart gateway. From this information patient gets notification what steps they need to perform further.

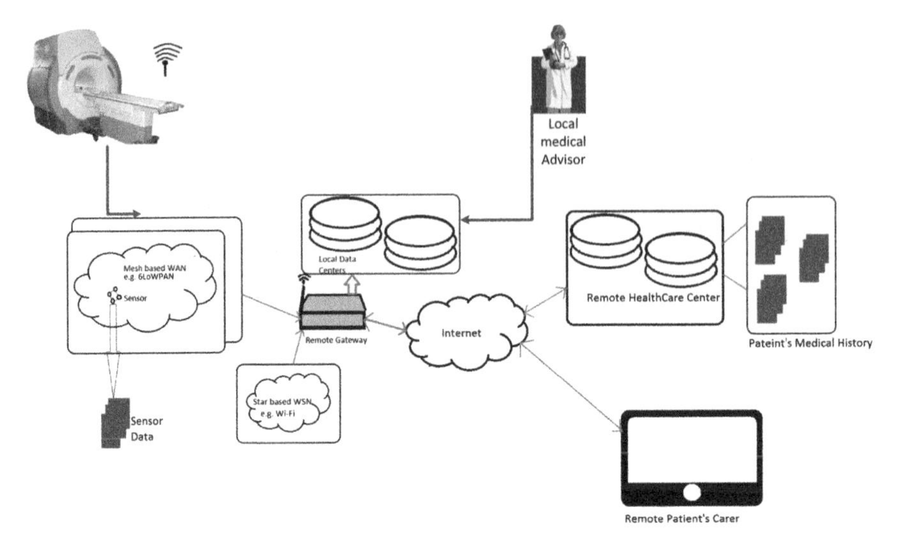

Fig. 2 Communication between devices

2.1.1 Medical Body Area Network (MBAN's)

Medical body area networks (MBANs), are networks of those devices which can be worn on the human's body communicates with a programmer and/or controller device that are unattached to the body via wireless communication link. The purpose of using Medical Body Area Network is to measure and to record physiological parameters along with patient's other information and/or for performing diagnostic/therapeutic functions. A lower power network which consist a programmer/control transmitter, one or more devices worn by patients which transmit or receive related device control commands, non-voice data in the purpose of recording and measuring patient's body parameters along with other patient information for performing therapeutic function (healing of dieses) via radiated uni-/bi-directional electronic signals.

Following are the **Restrictions** on Medical Body Area Network Operation:

- Medical Body Area Networks must be provided to a patient only under the guidance of professional and authorized health care professional.
- MBANs can be used only for diagnostic and therapeutic purposes.

The expectation with 5G communication technologies are: It will allow 100 times higher wireless bandwidth compared to last few years; high optimization; maximum amount of energy saving per service provide and storage and processing, variety of delivered services for communication and big data analytics; very dense deployments of wireless communication links to connect over trillions wireless devices serving over billions people; and to enable advanced user controlled privacy. Medical Body Area Networks (MBAN's) open the door for monitoring systems—which currently attach patients to machines using a mass of wires—to operate wirelessly using low-cost wearable sensors. Wired monitoring systems make it difficult for patients to move about, and they increase the chances for errors and hospital-acquired infections. MBAN's enable hospitals to monitor a much larger percentage of patient population and more quickly identify health events that require intervention. This, in turn, should lead to better patient care, improved outcomes and lower costs.

For example, a monitored hospital patient would have a roughly 39 % chance of surviving a coronary thrombosis, compared with a 7 % chance for unmonitored patients. FCC has approved a specific spectrum for wireless networks, used to monitor patient data within healthcare facility MBAN devices, in the 2360–2400 MHz band. The decision to open the use of this frequency range is part of an effort to lower the chances that other wireless devices such e.g. mobile phones could interfere with MBAN transmission. Examples: Philips, Qualcomm are developing MBAN devices for clinical diagnoses to deliver better patient care at lower costs. Which offer interoperable solutions to remotely monitor patients: diabetes, weight, heart rate, and blood pressure at their homes, and send the real time biometric information to healthcare providers onto PCs, tablets and smartphones.

3 Nanotechnology in Internet of Things

The recent researches in nanotechnology pushes the Internet of Things towards it. Internet of Things is the main concept through which all other devices are going to interconnect with each other. Example applications that can be supported by nanonetworks are smart drug administration, nanoscale surgeries, and epidemic spread detection and management. The architecture of Nano Technology Internet of Things includes the devices which size ranges from one to few hundred nano meters. Nanomechanics can perform various actions inside the body. It can create whole nano network inside of the body and directly communicate the outside devices. This communication happens with the help of nano routers, which acts as data sinks that will forward the data to micro-device or any smartphone or an access point.

There are many technologies that are used to provide communication medium between two nano devices. One of them is **Molecular Communication** which is Nano-electromagnetic communication consist of transmission and reception of electromagnetic radio frequency waves at Terahertz band. This communication type can be easily involved into nano device due to their size and domain of operation. It performs releasing and reacting to specific molecules to mirror the transmission and reception of the information.

3.1 Architecture Requirement: HealthCare Ecosystem in Nanotechnology

In order to provide the ubiquitous network for healthcare we have to bring various applications and services together and make them work as a single system so that patient can get access of it easily.

The Fig. 3 shows that various sensors placed at various places e.g. inside human body, inside the house, the information about human's health securely via gateway to the respective doctors. Same as the hospital uses the router as well as it maintains the record of the patients in distributed manner. That's how the doctors are able to access the patient's information. At patient's side one remote device/gateway works as intermediator to send the information to the database. Here sensors can be placed at so many place e.g. inside the human body, inside human's car, near the garden etc.

Various networks can be the part of the nanotechnology architecture of HealthCare Ecosystem. Which can be explained as Off-body Networks, On-Body Networks, and intra-Body Networks. On-Body Networks are clearly reside in body area networks and wearable devices that enable the mass customization of health monitoring and alert application and brings the health services closer to the patient's personal space. Off-body networks are deployed within a person's context e.g. hospital, street, home, vehicle. These networks can provide generic health and environment monitoring services as well as support application for comfort living. Lastly the intra-body networks are supposed to be deployed at different locations inside the human body itself either as connected, internetworked nano-devices or as

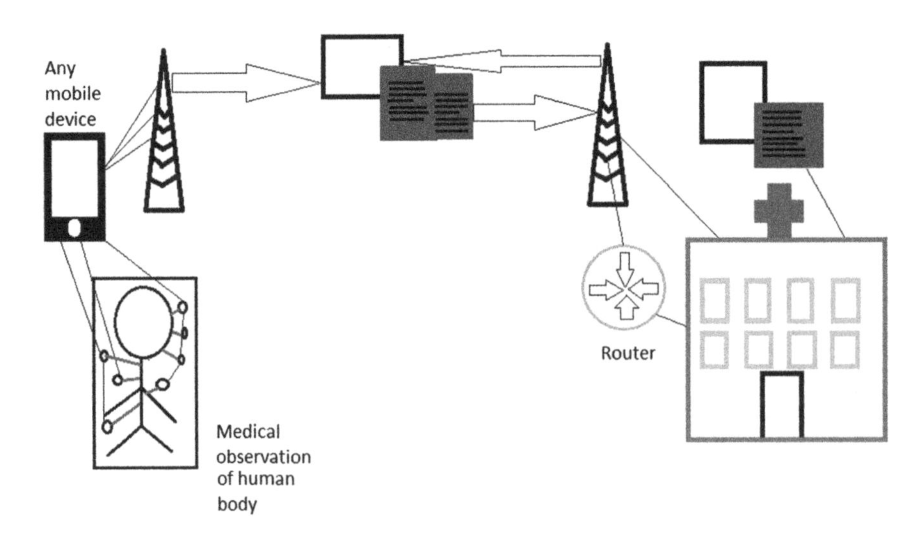

Fig. 3 Roughly overview of nanotechnology device working

embedded smart monitoring devices. The deployment of nanonetworks will not be limited to the human body only it can be deployed on to the human's body or within the patient's contextual environment. Few of the devices are already working like this. They monitor the patient's body routine and checks various conditions depending upon its ability.

In today's life few applications are developed which smoothens the human's life. Some of those applications are described in Table 1.

Table 1 Applications developed in the market with taking the concept of Internet of Things

Conditions	IoT roles/conditions
Diabetes	Non-invasive opto-physiological sensor connected using IPv6 and 6 LoWPAN protocol architecture
Wheelchair management	WBAN sensors (e.g. accelerometers and ECG and pressure); nodes process signals, realize the problem then it communicates with nodes wirelessly; smart devices and data center layers with heterogeneous connectivity
Eye disorder and skin infection	Smartphone cameras can be used for pattern matching and/or visual inspection with the standard library of images; cloud based app runs and helps on the software platform in the smartphone's SoC to drive the IoT
Rehabilitation system	A wide range of wearable and smart home sensors for tracking, coordination, event detection, cooperation, reporting and feedback to the system itself; interactive heterogeneous wireless network enables sensor device to have various access points
ElectroCardiogram monitoring	Electric activity which will check the rhythm of heartbeats at specific interval of time. It can give maximum information and can be used fullest extend various studies also have been performed
miPlatform	All-in-one platform which includes 3d images using cloud storage post processing and visualization and integrated telemedicine
Rejuven's Rejiva	Monitors the health by measuring their respiratory rate, ups and downs in heart rate, breathing index, sleep position, restfulness, and energy level. The device can also check for the automatic nervous system and ECG
Body temperature monitoring	A sensor that is wearable which measures body temperature; temperature measurement based on skin WBAN connects smart devices
Newsoft	Provides services to hospitals, public health facilities and health management
Alivcore	Company which have produced the phone cases which will predict your heart attack
Wound analysis for advance diabetes patients	A smartphone camera; image decompression and segmentation; the app run on the software platform in the smartphone's system-on-chip (SoC) to drive the IoT
BP monitoring	A wearable BP sensor; oscillometric and automatic inflation and measurement; WBAN connects smart devices

3.2 Internet of NanoTechnology Things: Health Application Requirements, Opportunities and Challenges

The Internet of Things in nanotechnology holds a very special place which will be changing phase for the development of various application and devices to detect various dieses. For this importance to be realised more requirements that restricts from IoNT's unique features need to be incorporated into its protocol design. As convention, here to summarize the requirements and challenges we will be following the conventional network layering approach.

(1) The Physical Layer (MAC)
The main requirement for the MAC layer is efficient coding schemes that will reduce the errors, a channel capacity that will guarantee reliable data delivery and an accurate channel model that accounts unique biological transmission medium and its associated noise.
Here we know that the capacity is less compared to conventional. For molecular communication the channel medium is molecules which have to propagate through biological channel. Channel characteristics of intra body network varies with the conditions of body. Ultrasonic communication was proposed as a more reliable and already operational paradigm to achieve internetworking of nanomachines for intra-body communication.

(2) The Network Layer
The communication range for IoNT system is expected 1 nm to 1 cm for molecular communication which shows that it has very limited amount of transmission range which makes routing a critical aspect and multi-hop communication for nanonetworks. Moreover, the direction of a communication route is not deterministic as the molecules inside the body may vary inside which can later led to communication delay. However this will require efficient schemes for multi-hop path creation and management.
The network topology inside the body can be random and dynamic due to the uncontrolled property of biological communication medium. This also affects cooperation between nanomachines which needs to be kept at minimum.

(3) The Transport Layer
The nanoscale of the IoNT makes impractical to have individual network addresses for the individual nanomachines. Addressing can be cluster based instead of nano based. This makes it possible to address a group of nodes based on the health functionality they perform or the biological organ or phenomena they monitor.
Nanomachines suffer from unreliable transmission due to the high level of biological noise. The projected dense deployment of nanomachines can make the nanonetwork as a whole more reliable. Dense deployment will make up for the potential packet loss since more nanomachines with the same functionality can report the same data.

(4) The Application Layer
The application Design for health care service needs to address requirements for real time, reliable and context aware operation. The criticality of health services makes real-time operation a fundamental requirement. The heterogeneous nature of nanomachines because of their use for different medical purpose inside the body will result in different data representation formats. That is why data fusion needs to be dynamic, optimal and more over delay tolerance. Here data aggregation and fusion are not always suitable for healthcare operation because of real time requirement and since many of those application depend on fine grained variations in the temporal domain that are lost in the aggregation or fusion process.

Context awareness is another challenging aspect for nanonetworks. Networks deployed outside of the body can be geographically tagged and can communicate with external environment in order to determine and update their context. Applications need to coordinate multiple contexts for more specific services that can benefit from the integration of intra body networks as well as external networks. For example an on body network can detect the change of context for patient and be alerted by an environmental network about the presence of certain allergen to which the patient is sensitive. The intra-body network is then notified and the proper drug is released in the body to control the allergic reaction.

Few applications that are developed in the area of Internet of Things are listed in Table 2.

4 Wearable Devices

4.1 The Concept of Wearable Device

Nowadays, internet connectivity is ubiquitous and has given birth to a whole new paradigm—The Internet of Things (IoT), namely the concept of interconnecting physical objects to each other or to the internet to create domain-specific intelligence through seamless pervasive sensing, data analytics and information visualization with cloud computing. Over the years, as we moved from basic internet services to social networks to wearable web, the demand for interconnecting smart wearables has increased (Fig. 4).

The Google search trend confirms that there is the concurrent growth and popularity of wearable technology and IoT over the past few years. This presence of wearable sensor devices is giving a new way to IoT by creating an intelligent fabric of wearable device or it can be kept near by the body sensors communicating with each other or with the internet. In other words, Wearable IoT (WIoT) can be defined as a technological infrastructure that interconnects wearable technology such as Bluetooth, used to exchange data with wearable sensors, and of heterogeneous networks, such as WIFI and GSM, used to send the data to the cloud.

Table 2 Application in the area of Internet of Things

Application	Description
Google fit	Keeps track of cycling, running and walking
Calorie counter	Keeps track of food consumed by the user as well as his/her weight and measurements
Pedometer	Records the number of steps user take and display related information such as burnt calorie
ElektorCardioscope	Displays ECG data through a wireless terminal
iOximeter	Calculates the pulse rate and SpO2
Health assistant	Keeps track of many health parameter such as body, water, weight, body temperature, fat, BP and various physical activities
Honda connect	Provides impact alerts, tracks the driver's position in real time and has emergency support features in case of an accident
Mayo Clinic Meditation	Helps the user in exercise and meditation
Calm	Helps user to mediate, relax and sleep
uHear	Allows for the self-assessment of hearing
My CF (cystic fibrosis)	Keeps track of user's cystic fibrosis status
Skin vision	It keeps track of the patient's skin health and enables the early discovery of any skin disorder
iFall	Detects a fall and responds accordingly
eCAALYX	Monitors several chronic diseases
Eye Care Plus	Tests and monitors vision
Noom walk	Serves as a pedometer to count user steps
Runtastic heart rate	Measure the heart rate on real-time basis
Asthma tracker and log	Keeps track of patient's asthma
Healthy children	Can search for pediatricians by locations
Instant heart rate	Measure the heart rate using smartphone's built in camera to sense the change of the fingertip which us directly related to the pulse
Finger print thermometer	It detects the body temperature from finger print
DoseCast medication reminder	Reminds the user of medication times, tracks the inventory and maintains a log for drug management

Some Gateway devices have the capacity to store data, to run some pre-processing algorithms evaluating whether the data is clinically relevant, and to send the data intermittently to remote servers.

To improve the performance and the battery life of smartphones, the paradigm of Mobile Cloud Computing (MCC) optimizes mobile computing and networking protocol to minimize the burden of computing for smartphones. WIoT can benefit significantly from MCC since it enables the data storage and the data analysis to happen on the cloud platforms. Research has shown that weight scales transmit data to a mobile smartphone that forwards the information to a cloud based server, so

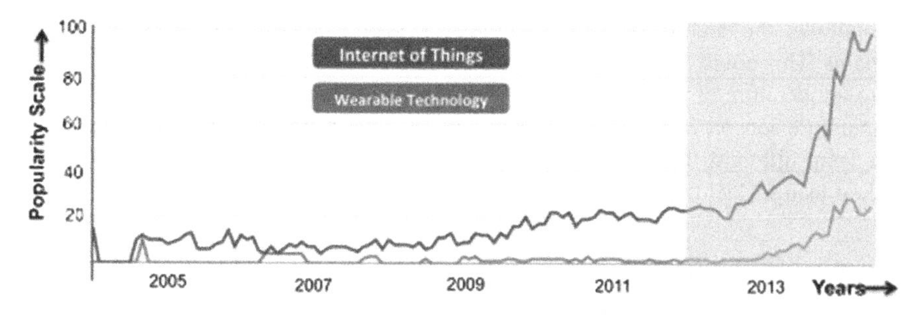

Fig. 4 Google statistics: increased use of wearable device

that clinicians can assess weight management in youth [4]. Smartphones sync with the cloud servers to monitor fall detection in elderly individuals [1]. These few examples show that how wearable or devices used by the person interact with smartphone or phones to send information to remote servers.

Cloud and Big Data support

The congruence of close companions—wearable sensors and smartphones—will flood the cloud centers with medical data at an unprecedented rate. Gaining knowledge from this data is as important as acquiring the information from the body. Patients only benefit from wearing sensors when intelligent algorithms process the data and offer some actions to take.

A cloud computing infrastructure can facilitate the management of wearable data and can support advanced functionalities of data mining, machine learning, and medical big data analytics. Cloud-assisted BAS (CaBAS) is emerging as a promising technology that provides integration of MCC and WBAS to facilitate the growth of scalable, data-driven pervasive healthcare.

Benefits from CaBAS are as follow

- Energy efficient routing protocols that can network smartphones and wearable sensors for handshaking and seamless data transfer
- Event-based processing that can reduce unwanted data processing on resource constraint wearable sensors
- Annotated data logs that can add activity-level information on top of clinical data for enhancing the accuracy of machine learning algorithms on the cloud
- Person-centred databases that can store the personalized data of patients securely for longitudinal analysis
- Data visualization that can channelize the data to end-users such as physicians and patients to provide decision support and patient-physician interactions.

IoT architecture that enables smarter, connected and personalized healthcare and wellness services to the persons in smart homes. Continuous monitoring of physical parameters through wearable sensors is highly necessary. These sensors correspond to the eHealth domain. We also consider the sensors deployed in smart home domain in order gain deeper understanding of the person's environment. This in turn allows the architecture in combining sensor measurements from different domains. This could be utilized to provide solutions like automatically adjusting the room temperature of a person having fever which is deduced from (wearable) body temperature sensor. Semantic web technologies have been used to combine sensor data from different domains and generate actionable intelligence. This is accomplished using Machine-to-Machine Measurement (M3) framework.

4.2 Internet of Things for Personalized HealthCare

This description initially demonstrates on consumer centric and architectural requirements for IoT based smarter, connected and personalized healthcare services. These requirements are then translated into a functional architecture and a mapping of its components on physical infrastructure is provided.

The Requirement Analysis

- The first requirement of personalized healthcare architecture is availability and integration of a data generation subsystem from where the physical parameters will be collected.
- The overall architecture system requires a processing and storage system since the data generating devices cannot support these functionalities due to limited resources.
- The processing and storage system should be able to access the data generation system regardless of communication technologies used in a network subsystem.
- The architecture also requires a consumer subsystem which will receive the personalized healthcare solutions.
- The consumer subsystem should support resource discovery to discover M2M devices present at data generation subsystem and select appropriate ones for data collection.
- A device management framework is necessary to keep track of the registered devices and their configurations.
- The processing and storage subsystem must incorporate mechanisms for generating high level abstraction from raw data. This forms the stepping stone for smarter, connected and personalized healthcare.
- Depending on the consumer's demand, the processing and storage subsystem should be able to communicate raw data or processed data (high level abstraction).
- The interaction between the mentioned subsystems should occur in a stateless manner using RESTful principles.
- Proper access control policies should be enforced to allow authorized users avail the personalized healthcare solutions.
- The overall system should be able to provide subscription service for occurrence of a list of events which is notified using push notification.

- The architecture should allow the consumer to react to the smart home environment based on the received push notification. This requires the presence of an actuation subsystem.
- From the consumer aspects, the architecture must ensure low latency, high QoS, easy user interface and social network integration. Usability, recovery from errors and timely feedback are very necessary for AAL based systems.

4.3 Wearable Device Characteristics

The prevalence of chronic diseases, such as diabetes, obesity, or cardiovascular disorders, affects the lives of millions of people around the world. Therefore, there exists a stringent demand to provide a solid foundation for creating wearable IoT technologies to deploy large-scale wearable sensors that are networked with remote medical infrastructure. To increase the treatment outcomes' efficacy and effectiveness. Below, description presents a new system for WIoTs to suggest future directions encompassing operational and clinical aspects:

Patient-Friendly Wearable Design Consumer usability studies have changed the design of new wearable devices (e.g. wrist accelerometer in the form of a jewelry), the development of interactive interfaces with which any nontech user even use it easily, and the abstraction of the information presented to the patient. Patients can interact with these systems, Moreover preventive healthcare initiatives by both publicly funded health systems and private health insurances are interested to increase the health and activity levels of patients. Some private insurance companies may provide incentives to encourage the use of pedometers and to reward good health results in annual check-ups.

Patient-Physician Interaction Nowadays whenever doctors desire to monitor patients beyond the physical boundaries of the clinic. Additionally, physicians intend to make their patients more proactive with respect to their health and medical conditions. Interconnections found in WIoTs among wearable sensors, mobile phones and medical infrastructure enable efficient communication between physicians and patients, allowing them to discuss digitally about micro-managing interventions, feedback on symptoms, and ability to adapt to new treatments. The level of information provided to the patient can vary depending on the individual's interest:

- The table heading
- The actual table
- An application may only provide one line actions such as "walk fast" or "run for 45 min today,"
- An application can be made more detailed in terms of asking the patient to do an aerobic activity of 40 min, an anaerobic activity of 15 min

- In second option additional reading material or online education material can be shared with the patient to inform them about the clinical practice or recent research
- Provide a contact to chat with a clinical support person or talk to a physician in an emergency situation
- On the clinician's side, the information about a certain patient can also be varied to provide brief and then detailed case information for the clinician to help the patient make a decision on an intervention or treatment. Clinical guidelines and range of acceptable values can be provided to the clinician in real-time to assist the clinician when offering treatment.

Treatment Personalization WIoTs can play a key role in personalizing treatment. Each disease clears a unique set of symptoms that differ in intensity and in their pattern based on the patient. For example, in the treatment management for chronic diseases, physicians face challenges when evaluating medication plans, because their patients may respond to prescribed medications differently. Future research can focus on health pattern identification, where the algorithms in the wearable sensors and the gateways can detect a health aberration or an impending emergency. This is possible as the WIoT are in the vicinity of the patient.

Management and Maintenance of Wearable Systems Elderly citizens who face major health related challenges are projected to become first target users of WIoT. New technologies such as inductive fast charging may reduce the burden of remembering to plug and unplug the devices on a regular basis. Also, new methods of intelligently sampling the sensors may prolong the devices' life. As we know that the wearable sensors are powered electronic systems that are worn by humans, regulatory standards will be derived from large-scale clinical trials. The regulations imposed by US Food and Drug Administration (FDA) are applied to mainstream medical devices and, therefore, wearable sensors are classified as wellness/lifestyle tracking devices in order to circumvent FDA's rigid standards. However, the trend is changing, and-wearable sensors are approved by the FDA for their use in consumer industry. FDA issued guidelines for wireless medical devices to ensure they address short and long range communication, major safety critical risks associated with radio-frequency wireless systems, and secure data transmission. Standards and Regulations WIoT need to meet international quality standards to cross the boundary from consumer gadgets to medical devices. Efficient management of wearable sensors on daily bases is an inherent issue due to their limited battery life that requires recharging periodically.

Security and Privacy As the internet evolves, it continues to pose issues of privacy and security. Earlier, desktop PCs were prone to cyber-attacks. While, mobile phones and wearable devices are now under constant threat of highly-skilled, organized hackers. WIoT deal with data collected from, and provided to humans. Collected from non harmful wearable sensors, such data is vulnerable to top privacy concerns. For example, some wearable devices collect sensitive information e.g. the user's absolute location and movement activities that compromise the user's privacy if this information is not safeguarded during the processes of storage or communication. To mitigate the risk of cyber-attacks on WIoT, we need strong network security infrastructure for all range of communication. In each passing layer in WIoT, from the wearable sensors to the gateway devices to the cloud, careful precautions are desired to ensure users' privacy and security.

The wearable device concept is applied into real life also. Stanley Healthcare's Experience Center in Waltham, Mass., which has simulated hospital rooms such as the emergency department, and medical-surgical intensive care unit post-anesthesia care unit (PACU) for the company to demonstrate its Internet of Things (IoT) offerings.

Joel Cook, senior healthcare solutions director at Stanley Healthcare, described the ways in which many of Stanley's customers use IoT in healthcare. For example, hospitals take advantage of the technology for real-time location services with badges that can track patients, staff and medical devices. "Many of our customers are using this equipment for asset management," Cook said. Such assets include infusion pumps, wheelchairs, defibrillators, scales and other items that employees tend to tuck into out-of-sight corners yet are needed frequently for treating patients. Another area in which many of Stanley's customers look to IoT in healthcare is patient flow.

With Internet of Things devices, clinicians "in the PACU can see what's going on in the ORs, where they are in the case, and can therefore interpret when people are going to arrive in PACU," Cook explained. "And likewise, people up on the med-surg floor can see what's going on in PACU" and prepare for new patient arrivals.

In addition to real-time location services, Stanley's IoT devices also help with environmental monitoring—for example, checking the temperatures of refrigerators or IT closets—and hand hygiene compliance.

In North America, the lack of hand hygiene in hospitals has been a longtime problem. Cook said that about 100,000 people die from hospital- or healthcare-related infections in North America every year. Greater hand hygiene can help decrease hospital-acquired illnesses.

As hospitals struggle to lower operating costs and remain competitive, IoT in healthcare may offer a way to tighten budgets and improve a patient's journey through a medical facility. "Have to have better patient experiences, better outcomes for those patients," Cook said. "They have to manage populations of people, and they have to do that as efficiently and effectively as possible" [5].

Depending upon different expectation vs requirements of a home remote monitoring system for patients that are having chronic dieses which are not curable easily, few devices have been selected to be used to monitor patient's health. Device that have wireless interface and characteristics that allows interoperability and data transmission. Devices selected for use in the project are:

- A Panasonic BL-C230A Wi-Fi IP camera to capture the movements of patients. Based on the day by day activity and the movements in patient's activity one can make sure that whether the patient is all right or not. All these things of monitoring patients and capturing movements are observed remotely by medical expertise. The device captures the movements in three different services for data (1) Images (2) Sound (3) Body heat. Every movements that are detected is captured as image and to be sent through an email or to FTP server.
- Another wireless body scale fitted with a Wi-Fi interface. It calculates patient's body fat, muscle mass and body mass in percentage. The working of this device connects to the wireless network, it calculates the mass lastly send the data to URL which is ultimately manufacturer site.
- The device to measure blood pressure, has one limit that its operation depends only after the connection is established to Apple device (iPod, iPad, iPhone etc.). The working of this device is similar to scale with one difference that is this device operates via Apple application. All operation is based on the application e.g. sending the collected data to remote server, informing the patient about its blood pressure statistics. The warning of how to handle device to get the correct measurement. The reading of data can be sent from monitoring device and patient's information can be read through web browser. These information is accessible to only authorized medical staff. Patient can communicate with medical staff too. To get the guidance about their regular dose of medicine. The device is responsible for centralizing the data transmission of selected devices is a wireless Access Point (AP). It supports Linux (DD WRT/Open WRT) operating system. This approach enables the development and deployment of additional software, supports IPV4, IPV6, NAT, SNMP, Proxy and server as a gateway to other monitoring device (Fig. 5).

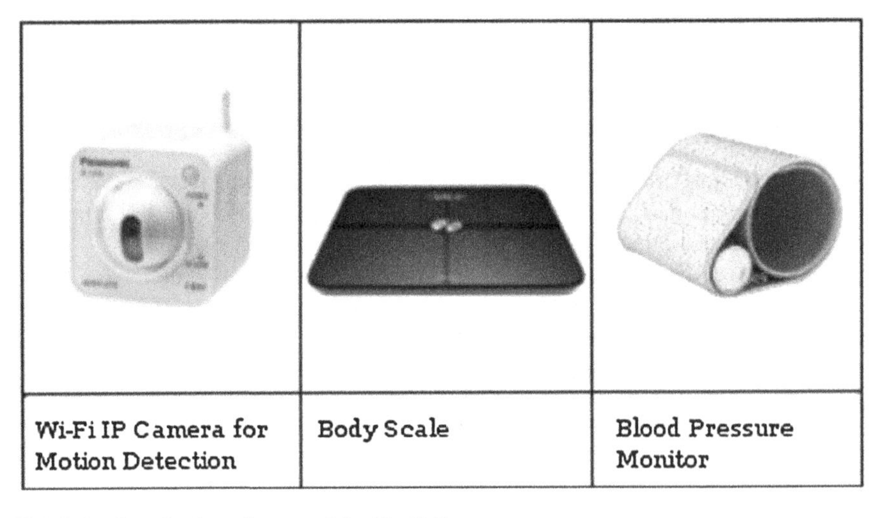

Fig. 5 Devices that have been used for HealthCare

4.4 Interoperability Issues

By understanding all the mechanisms firstly it was assumed that the communication to remote services will be possible with just Wi-Fi. Here in this architecture, the Wi-Fi would serve as a gateway between server (the Internet) and the supervised environment. This approach is applicable but it has restriction on availability of plenty of medical device. Mainly because of Bluetooth technology is widely used in medical devices. This is because of the cheaper cost of Bluetooth technology. Despite of major availability of different technologies in the market we tend to use Bluetooth (802.14) and Zigbee (802.15.4) networks and Internet. This point was adding difficulties in sending data collected by the device to remote server over Wi-Fi connectivity. Interoperability problem can be solved using providing all management capabilities desired Wi-Fi/Bluetooth gateway by either Simple Network Management Protocol or webservices. Healthcare devices built with Wi-Fi interfaces aren't 100 % suitable for use in a flexible monitoring environment. Most of the devices work under server communication for the case of withings body scale. This problem requires a solution to be implemented in the communication infrastructure. This solution is centered in a Access Point (AP) running on Linux (DD WRT/Open WRT) operating system. So it allows extra software to be added to Access Point. The transmitted data is protected in most cases but the traffic analysis reveals that the transmitted data is in JSON format. This simply shows us the flow in security as it allows eavesdropping.

While the wireless network will be implemented for healthcare the following challenges that will be faced:

- Need to understand the problem first. e.g. if we are developing any application for one person's comfort zone then a person should be able to connect to it via home not by going to any particular station.
- Understand the nature of end user. Who will use the solution for long time? What are their limitations or what should be taken consider for them. If this type of solution is invented then who is going to be the user for longer duration of time.
- What type of data is required? For healthcare some diseases shows some of same type of symptoms so to detect particular diseases we need to have specific symptoms. How that data will be transmitted to the other end? The second important aspect of it is how much a sensor read the data rather than focusing on what type of technology it uses.
- The understanding of environment is important. A sensor must be able to differentiate between clinic/hospital (because it does fail to provide that type of data). Moreover the other equipment of home might interfere.
- The noisy environment around, the smart phone complexity, the power management of device all are important things which needs to be focused on.
- Where the sensor should be placed? It should be embedded into walls, a person should wear it, or the sensor should be placed inside human body. What change will it bring into human's day to day life?

- The parameters related to sensors that need to be taken care of are its power, radio computation, weight, computation capacity, antenna type, radio frequency, communication etc. we do need to take one thing in mind that we want low cost with high throughput while designing it.
- The information should be accessed in appropriate manner. Authorized person only be able to access it in manner. Moreover authorized person should also access the data in authorized way.
- The devices should support chronic diseases (the diseases which are generally progressive in nature), medical emergencies (heart attack), real-time monitoring, early diagnosis.
- There are many situations where we need the help such as weather conditions, site collapse, fire. But no major studies have been carried out in this situation so more research is required in this area.
- It is difficult to manage the device diversity and interoperability.
- The data integration is difficult.
- To scale data volume and performance.
- The expected facility is difficult to provide within specific amount of time period and evolution of that facility.
- The data privacy is one of the important and challenge.
- After collecting the bunch of data while we send the data to other end we need a medical expertise at the other end.

The future of Internet of Things in HealthCare can be predict as below:

- Skin disease.
- IoT in healthcare will improve the quality of services than today's.
- By providing personalized and optimized services Internet of Things in healthcare will envisions a better standard of living.
- The IoT will add $1.9 trillion to the world economy by 2020.
- HealthCare IoT will be of $117 billion.
- Age disorder.
- The device for cancer treatment.

5 Conclusion

The Internet of Things still needs the research in healthcare industry. Because as we know now many people die due to lack of treatment or delay in treatment. The Internet of Things aspect in HealthCare industry will bring revolution. It will bring the services at the lower cost to the user who easily cannot afford big treatments like cancer cure. With the help of various devices RFID and sensors it is easy to connect patient with hospital but yet many thins to be considered e.g. interface, connectivity etc. HealthCare in Internet of Things is yet to be in development phase.

References

1. Bhayani, M., Patel, M., Bhatt, C.: Internet of Things (IoT): in a way of smart world. In: Proceedings of the International Congress on Information and Communication Technology, ICICT 2015, Vol. 1, pp. 343–350
2. Bhatt, C., Shah, T.: The Internet of things: technologies, communications and computing. In CSI Communications, April 2014
3. Fernandez, F., Pallis, G.C.: Opportunities and challenges of the Internet of Things for healthcare systems engineering perspective. In: 2014 EAI 4th International Conference on Wireless Mobile Communication and Healthcare (Mobihealth), 3–5 November 2014, Athens
4. http://www.cio.com/article/2981481/healthcare/how-the-internet-of-things-is-changing-healthcare-and-transportation.html
5. http://internetofthingsagenda.techtarget.com/video/Emerging-IoT-technologies-in-healthcare
6. Federal Communications Commission Washington, D.C. Medical Body Area Network. https://675apps.fcc.gov/edocs_public/attachmatch/DA-15-547A1_Rcd.pdf. Accessed 6 May 2015

Energy Efficient Network Design for IoT Healthcare Applications

P. Sarwesh, N. Shekar V. Shet and K. Chandrasekaran

Abstract Internet of Things (IoT) is the emerging technology, that holds huge number of internet enabled devices and allows to share the data globally. IoT technology provides effective healthcare service by constant monitoring and reporting the chronic conditions of patients. IoT is highly greeted by healthcare sectors. IoT devices are smart in nature but constrained by energy, because most of the IoT applications uses battery operated smart devices. Hence energy is considered as valuable resource in energy constrained IoT environment. In this chapter energy efficient network architecture is proposed for IoT health care applications. Proposed network architecture describes the suitable combination of two different techniques such as, routing technique and node placement technique. In routing technique energy level of the nodes are monitored, to transmit the data in energy efficient path. In node placement technique, data traffic is balanced by varying the density of the nodes. This chapter describes the major factors that affect energy efficiency and it elaborates the suitable techniques to improve energy efficiency in IoT network.

Keywords IoT healthcare · Energy efficiency · Reliability · Routing · Node placement

P. Sarwesh (✉) · N.S.V. Shet
Electronics and Communication Engineering, National Institute
of Technology Karnataka, Mangalore, India
e-mail: sarweshpj@gmail.com

N.S.V. Shet
e-mail: shekar_shet@yahoo.com

K. Chandrasekaran
Compute Science Engineering, National Institute of Technology Karnataka,
Mangalore, India
e-mail: kchnitk@gmail.com

C. Bhatt et al. (eds.), *Internet of Things and Big Data Technologies for Next Generation Healthcare*, Studies in Big Data 23,
DOI 10.1007/978-3-319-49736-5_3

1 Introduction

Internet of Things is smart technology, which utilizes the resource in efficient way. It converges physical objects with Internet to form cyber physical systems. Smart devices plays a major role in IoT health care applications, medical instruments with IoT features works autonomously with its basic capabilities, such as sensing (collecting health related information), processing and communication [1, 2]. Medical instruments collect the health related information of patients and report to the server through data acquisition boards. In Health care Bio-sensors plays a major role. Bio-sensor is a medical instrument that converts bio-signals into electrical signals. Bio-sensors serve the health care industry by monitoring the patients chronic condition and reporting to medical supervisors. Wearable bio-sensors monitors the metabolic activities of human body and changes the human behavior by instructing to them, it is more useful for elder people who stay in home alone. Designing bio-sensor involves various research areas such as, bioreactor science, spanning biochemistry, electrochemistry, electronics, physical chemistry and software engineering. Bio-sensors consist of transducer that converts bio signal into electrical signals, processing unit, storage unit, data transmission unit and battery source [3]. Most of the bio-sensors uses smart antennas for transmission and reception and radio links such as, IEEE 802.15.4, IEEE 802.11, IEEE 802.15.1, etc. The data generated by bio-sensors need to be retrieved, hence servers such as SQL server can be used for storing the patients health information. In health care applications, edge devices (medical instruments equipped with sensor devices) and data acquisition boards are operated by battery source. Hence energy wastage should be highly prevented in IoT network [2]. Balanced energy utilization in energy constrained network is the major challenge in low power IoT networks. The network is said to be energy efficient, when it provides effective communication between IoT devices with better reliability [4]. Design IoT application involves various technologies such as, communication, embedded systems, cloud computing, network design, devices design etc. In these technologies, energy efficiency can be improved by communication technology (by adjusting physical parameters), network design (by constructing energy efficient protocols) and device design (designing less power consuming devices). Providing effective service to patients is the major goal in healthcare sectors, to provide effective service, Quality of Service (QoS) parameters need to be satisfied. QoS parameters can be achieved by transmitting data in stable and reliable links, Stability of the data transmission links depends on the transmission power of antenna. Hence effective power utilization improves the reliability as well as QoS of the network [5].

In health care applications, health conditions of patients will be constantly monitored by the health care instruments and transmitted to data acquisition boards. If these devices run out its battery short span, it severely affects the service [5]. Frequent battery replacement will degrade the entire system performance. Hence necessary steps should be taken care for balancing energy consumption in IoT networks. Non uniform energy consumption decreases the network lifetime and QoS; hence it affects service provider as well as customer. To improve the energy utilization, the factors that affect the energy efficiency need to analyzed and rectified. The major factors that affects energy efficiency are uneven data traffic, energy hole problem, multi data retransmission and delay [6]. The energy efficient techniques such as, routing technique (network layer technique), node placement technique (physical layer technique), power control techniques (MAC layer technique) etc., are suitable techniques to improve energy efficiency in low power networks [6].

In many research papers it's mentioned that, nodes which are far from base station not utilized its battery power more than 50 %. The reason behind ~50 % un-utilized energy is communication block to sink, where nodes near to the sink will be overloaded and drains its energy quick, which stops entire communication to sink, this issue is referred as energy hole problem [2]. Data re-transmission is another issue which severely affects the energy efficiency of the network. Transmitting data through poor quality links/unstable links leads to packet loss, which increases the data re-transmission. When re-transmission increases, nodes drain out its battery in quick span of time. The other major issue which affects the energy efficiency and lifetime of the network is collision [7]. Source node transmits data to destination node in particular channel and a new node transmits data through same channel, it leads to collision of data. Once collision occurs, receiver and transmitter re-establishes the connection to recover the lost packets, connection re-establishment increases the congestion as well as energy consumption. Collision severely affects the latency and energy efficiency of the network [7]. Collision occurrence is more in carrier-sense multiple access technique (CSMA). In time division multiple access (TDMA) collisions can be avoided, TDMA allots particular time slot to each node for accessing the channel, which prevents the collision. In some cases, allotting time slots to every node may increase the control overhead and wastage of energy.

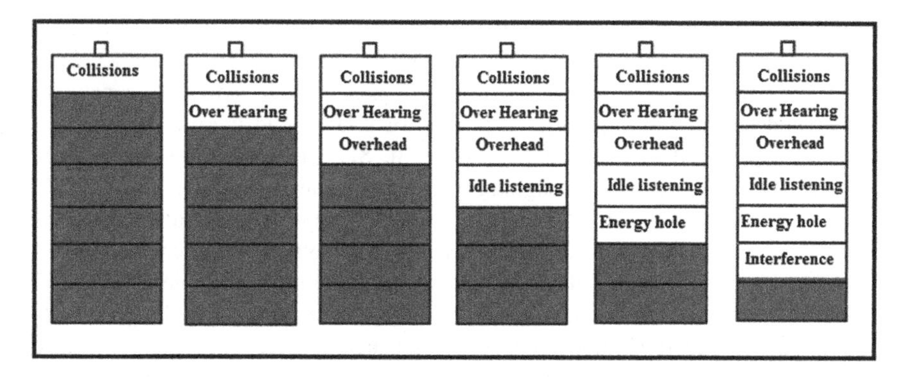

Fig. 1 Factors that affects energy efficiency

Figure 1, describes the major factors that affects the energy efficiency of the network. The other major factors that influence energy efficiency is overhearing and idle listening [8]. Unwanted packet reception of a node is referred as overhearing; it severely affects the performance and lifetime of the network. Chance of overhearing is more in unicast communication, when multi receiver receives un-wanted packets in their active state; it leads to huge energy wastage [8]. In low power networks, receive board and transmitter board almost consumes same amount of energy. So receiver energy is also more considerable in low power networks. Compared to TDMA-based schemes, occurrence of overhearing is more in CDMA-based schemes [8]. Reducing the overhearing reduces the energy wastage in receiver; effect of overhearing is more in large scale applications. Idle listening is similar to over hearing issue, when a node is in active state with idle job (without receiving any data) is referred as idle listening. Effect of idle listening is more in monitoring applications, because in monitoring applications nodes will be in active state without receiving any data, to detect the event. In some research work, sleep and awake mechanism is implemented based on event occurrence, if event occurs the nodes will be turned to active state else it will be in sleep state, but switching the nodes to different states consumes energy [8]. Hence overhearing and idle listening issues need to be addressed to improve the lifetime of the network.

Control packet overhead is the major factor that is increases the energy consumption in the network. To establish the connection in the network (nodes need to identify the neighbour nodes and base station in the network), control packets need to be flooded in the network, which consumes significant amount of energy. Control packets are referred as hello packets or rout request and route replay packets, which is used for connecting nodes and computing paths. Hence control overhead is required for a network to establish effective connectivity, but it should not exceed it limit, which leads to huge energy wastage [8]. Interference is the other major issue in low power and lossy networks, interference occurs when unwanted signal interfere the original signal. The major reasons for interference are noise, environmental conditions, more number of radio signal sharing the same bandwidth, etc. The interference that occurs during channel overlaps is called as co-channel interference. The chance of interference is more in network, which have low power devices connected by unstable links [8]. This are the major factors that influence the energy efficiency in low power network (IoT network), it reduces the network lifetime and degrades the performance of network. To avoid these issues, various layers are optimized in research filed [2, 5, 6, 8]. One of the possible way to implement IoT applications is designing IoT network with battery operated devices. Most of the zone or sensing environment, where IoT network implemented will be remote environment. Providing electrical wires in remote environment is impossible. Hence battery operated devices are possible solution for implementing IoT devices, which operates wirelessly. So the possible solution to prolong network lifetime and reduce implementation cost is balancing energy in battery operated devices.

There are several factors that affect the energy efficiency in wireless network. The major factor that affects the energy efficiency in IoT health care applications are re-transmissions and uneven data traffic. Transmitting data through poor quality links leads to re-transmission which severely affects energy efficiency and reliability. Uneven data traffic occurs due to improper node placement; hence these issues are mainly focused in proposed network architecture.

In further sections the optimization techniques to improve the energy efficiency in IoT network is elaborated. The sections of this chapter is organised in following way, Sect. 2 describes the importance of energy efficiency in IoT health care applications, Sect. 3 elaborates the techniques which are used to improve the energy efficiency, Sect. 4 explains the proposed network architecture for IoT health care applications, results are discussed in Sect. 5 and Sect. 5 concludes this chapter.

2 Importance of Energy Efficiency in IoT Healthcare Applications

2.1 IoT World Forum Reference Model

Internet of Things is considerably attracting many applications such as, e-health, smart home, smart city, smart grid, smart environment, industrial automation, smart market etc. Network architectures of these applications are referred from IoT world forum reference model [9], it is the seven layered architecture model, which gives the clear idea about IoT architecture. In Figure, first three layers (devices and controllers, connectivity, edge computing) of the IoT world forum reference model refers the data aggregation and processing (real time data) of real time events, last three layers (data abstraction, application, collaboration and process) refers data aggregation and processing (non real time data) of query based events and middle layer refers the storage of data, which is generated by all other layers.

The devices used in higher layers and middle layer are referred as higher end devices, which are operated by main power lines. So energy utilization is not a major challenge in these layers, the major challenges of these layers is data management and processing, because it handles huge amount of data (Big Data). Devices used in lower layers are referred as edge devices, which are operated by battery power. Hence balanced energy utilization is the major challenge in lower layers. Figure 2, describes the features of various layers and challenges of higher layers and lower layers. Based on the real time challenges various layers are optimized, energy is considered as important resource in lower layers, because it holds energy constrained smart devices. In many IoT applications, battery powered smart devices are expected to run for few years, when the battery drains out its power soon, it leads to frequent battery replacement, which severely affects the cost of the network. Hence improving the network lifetime is one of the major challenges in small scale IoT applications as well as large scale IoT applications.

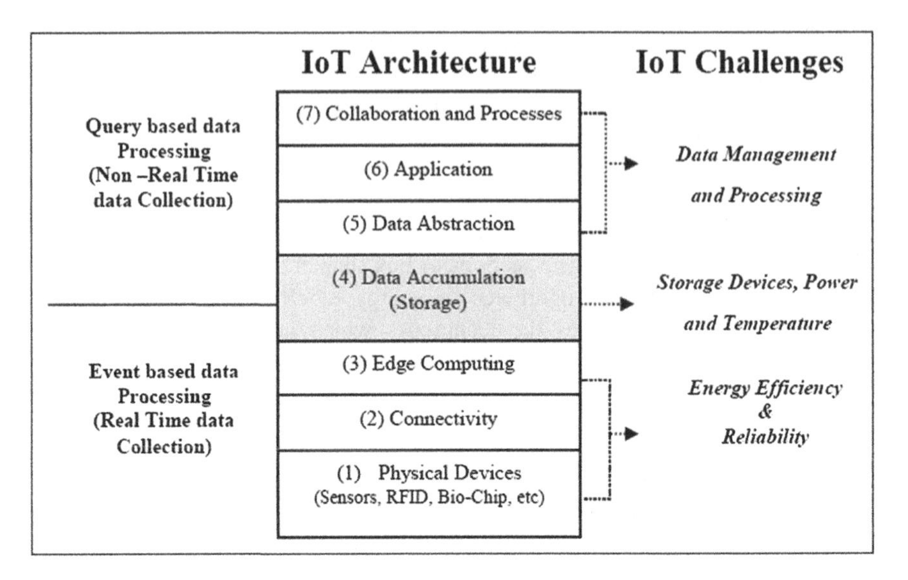

Fig. 2 IoT world forum reference model

2.2 *Energy Constrained Nature of IoT Network*

The term "energy constrained" refers the battery operated smart devices and low power radio links in the network. In IoT network device level challenges are cost, physical size, and power consumption, similarly network level challenges are bandwidth, transmission range and power (transmission power and reception power). To satisfy cost requirements and bandwidth requirements most of the IoT applications handles low power device and low power radio links [5, 6, 10]. Providing effective communication in low power environment with low cost and low bandwidth is the challenging task in IoT networks. Hence energy utilization is major concern in low power network environment. In environmental monitoring applications (land slide, flood monitoring, tsunami, etc.) frequent battery replacement is impossible, because the nodes will be deployed in harsh environment. In health monitoring applications (chronic conditions of patients) often battery replacement severely affects the health care service, because patients who are in critical conditions will be monitored continuously.

IoT network establishes connection to remote devices through unreliable links, which are low power radio links (IEEE 802.15.4, IEEE 802.11), which are unstable and highly lossy in nature. Where in Internet Ethernet links and SONET/SDH links are used for connecting devices, which are highly stable in nature, So reliability issues are less in internet and high in Internet of Things. Reliability issues (data re-transmission) give rise to energy efficiency issue (quick battery drains out). Routers and other devices used in Internet are operated by main power supply, where in IoT it is operated by battery power, Hence Internet highly differs from Internet of Things [10–13]. The

Table 1 Energy constrained nature of IoT

Features	Internet	IoT network
Nodes	Routers	Sensors/actuators, bio-chip etc.
Links	High power and stable links	Low power and unstable links
Nature of device	Non-constrained device	Constrained device (limited in battery)
Address	Internet protocol address	Internet protocol address
Routing	Non-application aware routing	Application aware routing
Power source	Main grid power	Battery (most of the applications)

Table 2 Energy constrained nature of IoT devices

Device	Signal type	Applications	Power
RFID tag	Low power radio	Tracking objects, etc.	Battery
Multimedia sensors	Low power radio	Wildlife monitoring, etc.	Battery
Bio-sensors	Low power radio	Healthcare monitoring, etc.	Battery
Sensors	Low Power radio	Household, Industry, etc.	Battery
Smart dust	Low power radio	Military applications, etc.	Battery

common feature for IoT and Internet is both uses Internet Protocol version 6(IPv6) address for establishing communication, which has large address spacing. Table 1 describes the energy constrained nature of Internet of things.

Providing main power lines to harsh environment is difficult task and Devices designed for health monitoring applications are battery powered. In low power radio are fairly unstable in nature and chance of packet loss is high, due to weak signal strength, interference and other issues. Low power links for low power devices cannot be neglected, it is the only possible solution, because only radio links like (IEEE 802.15.4, IEEE 802.11) can offers low duty cycle for smart devices [5]. So it is very important to monitor the stability of links and battery level of devices. Table 2 describes the energy constrained nature of IoT devices.

Over flooding is the other major issue, which severely affects the energy consumption. In low power network scenario, transmitting control packets frequently destroys the stability of the link, hence flooding need to be in controlled manner. Irregular data traffic may also reduces the signal strength and increases the dynamicity in link quality. So little variations in data traffic or network over load will reduce the stability of links. By considering the features of low power links and battery operated IoT devices, we can say IoT networks are highly constrained by energy.

2.3 Energy Constrained Nature of IoT Health Care Application

The technology is said to be successive technology based on how it provides effective service to the society. IoT technology is a successive technology, which plays a great role in resource utilization (smart grid, home automation, industrial automation etc.), service providing (e-health, smart market, smart city, etc.) and environmental friendly (pollution control in vehicles as well as industries, flood monitoring, garbage monitoring etc.). Hence it is highly greeted by many organizations (private as well as public). In these applications, smart health is one of the successive applications developed by IoT technology. The major challenges in e-health applications are energy efficiency and QoS, to achieve QoS the system should be energy efficient [5, 10, 12]. Hence energy efficiency is taken as major objective in this chapter.

In Healthcare organization verities of bio devices are used to monitor the health conditions of the patients, in that data acquisition boards plays a major role in e-health application. Data acquisition boards collect the health information of patients from bio-devices and transfers it to the sink and sink will forward it to storage systems, where the doctors can access the data. This entire process can be said as smart health or e-health. In bio-devices, some are operated by main power supply and some are operated by battery power. But most of the data acquisition boards, which collect the information from the bio-devices, are operated by battery power. In healthcare applications, sensitive data is collected and stored, if data loss occurs due to device failure (battery run out) it severely affects the service to the patients. The most data acquisition boards and medical instruments equipped with IoT features uses low power radio such as, IEEE 802.15.4, IEEE 802.11 for their communication, so there is a chance of reliability issues. Hence balancing the energy consumption and maintaining the energy efficiency with effective health care service is the major aim of this application. The following section describes the major techniques that are used to improve the energy efficiency.

3 Techniques to Improve Energy Efficiency

Internet of things and wireless sensor networks are the fast growing user friendly technology in emerging field. Production of low power and low cost devices by the MEMS technology and low power radio communication by efficient protocol design are the major reason for the development of IoT and WSN applications. Due to MEMS technology, low power and low cost devices works autonomously by its basic capabilities (sensing, processing communication etc.) and due to low power radio protocol design, network implementation became possible in all kinds of applications from wild life monitoring to patients health monitoring. Rapid development of low power device and protocol design, improves the resources utilization in efficient way. In every application from large scale to small scale, implementation cost and effective service need to be satisfied. In many application scenario providing main power line is difficult task, so the possible way is battery operated devices, when the battery runs out its energy frequently it affects both implementation cost as well as user service. Hence effective energy utilization in IoT network is considered as challenging task in research field [2].

3.1 Role of Hardware and Software in Improving Energy Efficiency

Many technologies and optimization techniques are developing, to improve the energy efficiency in low power networks. Energy can be efficiently balanced by the considering the device level power constraints of particular application. Designing an effective and low cost devices based on application environment improves the energy efficiency in the system. IoT devices consist of transducer (sensing unit), micro controller or micro processor (processing unit), antennas and transmission and reception circuit (communication unit) and kind of power source, either main power or battery operated (power unit). Configuration of all these parts (units) of device need to satisfy the implementation cost as well as its performance (device lifetime, reliability, etc.) of device. If the cost and performance decreases it affects the end users (consumers). Better device performance with better device lifetime is the major expectations from end users. Lifetime of device can be improved by constant monitoring of current leakage and efficient processor design, current leakage severely affects the power efficiency of the device similarly processor speed consumes significant amount of device energy, which should be regulated. Similar to hardware design software design also have a impact on the power utilization of the device. Efficient software design regulates the power usage of hardware components, software and operating system should switch the hardware components sleep state, whenever the data transmission and data reception is in idle state. Hence efficient design of hard and software design improves the lifetime of the device [5].

3.2 Role of Protocols in Improving Energy Efficiency

Efficient protocols play a major role in improving the lifetime of entire network. In many research works, it is described that 70–80 % of energy is consumed by communication unit (transmission unit and reception unit), processing unit also consumes significant amount of energy, when compared to sensing unit. Hence regulating the communication unit highly improves the performance and lifetime of the network. Efficient protocol design is the possible solution for regulating the communication unit of the system. Protocol design varies from layer to layer (from physical layer to application layer). Figure 3 describes the techniques to improve the energy efficiency based on TCP/IP layer structure.

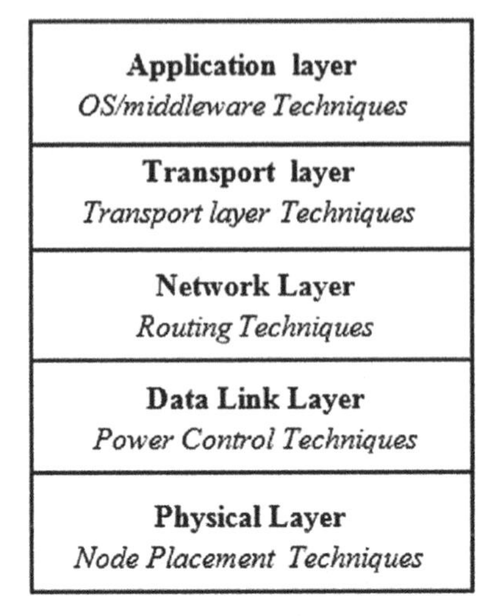

Fig. 3 Techniques to improve the energy efficiency

Figure 3 describe the various techniques in research field, that are used to improve the energy efficiency. The following sub section elaborates the features of the techniques.

3.3 Physical Layer Technique to Improve Energy Efficiency

Node placement technique is considered as effective physical layer technique to improve the energy efficiency in low power networks. Uneven data traffic can be highly regulated by node placement technique, balancing uneven data traffic reduces the node over burden, which avoids the quick node death and improves the network lifetime. Designing efficient node placement technique reduces the implementation cost and prolongs the network lifetime with better device connectivity. In any kind of node placement technique, Network lifetime and better connectivity are the major goals of researchers. In node placement technique one board transmission range will be assigned with respective to positions of nodes, which highly balances the energy consumption. Major node placement techniques uses as graph based optimization techniques to improve the performance of the network [14]. Various algorithms used to optimize the node placement techniques are Particle swarm optimization (PSO)-based algorithms, optimized artificial fish swarm algorithm (OAFSA), multi-objective optimization, bio-logical inspired algorithms, genetic algorithm (GA), territorial predator scent marking algorithm (TPSMA), virtual force directed co-evolutionary PSO (VFCPSO), artificial bee colony (ABC), etc. By the effective node placement technique, density of nodes can be significantly reduced, which highly reduces the implementation cost of the system.

In many research papers, it is proved that efficient node placement technique reduces the cost of network by reducing the node densities and improves the life time of network by balancing the energy consumption. Device connectivity is the major process in node placement technique, if the connectivity between the nodes are better with respectively densities then the communication will be established between the nodes. Varying the node density in network also improves the energy efficiency in the system. Most of the network application scenarios are many to one (sensors to base station), the nodes in such network scenario will forward the collected information to the neighbor nodes, which are near to base station [15–17]. Due to such kind of forwarding process the nodes, which are near to the base station will be over-burdened by huge data traffic and drain out its power soon. If the nodes are deployed in non uniform fashion, such as more number nodes near to base station and moderate amount of nodes little far from base station and less amount of nodes far from base station, it highly regulates the data traffic and improves the energy efficiency. In many literature it is described that varying the node density in network scenario, highly improves the life time of the network. In [16, 17] authors considered energy consumption per data collection round as lifetime metric and improved the lifetime of the network, they describe that, spreading the loads of nodes in balanced way highly balances the energy utilization in resource constraint network scenario. In [18, 19] authors analyzed relation between the node density and network lifetime and formulated one dimensional placement scenario analytically.

In node placement technique, many research works is done on relay node placement, relay nodes are special kind of nodes that are responsible for data aggregation from sensors. In Relay node placement technique nodes can be categorized into two types, relay nodes and sensor nodes. Sensor nodes are responsible for sensing, computation (processing) and communication (transmission and reception). Relay nodes are responsible for computation and communication. Sensor does sensing (collect the environmental data), processing the sensed data and transmits the data to base station. Relay collects the data from sensors and other relays, after data aggregation, relay node transmits the data to base station. Base station collects information from relays and sends the data to storage unit. By considering two verities of nodes, device complexity can be minimized, where sensor will be free from forwarding process and relays will be free from sensing process [19–22].

In smart health applications, sensor nodes can be considered as bio-sensors and can be considered as data acquisition boards can be considered as relay nodes. Suitable relay node placement technique with non uniform node density can highly improve the performance and lifetime of network, which can be implemented in healthcare applications. Hence implementing effective node placement in healthcare applications improves the energy efficiency and network lifetime in IoT healthcare networks.

3.4 Network Layer Technique to Improve Energy Efficiency

Routing is the well know network layer technique to improve the energy efficiency in low power networks. An efficient routing satisfies the network lifetime, reliability and QoS of the network. Many non-uniform energy utilization problems such as, uneven data traffic, multi-retransmissions, high latency, etc., can be solved by routing technique. In main power networks (grid powered network) like internet, routing mechanism will be designed to satisfy the reliability and QoS of the network. In energy constrained network (battery operated network) routing mechanism will be designed to satisfy the energy efficiency, reliability and QoS of the network. Hence power efficiency is more important in resource constrained network [23–25]. In previous section it is described that maximum energy utilization is done by communication unit of the system, routing will be the better choice to regulate the communication in the network. Efficient routing technique computes the energy efficient and reliable path to transmit the data, hence energy level of nodes will be in balanced way and packet loss will be prevented.

In low power networks, finding the stable link and transmitting the data in stable link prevents packet loss and re-transmissions can be avoided. Similarly energy level of nodes can be monitored and transmit the data to nodes with good energy level, balances the energy consumption, routing plays a major role in this operation. Routing protocols transmit the route request (control packet) with energy and reliability related information and receives route replay packet (control packet) with those information's and transmits the data in energy efficient and reliable path, this process is called flooding. When the flooding increases the packed overhead increases, which leads to huge energy consumption, hence over flooding need to be avoided while designing an efficient routing protocol. In current research field there are several routing protocol address the energy efficiency, reliability and QoS issues. Routing protocols are broadly classified into six different types, the following sub section elaborates the various classifications of routing protocol [26–29].

(a) Attribute-based protocols

It is the content based routing mechanism. In attribute-based routing mechanism, nodes are aware of the neighbor information, nodes transmits the content based data packet and receives the neighbor nodes information. In this type of routing mechanism nodes take its own decision to forward or drop the packet, they follow data centric routing approaches. The major protocols works in attribute-based routing are energy-aware data-centric routing protocol, directed diffusion protocol, constrained shortest-path energy-aware routing protocol, RUMOR protocol etc. This kind of routing approach is better in improving the energy efficiency of the network. The major concentration in these type of approach is over flooding need to be avoided [2].

(b) Flat protocols

In flat based routing huge number of node work together and collects the environmental data and transfer it to the destination. In this type of routing all the nodes will have same configuration and features. Flat based routing is more suitable in large scale applications. Many flat based routing protocols concentrate on parameters such as, hop-count, energy level, signal strength. This information will be stored in routing table of nodes and based on routing table, source node will select the intermediate nodes to destination [2]. The popular flat based routing protocols are sequential assignment routing protocol, minimum cost forwarding routing, gradient broadcast, etc. This protocols works better in low power large scale environment and improves the power efficiency.

(c) Geographical Routing

In geographic routing, nodes are aware of the neighbor location information and nodes priory finds the neighbor nodes location information and based on the location information nodes forwards the data packets to destination node. Due to exchanging the location information, source nodes transmits the data in shortest distance to destination. This improves the energy efficiency of network [2]. The well know protocols in this technique are stateless protocol for soft real time communication, geographic routing with no location in-formation, etc. Geographic based routing protocols reduce the packet overhead in network and improve the network lifetime.

(d) Hierarchical protocols

Hierarchical routing protocols are the efficient routing protocols, which improves the energy efficiency and lifetime of the network. In hierarchical based routing mechanism, nodes are classified into different types such as, sensor node, cluster-heads, and base station. Sensor nodes form a cluster and there will be cluster head for every cluster, sensor collects the environment information and transmits to cluster head, cluster head aggregates the collected information and forwards it to base station. This entire process is referred as hierarchical based routing [2]. Some of popular hierarchical protocols are power-efficient gathering in sensor information system, threshold sensitive energy-efficient sensor network protocol, low-energy adaptive clustering hierarchy, etc. These protocols are better in energy balancing.

(e) Multipath Routing

The major reason behind the development of multipath routing protocols is to avoid route failures and reduce packet re-transmissions. Alternating the data path in case of rout failures, highly improves the energy efficiency and reliability of the network. When route failures occurs in single path routing, control packets need to be generated additionally, which increases the overhead of the system. Hence multipath routing reduces the overhead of the system and improves the energy efficiency as well as reliability. The following common protocols used for multipath routing technique, energy efficient multipath routing in wireless sensor networks, reinForM, meshed multipath routing, etc. [2].

3.5 Data Link Layer Technique to Improve Energy Efficiency

MAC based optimization techniques, regulates the transmission range of antennas as well as schedules the data transmission to improve the energy efficiency. MAC layer is the sub-layer of data link layer. Scheduling is one of the efficient technique in MAC based optimization, in scheduling techniques transmission period of each nodes will be scheduled, during the allotted active (transmission) period nodes forwards the collected information to destination. The other important MAC based optimization technique is power control technique, based on the distance and signal strength of the neighbor, transmission power will be tuned. MAC based protocols majorly concentrate on effective channel allocation, sharing the channels in effective way highly improves the bandwidth utilization and prolongs the network life time. This technique adopts dynamic topology changes and its flexible for any kind of network scenario. Hence MAC plays the major role in regulating the transmission power of the system, Low power MAC protocols are used for IoT applications. The common MAC based optimization techniques are Scheduling-based mechanism, Power off mechanism, Power Control Techniques, Antenna-based mechanism and Multi Channel Mechanism [7, 8, 30].

(a) Scheduling-based mechanism

Scheduling is one of the efficient technique to address the collision and idle listening issues. By avoiding the collision and idle listening major amount of energy can be saved. The scheduling-based mechanism are majorly classified into three types they are time-division multiple access (TDMA), frequency-division multiple access (FDMA) and code-division multiple access (CDMA). In FDMA technique the frequency of the band will be divided, based on frequency values nodes can access the various frequency at same time period. In TDMA technique same frequency can be accessed by various nodes at different time slots. In CDMA node can access the same frequency at the same time based on different code values. In current research, hybrid scheduling protocols are emerging, for example combination of TDMA and CDMA, which improves the power efficiency of the system. Some of the standard scheduling based MAC protocols are IEEE 802.15.4, EC-MAC protocol, IEEE 802.11, PAMAS protocol, etc. [30, 31].

(b) Power Control Techniques

Power control techniques are more suitable solution for contention based mechanism. In contention based schemes topology of the network changes dynamically and they are robust in nature, which consumes energy for acknowledgement and retransmissions. Some energy reservation is required for balancing the energy consumption, which is done by power control techniques. Power control techniques reserves the energy by tuning the transmission range based on the distance and signal strength, hence it is more suitable for contention based techniques. The protocols used for power control techniques are Power Controlled Multiple Access (PCMA) Protocol, Power Control MAC (PCM), Power Controlled Dual Channel (PCDC), Dynamic Channel Assignment with Power Control (DCA-PC), Common Power (COMPOW) Protocol, etc. [old 29, 30].

(c) Power off mechanism

Power off mechanism controls the idle listening in low power network scenario. In many wireless network scenario, receiver will be in active state without sensing any data, this state is referred as idle listening state. In low power network, receiver board consumes approximately same power in which transmitter board consumes. Receiver power is more important in low power networks. When receiver is kept in active state for entire simulation period, it consumes huge energy and life of network will be severely affected. To avoid the energy wastage in network, receiver power should be kept in sleep mode when it is in idle state, which is done by the power off mechanism. Some of the efficient power off mechanisms is MACA protocol, synchronization-MAC, Power-aware Multi-access Protocol with Signaling (PAMAS), Power management using multi sleep states, Pico Node Multi-Channel MAC, etc. [30, 31]. Hence power off mechanisms are improves energy efficiency by avoiding idle listening.

(d) Multi channel mechanism

Multichannel mechanism outperforms various other techniques in channel utilization. Multi channel mechanism basically uses two different channels for communication establishment; it uses one control channel and multi data channel from overall bandwidth, which prevents the collisions in network. In this scheme control channel carries contention based data and data channel carries data and acknowledgement. Hence it is more suitable for contention based schemes. Multi channel mechanism is categorized into two types one is multichannel scheme and other is busy tone scheme. Both schemes are designed to avoid collision occurrence. The common protocols used in multichannel mechanism are Dual Busy Tone Multiple Access protocol (DBTMA), Dynamic Channel Assignment (DCA) protocol, etc. [30, 31].

(e) Antenna-based mechanism

Antenna based mechanism highly improves the energy efficiency by optimizing or regulating the transmission and reception power of the antennas. The major source of power consumption in wireless network is transmission and reception antenna power. Hence fine tuning the transmission and reception power of antennas, reduces the energy wastage and improve the life time of the network [8, 30]. Some of the popular antenna based schemes are directional antenna (smart antenna) and Omni-antenna, which improves the power efficiency of the system in effective way.

Many research work is carried out in antenna design for optimizing antenna structures such as, maximum gain, minimal size and minimum consumables. Designing antenna for wireless devices which are randomly deployed in harsh network environment is challenging task. The adaptive antenna generally has degrees of freedom in the form of amplitude and phase or time delay weighting of multiple channels to adjust its radiation pattern, which are more suitable for WSN and IoT applications. Planar inverted F-antenna, Chip antennas, Whip antennas, Patch antenna, Dual-band dipole antenna, Bowtie antenna, Bowtie-Shaped Folded Dipole antenna are some of common antennas used for low power sensor devices [32].

By optimizing the MAC layer technique, issues such as collision. Idel listening, over hearing, re-transmission can be avoided and energy efficiency can be improved. Implementing the efficient MAC protocol technique in healthcare applications increases the reliability and energy efficiency of the IoT healthcare system.

3.6 Transport Layer Technique to Improve Energy Efficiency

Transport layer techniques concentrate on optimizing the reliability of the network. By improving the reliability, parameters such as overhead cost and frequency utilization can be improved and link failures and data retransmissions can be avoided. These parameters are directly related to the energy efficiency of the network. Hence transport layer techniques indirectly improve the energy efficiency of the network [7]. Some of the versions of TCP concentrate on energy related parameters.

3.7 Application Layer Technique to Improve Energy Efficiency

OS/middleware Techniques plays a major role in increasing the performance of the network. High mobility is the major reason for power reduction in devices, which can be optimized by OS/middleware techniques. An efficient processor with good processing capability can utilize the bandwidth and power in optimized way, but in current market processor with high processing capability are quite expensive. Implementing expensive processors for large scale application is impossible. The alternate way of achieving energy efficiency in device level is designing a efficient operating system, which balances the CPU usage and scale down the supply voltage. Predictive shut down technique is one of the efficient OS/middleware techniques to improve the power efficiency of the system. This technique works in different modes such as, active mode, standby mode, nap mode and power down mode. It highly reduces the power consumption of device [7]. Particularly for health care applications Energy based and QoS based algorithms such as sequential assignment routing protocol, minimum cost forwarding routing, gradient broadcast, stateless protocol for soft real time communication, geographic routing with no location in-formation, power-efficient gathering in sensor information system, threshold sensitive energy-efficient sensor network protocol, low-energy adaptive clustering hierarchy, multipath routing technique, energy efficient multipath routing in wireless sensor networks, reinForM, meshed multipath routing can be suitable for IoT Health Care applications.

The techniques which described in this section, does the efficient task to improve the energy efficiency, but still there is a tradeoff between cost and lifetime of the network in present low power network scenario. The following section describes the proposed network architecture for IoT health care applications.

4 Proposed Network Architecture

Most of the IoT applications run by IoT and WSN technology are low power network. Many optimization techniques are emerging to prolong the network lifetime in low power networks. In low power network design, particular technique (single layer) is optimized by concentrating particular parameter to improve the performance of network. It is complex to satisfy multiple parameters by single optimization technique, when complexity of algorithm increases the performance of network decreases. In proposed network architecture, we used two different techniques to improve the performance of network. The basic idea to optimize two different layer techniques in single network architecture is to split the parameters and reduce the complexity of particular layer. In proposed network architecture routing technique and node placement techniques are optimized to improve the energy efficiency of the network [33].

4.1 Adopting Real-Time Healthcare Scenario to Proposed Network Architecture Scenario

In real time health care applications, bio-sensors with transmission and reception features and data acquisition boards are used with data storage systems. In proposed network scenario, we consider sensor nodes as bio-sensors and relay nodes as data acquisition boards and sink node as base station. Based on the assumptions, we designed network architecture in NS-2 simulator and analyzed the performance of the network. In [34] EOROTECH real-time healthcare scenario is described, based on [34] EUROTECH architecture, we designed the simulation scenario for IoT health care applications.

Figure 4 describes the proposed network architecture with relay nodes and sensor nodes, in proposed work node placement is done in setup phase and routing is done in initialization phase. Node placement and routing technique holds two different parameters. In proposed work two parameters such as data traffic and SNR are optimized by using node placement and routing technique. Data traffic is taken care by node placement technique and SNR is taken care by routing technique. Burdening to parameters in single technique increases the complexity of the algorithm, hence two parameters are split to two different techniques (Fig. 5).

The following sub-section elaborates the overall features of proposed network architecture. Hence proposed architecture will be good in load balancing, energy balancing and link quality balancing, which will be suitable for most of the IoT and WSN applications.

4.2 Proposed Node Placement Technique

Node placement technique improves the energy consumption, node placement technique is chosen for regulating the data traffic in proposed network scenario. Node placement technique is done in network setup phase, in proposed network architecture density of nodes are increased towards the sink, because the nodes near to the sink carries huge amount of data traffic, when compared to other nodes in the network. The density variation of sensor nodes and relay nodes are done based on the following assumptions.

Basic node placement Assumptions

(1) *For every sensor node, one relay node is assigned in high traffic area (red circle).*
(2) *For two sensor nodes, one relay node is assigned in medium traffic area (blue circle).*
(3) *For three sensor nodes, one relay node is assigned in low traffic area (green circle).*

In Fig. 6, red circle indicates high data traffic area, blue circle indicates medium data traffic area and green circle indicates low data traffic area. By considering the traffic area, the relay nodes are assigned to sensor nodes.

4.3 Proposed Routing Technique

In proposed architecture AODV routing protocol is used for data transmission. The reason for choosing AODV protocol is its reactive nature, no topology messages exchange is required for communication along the links, which reduces bandwidth

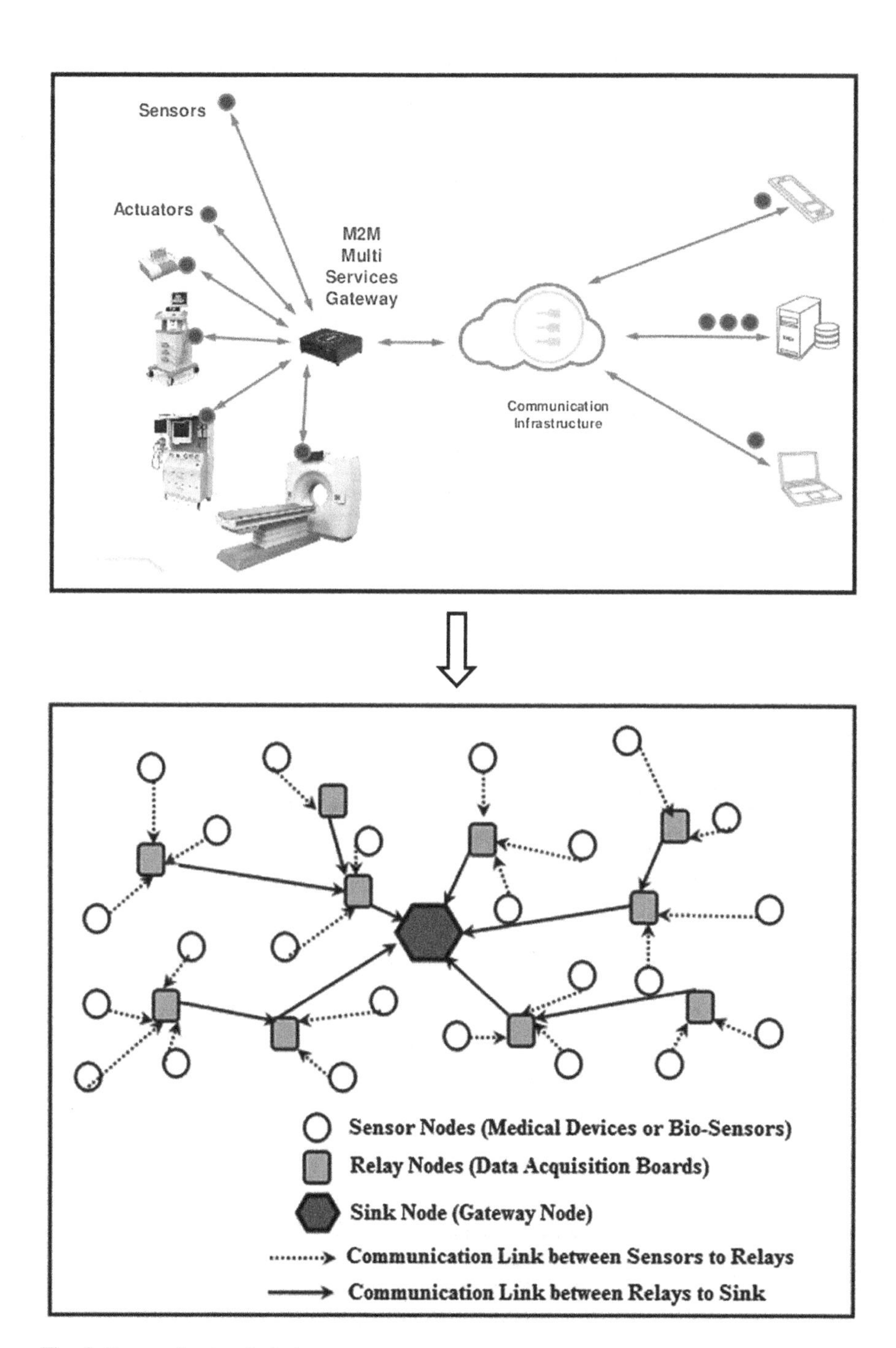

Fig. 4 Proposed network design

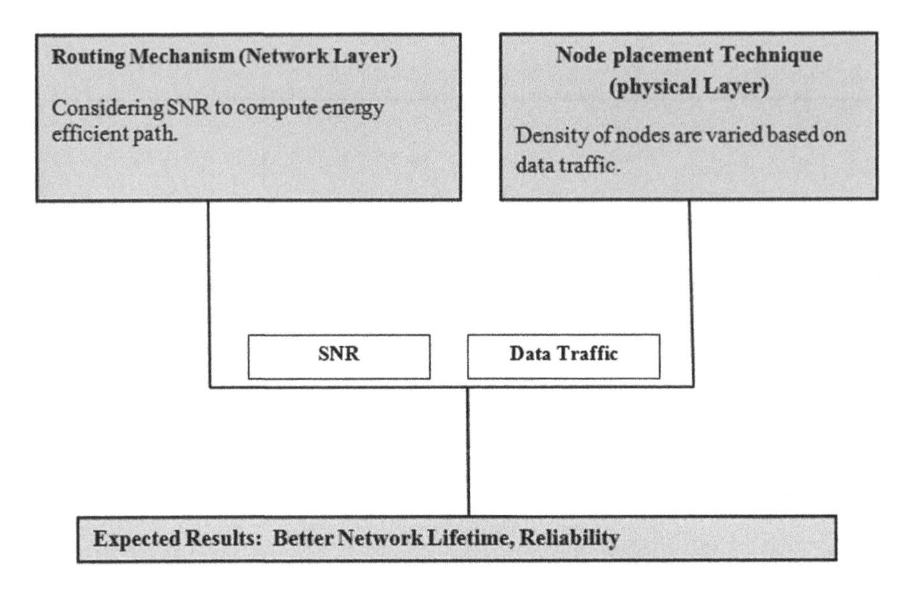

Fig. 5 Proposed work

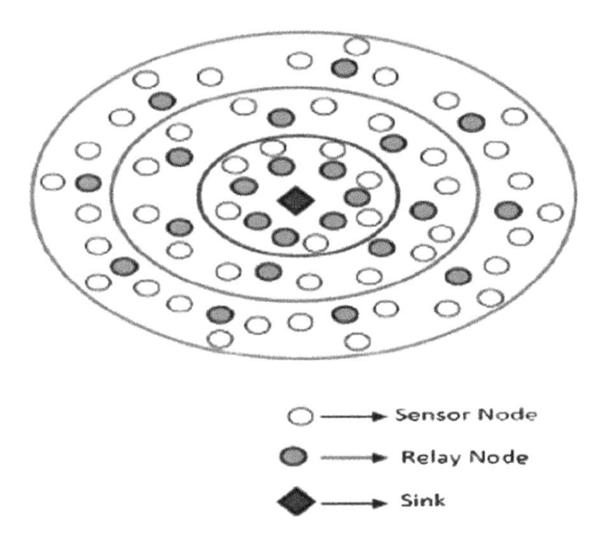

Fig. 6 Hierarchical node placement

utilization. The most important advantage of AODV is its ability to heal itself in case of node failures. It finds the shortest path from source to destination, based on the hop count [old 27]. Most of the resource constrained wireless sensor network uses low power links, because it holds low power devices (battery operated). Low power links will be unstable and lossy in nature. If a node sends the data through poor quality links, packet loss may occur and number of retransmission a increase, which leads to uneven energy consumption and quick node drain out, so an efficient routing metric is required to measure the link quality. Signal to Noise ratio (SNR) is one of efficient routing metric for link quality estimation. Hence we consider SNR based path computation. In proposed work SNR is considered for route discovery process. The nodes with good SNR value can be considered as next hop neighbor to the source node.

4.4 Packet Format

RREQ packet format: AODV protocol use Route Request (RREQ) packet for route discovery from source node to destination node. To implement the SNR in AODV, it should be added in RREQ control packet.

Figure 7 describes the RREQ packet format with SNR information. By adding this information in control packet, AODV selects the path based Hop Count and SNR.

4.5 Route Selection by Destination Node Based in SNR Value

Route selection of AODV protocol is done by destination node. When the destination node receives route request, it discards further route request and starts sending the route replay to the source. In Fig. 5, (flow chart) refers the route selection procedure of destination node [35].

Figure 8 explains the route selection of destination node based on SNR. It selects the node, which has good SNR. After starting RREP timer, destination node

<table>
<tr><td>Type</td><td>Flags</td><td>Reserved</td><td>Hop count</td></tr>
<tr><td colspan="4">RREQ (broadcast) ID</td></tr>
<tr><td colspan="4">Destination IP Address</td></tr>
<tr><td colspan="4">Destination Sequence Number</td></tr>
<tr><td colspan="4">Original IP Address</td></tr>
<tr><td colspan="4">Original Sequence number</td></tr>
<tr><td colspan="4">SNR</td></tr>
</table>

Fig. 7 Control packet format

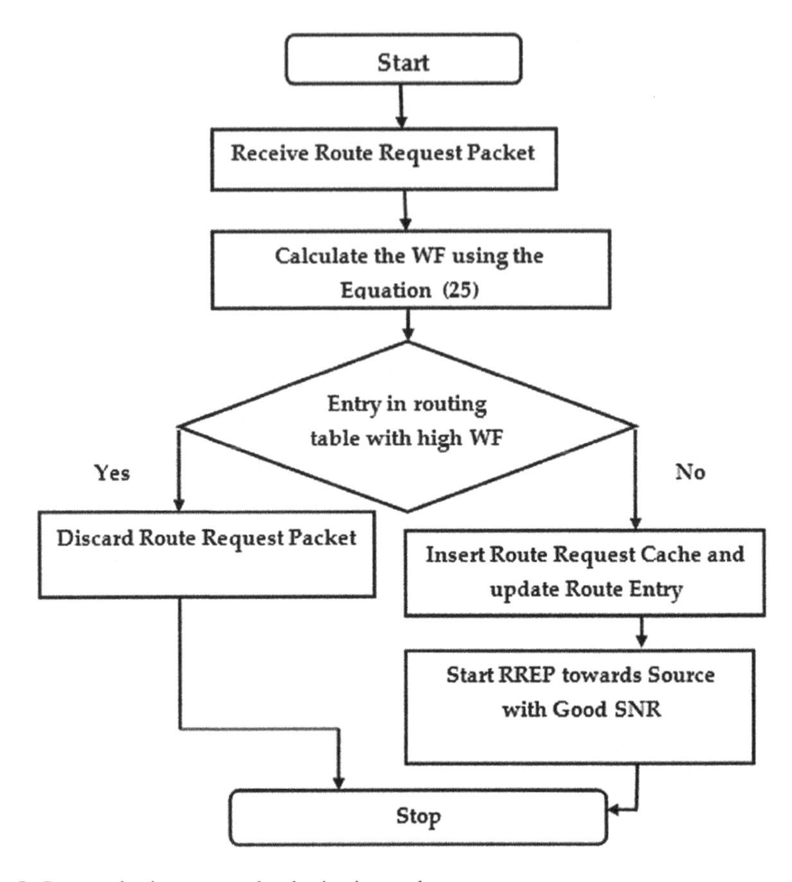

Fig. 8 Route selection process by destination node

sends reply RREP to each RREQ packet stored in cache. After data transmission it removes all the entries in the cache [36].

4.6 Basic Assumptions in Proposed Network Architecture

- Stationary nodes (relays and sensors) are placed.
- Nodes are aware of SNR information.
- The battery levels of relay nodes are high, when compared to sensor nodes.
- Relay nodes are placed one hop neighbor to sensor node and relay node.
- Relay nodes does Path Computation process.
- Sink is not limited by energy.

Table 3 Simulation setup

Routing protocol	AODV, AODV (SNR)
MAC layer/physical layer	802.11
Channel type	Wireless
Radio propagation model	Two ray ground
Traffic type	Constant bit rate
Antenna model	Omni directional
Initial energy (sensors)	50 J
Initial energy (relays)	60 J
Total number of nodes	68 (28 relay nodes and 40 sensor nodes)

4.7 Performance Evaluation

The proposed network architecture is implemented in NS-2.35 simulation tool and following results are obtained (Table 3).

(a) Network lifetime

The network is said to be energy efficient network based on its network lifetime. The lifetime of the network is estimated based on first death node, because when first node starts drain out its energy, within a short span of time all other nodes will drain out its energy. The reason for quick node death after first node death is, after first node death the second node will carry the data load of fist node, hence it will be overloaded and leads to battery drain out. After second node death, the data overload of first and second will be given to third node. Similar to that all the nodes in network drain out its battery.

Figure 9 describes the first node death in uniform node density occurs at 135th second, in proposed network architecture first node death occur at 200th second. In uniform node density, all the nodes lose their energy in 500 s. In proposed architecture, only 15 nodes losses its energy after entire simulation period. This shows, the proposed network architecture performs uniform energy consumption and gives better network lifetime.

(b) Throughput

Throughput is a parameter, which measures the reliability of network. Throughput of network depends on the link quality and data transmission (Fig. 10).

The throughput of proposed method is high, when compared to random node placement. The reason for obtaining good throughput is SNR based routing mechanism. From above results it is understood that, the effective combination of node placement and routing mechanism gives energy efficient and reliable network. Implementing the same architecture in real-time IoT healthcare applications will increase the performance of the network.

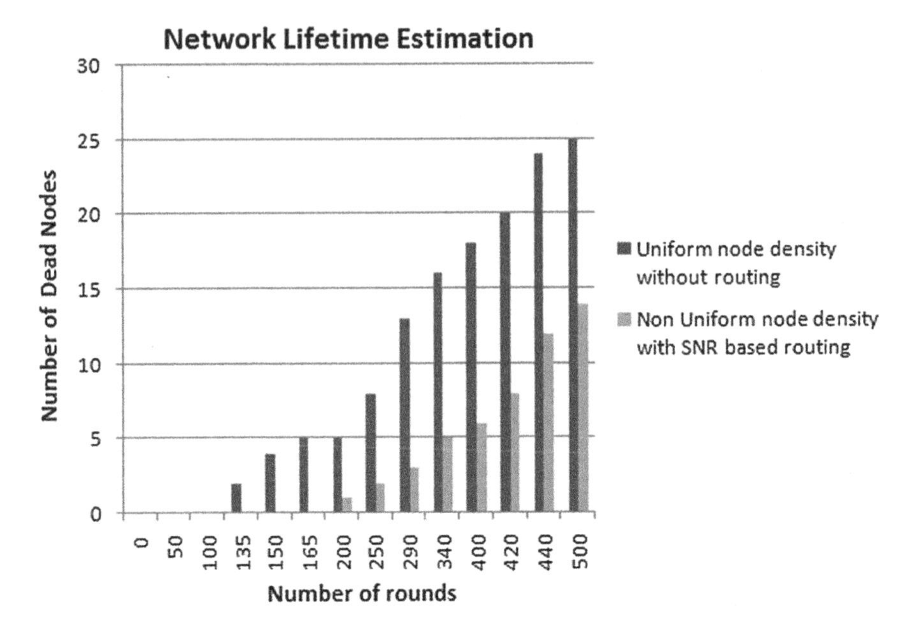

Fig. 9 Network lifetime estimation

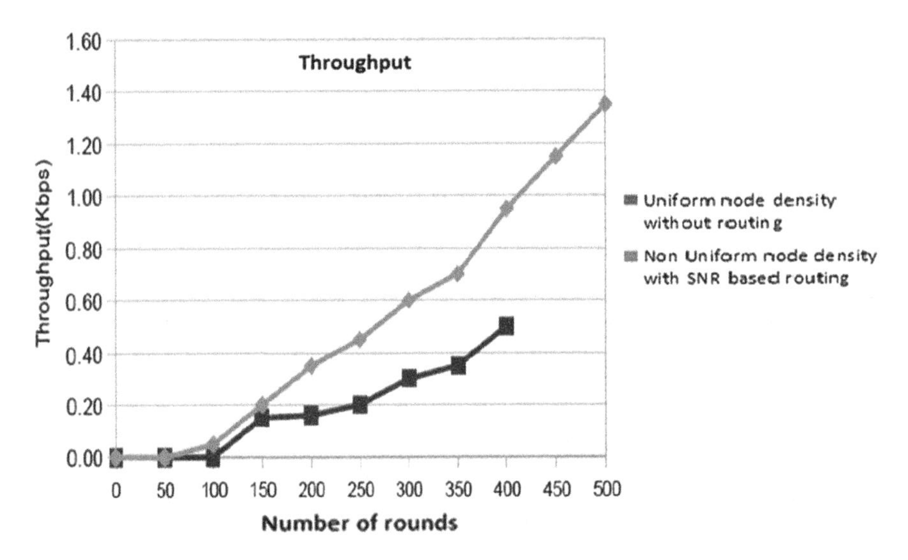

Fig. 10 Network lifetime estimation

Similar to the above architecture various network architectures can be proposed with effective combinations two different techniques, to improve the energy efficiency of IoT network.

5 Conclusion

Internet of Things technology is highly greeted by health care applications. Providing the wearable bio-sensors to old-age peoples and monitoring their health conditions is the most appreciable feature of IoT technology. Gartner's hype cycle says IoT is in peak of inflated expectations, it can be used in any kind of applications in centralized manner. Energy, reliability, QoS and Security are major parameters need to be concentrated in low power IoT environment. Utilizing the energy in efficient way and transmitting the data in reliable path (good quality links) are the two main goals in energy constrained IoT. In this chapter, hierarchical network architecture is proposed to solve the energy hole problem and suitable routing mechanism is implemented to handle Low power devices (battery operated) and low power links (Lossy links). Our simulation result shows, the proposed architecture gives b better network lifetime and efficient throughput. Hence it is concluded that, proposed network architecture is more suitable for energy constrained IoT networks.

In proposed network architecture, SNR is included in routing technique to find the reliable path. In future work various parameters can be included with efficient nodes placement technique. Similarly in node placement technique various types of node placement strategies can be implemented based on application requirements.

References

1. The Internet of Things. ITU Internet reports (2005)
2. Boukerche, A.: Algorithms and Protocols for Wireless Sensor Networks. Wiley-IEEE Press (2008)
3. Enzyme Technology. www.lsbu.ac.uk/water/enztech
4. Lee, G.M., Park, J., Kong, N., Crespi, N., Chong, I.: The Internet of Things—Concept and Problem Statement. Internet Re-search Task Force (2012)
5. Vasseur, J.-P., Dunkels, A.: Interconnecting Smart Objects with IP. Elsevier (2010)
6. Ko, J., Terzis, A., Dawson-Haggerty, S., Culler, D.E., Hui, J.W., Levis, P.: Connecting low-power and lossy networks to the Internet. IEEE Commun. Mag. **49**(4), 96–101 (2011)
7. Jones, C.E., Sivalingam, K.M., Agrwal, P., Chen, J.C.: A survey of energy efficient network protocols for wireless networks. Wireless Netw. 343–358 (2001)
8. Rajendran, V., Obraczka, K., Garcia-Luna-Aceves, J.J.: Energy-efficient, collision-free medium access control for wireless sensor networks. In: Proceedings of the ACM SenSys 03, Los Angeles, California (2003)
9. IoT World Forum Reference Model. https://www.iotwf.com/resources
10. daCosta, F.: Rethinking the Internet of Things—A scalable Approach to Connecting Everything. Apress (2013)
11. Chase, J.: The Evolution of Internet of Things. Texas Instruments, white paper (2013)
12. Webera, R.H., Weber, R.: Internet of Things the Legal Perspectives. Springer (2010)
13. Smith, I.G., Vermesan, O., Friess, P., Furness, A., Pitt, M.: Internet of Things European Research Cluster, 3rd edn. (2012)

14. Zainol Abidin, H., Din, N.M., Yassin, I.M., Omar, H.A., Radzi, N.A.M., Sadon, S.K.: Sensor node placement in wireless sensor network using multi-objective territorial predator scent marking algorithm. Arab. J. Sci. Eng. (Springer) **39**(8), 6317–6325 (2014)
15. Younis, M., Akkaya, K.: Strategies and Techniques for Node Placement in Wireless Sensor Networks: A Survey, pp. 621–655. Elsevier, Ad Hoc Networks (2008)
16. Cheng, P., Chuah, C.-N., Liu, X.: Energy-Aware Node Placement in Wireless Sensor Networks, pp. 3210–3214. IEEE Communications Society, Globecom (2004)
17. Dasgupta, K., Kukreja, M., Kalpakis, K.: Topology–aware placement and role assignment for energy-efficient information gathering in sensor networks. In: Proceedings of the Eighth IEEE International Symposium on Computers and Communication (ISCC'03), pp. 341–348 (2003)
18. Dhillon, S.S., Chakrabarty, K.: Sensor placement for effective coverage and surveillance in distributed sensor networks. In: International Conference on Wireless Communications and Networking, pp. 1609–1614. IEEE (2003)
19. Kirankumar, Y.B., Mallapur, J.D.: Energy aware node placement algorithm for wireless sensor network. Adv. Electron. Electr. Eng. 541–548 (2014)
20. Bari, A.: Relay Nodes in Wireless Sensor Networks: A Survey. University of Windsor (2005)
21. Tang, J., Hao, B., Sen, A.: Relay node placement in large scale wireless sensor networks. Comput. Commun. (Elsevier) **29**(4), 490–501 (2005)
22. Cheng, X., Dingzhu, D., Wang, L., Baogang, X.: Relay sensor placement in wireless sensor networks. EEE Trans. Comput. **56**(1), 134–138 (2001)
23. Renu, B., lal, M.H., Pranavi, T.: Routing Protocols in Mobile Ad-Hoc Network: A Review. Quality, Reliability, Security and Robustness in Heterogeneous Networks, pp. 52–60. Springer (2013)
24. AlKaraki, J.N., Kamal, A.E.: Routing techniques in sensor networks: a survey. IEEE Commun. **11**(6), 6–28 (2004)
25. Gao, J.L.: Energy efficient routing for wireless sensor networks. Ph.D. thesis, Electrical and Computer Engineering Department, UCLA (2000)
26. Akkaya, K., Younis, M.: A survey on routing protocols for wireless sensor networks. Ad Hoc Netw. J. 325–349 (2005)
27. Youssef, M.A., Younis, M.F., Arisha, K.: A constrained shortest-path energy aware routing algorithm for wireless sensor networks. In: Proceedings of WCNC, pp. 794–799 (2002)
28. Ye, F., Chen, A., Liu, S., Zhang, L.: A scalable solution to minimum cost forwarding in large sensor networks. In: Proceedings of the Tenth International Conference on Computer Communications and Networks (ICCCN), pp. 304–330 (2001)
29. Sohrabi, K., Gao, J., Ailawadhi, V., Pottie, G.J.: Protocols for self-organization of a wireless sensor networks. IEEE Personal Commun. Mag. **7**(5), 16–27 (2005)
30. Liu, F., Xing, K., Cheng, X., Rotenstreich, S.: Energy Efficient MAC Layer Protocols in Ad Hoc Networks. Resource Management in Wireless Networking. The George Washington University, Washington, D.C. (2004)
31. Willig, A.: Wireless sensor networks: concept, challenges and approaches. e & i Elektrotechnik und Informationstechnik (Springer) **123**(6), 224–231 (2006)
32. Miguel, T., Parra, C., Gao, J.L.: Antenna design for a wireless sensor network node. Master thesis, Electrical and Computer Engineering, Tecnico Lisboa (2014)
33. Sarwesh, P., Shet, N.S.V., Chandrasekaran, K.: Energy efficient network architecture for IoT applications. In: IEEE, International Conference on Green computing and Internet of Things, pp. 784–789 (2015)
34. http://image.slidesharecdn.com/ethiotm2mmedicalhealthcare20150502-150518132645-lva1-app6891/95/medical-healthcare-iot-m2m-solutions-4-638.jpg?cb=1431956058
35. Farooq, H., Jung, L.T.: Energy, traffic load, and link quality aware ad hoc routing protocol for wireless sensor network based smart metering infrastructure. Int. J. Distrib. Sen. Netw. (Hindawi Publishing Corporation) (2013)
36. Chang, L.-H., Lee, T.-H., Chen, S., Liao, C.-Y.: Energy efficient oriented routing algorithm in wireless sensor networks. In: IEEE International Conference on Systems, Man and Cybernetics, pp. 3813–3818 (2013)

37. Xia, F., Rahim, A.: MAC Protocols for Cyber-Physical Systems. Springer (2015)
38. Chakraborty, S., Dey, N., Samanta, S., Ashour, A.S., Balas, V.E.: Firefly Algorithm for Optimized Non-rigid Demons Registration. Bio-Inspired Computation & Applications in Image Processing. Elsevier, London (2016)
39. Kaliannan, J., Baskaran, A., Dey, N., Ashour, A.S.: Ant colony optimization algorithm based PID controller for LFC of single area power system with non-linearity and boiler dynamics. World J. Model. Simul. **12**(1), 3–14 (2016)
40. Samanta, S., Choudhury, A., Dey, N., Balas, V.E.: Quantum Inspired Evolutionary Algorithm for Scaling Factors Optimization during Manifold Medical Information Embedding. Book: Quantum Inspired Computational intelligence: Research and Applications. Elsevier (2016)
41. Jagatheesan, K., Anand, B., Samanta, S., Dey, N., Santhi, V., Ashour, A.S., Balas, V.E.: Application of Flower Pollination Algorithm in Load Frequency Control of Multi-area Interconnected Power System with Nonlinearity. Neural Computing and Applications, pp. 1–4. Springer (2016)
42. Kaliannan, J., Baskaran, A., Samanta, S., Balas, V.E.: Particle swarm optimization based parameters optimization of PID controller for load frequency control of multi-area reheat thermal power systems. Int. J. Adv. Intell. Paradigms (2015)

Exploring Formal Strategy Framework for the Security in IoT towards e-Health Context using Computational Intelligence

Youcef Ould-Yahia, Soumya Banerjee, Samia Bouzefrane and Hanifa Boucheneb

Abstract This chapter proposes a novel strategic framework and computationally intelligent model to measure possible vulnerabilities for security context in e-health. In order to keep track of security of e-health paradigm, the chapter conceives a bio-inspired model comprising the collective intelligence of social insects e.g. ant colony. Ant colony optimization is a computationally intelligent meta-heuristics, which takes care-off the different random and uncertain behavior of different sensors deployed towards e-health measures. The essential input is provided from interconnected wireless sensors under Internet of Things (IoT) paradigm and intelligent social insects that could sense the possibility of threats for a patient moving in different physical locations during his medical diagnosis. Social insect ants can sense and communicate through a chemical, known as pheromone, remotely from their nest towards collection of food. The intensity of pheromone measured for different interconnected graphs of e-health could lead to a consolidated algorithm and finally the differences of intensities can infer on the affected or safe path for propagation of medical information. Modelling the pheromone dynamics can be a precise measure to quantify the different e-health security issues like Sinkhole threat or sybil attack under IoT environment. The proposed pheromone alert is presented and compared statistically in terms of precision to identify the classification of possible vulnerabilities.

Y. Ould-Yahia · S. Bouzefrane (✉)
Conservatoire National des Arts et Métiers, Cedex 03, Paris, France
e-mail: samia.bouzefrane@lecnam.net

S. Banerjee
Birla Institute of Technology, Mesra, India

H. Boucheneb
École Polytechnique de Montréal, Montreal, Canada

C. Bhatt et al. (eds.), *Internet of Things and Big Data Technologies for Next Generation Healthcare*, Studies in Big Data 23,
DOI 10.1007/978-3-319-49736-5_4

1 Introduction

The emphasized growth of computational and web based resources improvise the different contexts of smart environment. Hence, emerging applications of smart and connected devices and IoT (Internet of Things) can be made more pervasive with respect to diversified applications. E-health incorporated with IoT is one of the recent vertical applications of smart environment [1, 2].

IoT under e-health paradigm can be targeted to track objects and people (staff and patients). In addition, the combination of e-health and IoT could detect and authenticate people, acquire and sense data automatically. Conventionally, e-health provides a new method for using health resources—e.g. information, communication, expenses and medicines. Hence, optimized utilization of resources also becomes significant. Although, there is a legitimate concern that security vulnerabilities could pose a significant risk as opposed to the popular usage of Machine to Machine communication (M2M) or IoT towards efficient optimization of resources. M2M elaborates synchronization of devices being connected to the Internet. They basically utilize different static and wireless network components and interact with each other as a part of intra-level communication. There are various active components, data units and sensing elements that persist to execute successful deployment of IoT orientation for e-health applications. They include sensor devices and actuators, networking, processing and storage [3, 4]. The overall level of security is upper-bounded by the weakest component in this interactive system. Hence, each component, and the holistic system must be designed with security measures. There are three basic attack vectors, and a corresponding attack surface to each vector. Data is the first attack surface, followed by the communication channels. There could be even malicious attacks to compromise the insulin pump of specific patients. The several aspects solicit to develop an application control comprising of sound alert system with continuous monitoring for all health related IoT devices. The expected behavior to be analyzed from such security framework could be the basis for building a tampering-resistant device in implementations [5]. Considering such manifold parameters of security measures, this chapter contributes to a novel architecture to define normal model of security components of e-health in IoT paradigm, primarily utilizing computational intelligence. Broadly, the term of computational intelligence is defined as a set of evolutionary-inspired computational methodologies and algorithms to address complex real-world problems, where mathematical or generic modelling cannot be adequate. The reason to justify computational intelligence could be bi-focal: firstly, the security strategy for IoT in the context of e-health applications can be made adaptive to tune with the specific patient and requirement. For example, insulin or monitoring concerned remedies could be different for different patients and a generic framework of medical records cannot be appropriate. Secondly, to interact with data and different medical agents, they can learn from environment. The chapter coins an application envisaging bio-inspired algorithms to measure, monitor and update the security alerts in the IoT framework. Bio-inspired elements mimic the natural insects, their dynamic and formal model could assist to develop an application interface for security context in IoT environment. Specifically, the collective behavior and pheromone mapping of social insects can be an interesting proposition to model the ant colony metaphor [6] in the form of mobile and connected devices as IoT. The strategy framework of security measures has been defined as a formal model of dynamic digital pheromone followed by their deposition, evaporation and reinforcement processes. The contribution of ant colony algorithm in defining security of IoT incorporated in the model could be briefed as follows.

The social insects, ants can randomly move towards the interconnected graph of sensor devices, following basic principle of shortest path from their nest (initial position) to final destination of food source and vice versa. Interestingly, the deposition of pheromone for a safe path and vulnerable path across that graph could be detected on the basis of differences of certain standard medical parameters of sensors. Finally, the path is marked up as free from threats and this alarm of pheromone signal could be commissioned as control panel of interconnections of IoT and sensor devices. However, to incorporate pheromone deposition and evaporation as security control components, it becomes mandatory to establish a directed or undirected graph as interconnection of IoT and sensor devices operational for dynamic data collection of patients under their different physical locations.

It is significant that whenever an IoT environment expands, the level of pheromone differs and compared to exact value across the sensors under the sensor graph. A certain deliberate tampering, of patient on-line data, could be vulnerable with respect to the patient medical history. Thus, the treatment to be solicited could be wrong. At present, the model considers only single graph yielded from IoT, later more parallel such graphs could be tested and more secure e-health IoT applications can be invoked. The Fig. 1 is relevant to visualize the interconnected complex network architecture of sensors with different nodes. The ants are placed randomly to traverse the graph and inherent with their properties they follow the shortest path, while depositing the pheromone across the well accepted path of other follower ants. The interconnected path traversal time could be higher, if there is a possibility of security threats in terms of delayed access of test data contents of patients. The movement of patients are being tracked with sensor devices and based on their

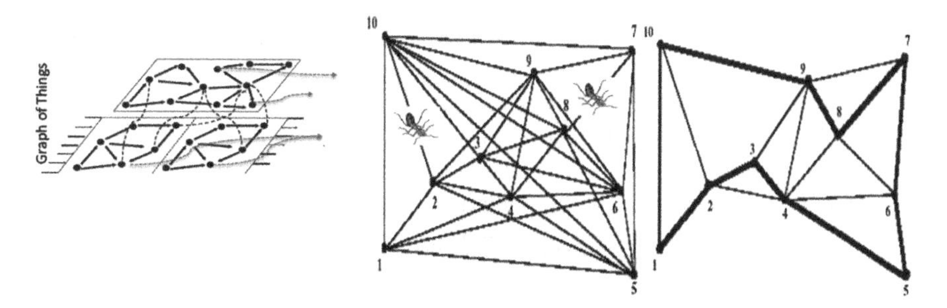

Fig. 1 Visualization of GoT and ants

physical locations the connected graph is produced dynamically. Ants can traverse the yielded graph and could raise the alarm of vulnerability, if it exists.

The relation between security threats and colony of ants are not directly related. However, the ants can act as security agents to disburse the information of alert under IoT environment, where multiple-health sensors are being connected. They also can formulate the interaction process during the acquisition of sensor data. The incorporation of ants injects computational intelligence in the control of IoT, and relevant heath sensor devices and importantly the dynamics of ant colony are computationally programmable.

The major contributions of the chapter have been depicted as follows:

- Comprehensive mathematical parameters as objective function are defined to measure the degree of risks or threats for health IoT.
- The deployment of pheromone marks up as computationally intelligent tool across IoT environment.
- The validation of the empirical parameters of existing standard IoT security benchmark protocol with the proposed model.

The remaining part of the chapter has been organized as follows: Sect. 1.1 describes the basic motivation and need for applying computational intelligence in IoT interaction. Section 2 discusses similar works followed by a formal model, parameters and relevance in Sect. 2.1. Section 3 introduces a generic algorithm of pheromone alert, envisaging computational intelligence. Section 4 discusses the post implementation scenario and data set where the e-health IoT behavior could be tested. Section 5 finally summarizes the results and mentions the relevance of further prospects of such application development. A brief glossary of essential definitions is provided at Appendix for readers.

1.1 Motivation

The e-health system provides new opportunities and improves the quality and efficiency of care while reducing costs. The purpose of the e-health is to make available to health professionals and patients' tools to collect, process, store, return and exchange of health data in automated, convenient, reliable and secure way. To illustrate the contribution of e-health, we consider the example of patient monitoring. Indeed, traditionally to monitor a patient (heart rate, blood pressure, etc.), hospitalization is mandatory, which is constraining and expensive. However, with the Internet of Things (IoT) this monitoring can be extended easily to the patient's daily environment (home, workplace, etc.). This model allows considering a broad spectrum of application for self-care with medical measurements [7]. And in turn a reduced cost effective health assistive model could be invoked. In other words, there could be many relevant applications concerning e-health with IoT environment.

Internet of Things (IoT) ideally resembles to the linked and chained data representation among its various components like actuators, sensors and associated hardware. It is a common practice to represent, wireless sensor network and any variation of ad-hoc network as a directed graph. Here, any graph and its vertices are analogous to the linked and interconnecting nodes. The vertex of a directed edge from one node to another will allow transmitting the data directly to the node. Potentially, it becomes too generic that embedding conditions of propagation depends on the range of transmission. If all nodes have homogeneous capacity of communicating to each other, then the graph becomes undirected. A connected network ideally has to be expressed as an associated graph, which is connected by itself. A graph G is inter-linked or directed if and only if vertices are traced by a pre-defined path [8]. Whenever a network is interconnected, then any pair of nodes can interact with each other, most likely considering multiple iterations through indirect nodes. In some cases, it becomes useful to justify stronger forms of connectivity. It is known as k-connectivity. In this case, the network still remains live, even if $(k - 1)$ nodes are removed from the network. If a network is k-connected $(k > 2)$, it demonstrates better fault-tolerance capability. Asserting, k-connectivity extends the lifespan of networks, if nodes become non-functional at random times [3, 4]. The essential parameters of IoT visualization of an entity abstraction layer, and the associated parameters for configuring IoT and device can converge into:

- Capturing invariants and relevant complexity of environments shared by different IoT applications like smart home
- Entity models (nodes of the graph) capture real-time behavior
- Entity to entity and entity to device relationships
- Entity to entity group relationships.

Figure 1 could be the visualized form of Graph of Things (GoT) and also ants are placed at random nodes of connectivity of IoT sensors.

These features are responsible for using substantial number of object oriented graph data bases like neo4j. Considering the baseline of IoT orientation, the present model converts the real instant into graph, on which the social insects e.g. ants are placed. The advantage of ants is their flexibility to navigate and reinforce any path while enhancing the population towards that specific path. Ants use pheromone as their primary communication media and most importantly the dynamics of ant colony is programmable and formal mathematical models are available. Any type of security lapses and vulnerable events can be measured.

The flow of the proposed model can be given as:

- Step 1: Conversion of IoT graph, to be known as Graph of Things (GoT) or G
- Step 2: Positioning the ants on random nodes on the graph
- Step 3: Depending on sensors interaction, physical positions of a patient, the node(s) will be reiterated and particular threshold values of nodes are predefined. The value is based on time to access the minimum intra communication link, access point and termination criteria (See Fig. 3)

- Step 4: Deposition of pheromone across the nodes, where connectivity and interaction are present
- Step 5: If the value of pheromone differs from the threshold value of a particular sensors-connected path, alert message/signal will be initiated anticipating vulnerable points across IoT connection.

The choice of ant colony optimization algorithm is obvious amongst the other bio-inspired approaches for its capability to avoid local minima while traversing the graph. As if the solution is trapped in local minima, then the solution becomes harder with hard sample of data. ACO can perform considerably efficient in such complex cases and also in e-health and IoT several activities and sensors will be required to synchronize. Multiple ant colonies in parallel can serve this purpose. Presently, a pure multi-objective optimization problem has not been presented here, as only quality of service has been investigated. Subsequently, cost and energy efficiency of sensor devices can also be considered as the components of optimization effort.

Following the above mentioned steps, a pheromone alert algorithm and a model are presented. Relevant background and scope are also discussed.

1.2 About the Health Sensors

There are different heath sensors for e-health (referring Shield v2.0 Arduino and Raspberry Pi). Categorically, Patient Position Sensor (Accelerometer), Glucometer Sensor, Body Temperature Sensor, Blood Pressure Sensor (Sphygmomanometer) V2.0, Pulse and Oxygen in Blood Sensor (SPO2) are crucial for the simulation of physical locations and data accusation from patients. The gestures of patients denote the physical positions like standing, seating, left and right. Standard e-health library for Ardunio and Raspberry Pi supports to pass a function for retrieving the behavioral position of patients. More treatments with physical coordinates can be plugged as the following structural syntax:

```
{
        eHealth.initPositionSensor();
}
```

Patient may utilize a smart phone application, which bridges to the database with location information and category of specialist needed by a patient. This will be an additional feature.

Fixation of threshold values of sensor node could depend on test cases of the actual physical and behavioral status of patients. For example, normally heart rate is measured in beats per minute (bpm), and the usual heart rate is within the interval (60–100) for a healthy adult at rest. If the adult patient moves, the heart rate may differ, and the access of rate could be delayed too through the sensors. However, the rate cannot exceed more than 200 and if the access delay is beyond the standard sensing time, then the chances of data tempering prevails. The pulse is measured in beats per minute (bpm) and BP is measured in millimetres of mercury (mmHg). The average respiration at rest for adults is 12–20 breaths per minute and the normal SpO2 (peripheral capillary oxygen saturation, an estimate of the amount of oxygen in the blood) rate must be within the range (95–100 %) [9].

2 Similar Works

There are significant developments of e-health applications with IoT environment. The authors of [10] demonstrate the implementation ease of such models. In Taiwan, a telemedicine platform is deployed for monitoring elderly [11].

Karunarathne et al. [12] proposed a contemporary application for monitoring people pre-disposed to cardio-vascular mishaps with motion and acceleration sensors. The public health research provides a platform for the acquisition of epidemiological data [13]. In Spain, a national R & D project was initiated to create innovative health services for addiction based and chronological diseases, incorporating software verticals related to the Internet of Things and Cloud Computing [14] (Fig. 2).

There are technological and commercial benefits of e-health by harnessing the opportunities offered by IoT. However, the main challenge of using these technologies in the field of healthcare is the protection of patient data and privacy, because the loss of the security properties may have a negative impact on the patient and the health systems in general. These impacts can be legal, ethical or financial and even can be responsible for the associated damage to the patient's health. According to HIPAA general rule, which is known as Standards for Privacy of Individually Identifiable Health Information in United States, a covered entity (Health Care Providers, Health Plans, etc.) must distinguish and protect against logically and probabilistic threats to the integrity of the information. This can

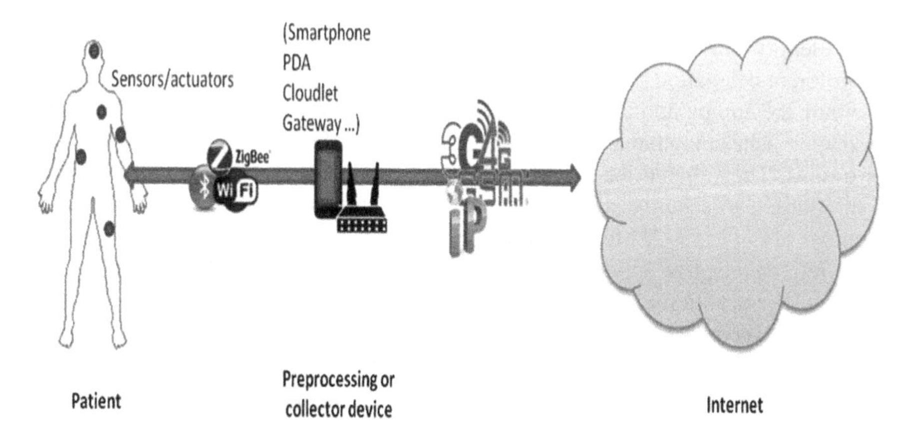

Fig. 2 Conceptual representation of IoT and e-health

protect some anticipated imprecision about the integrity of medical information content [15]. It implies that an application that collects processing and stores patient's data must ensure the confidentiality and integrity of data and performs access restrictions. Furthermore the service provider must deploy a solution to measure, monitor and update the security alerts. Gope and Hwang, in [16], refer to several sample applications and research projects on e-health where security has deficiency or pending aspects. An additional challenge for this application is the limitation of connected objects, in terms of energy, computation and memory capacity. In case of e-health using IoT technology, we must deal with strong security requirements and physical constraints of IoT devices. The research community proposes a wide range of security solutions for e-health that take into account the constraints of IoT. These solutions aimed towards two directions, those are categorical to e-health systems and those customizing the relevant protocols for the IP-driven IoT and its security framework [17], to protect data and communication channels. However, malicious attacks that may compromise the IoT devices are serious threat in e-health applications. Regarding IoT communications security, in traditional network communications, security is assured by transport (e.g. TLS/SSL) or network (e.g. IPSec) layers technologies, providing all the security features. In the context of IoT, the resource limitations of things make it difficult to deploy traditional security technologies, such as update, control and management of authentication and access privileges. A review of the paradigm of security solutions for IoT is presented by Keoh et. al. [18]. The authors focus on solutions that will be used in conjunction with the Constrained Application Protocol (CoAP), the equivalent of http in constrained networks. The most promising solution is Datagram Transport Layer Security (DTLS) that is derived from TLS. This solution is promoted by IETF. Hence, many researchers consider IPsec combined with minimal IKEv2 as desirable security solutions for IoT [18]. This approach is reinforced by using 6LoWPAN (IPv6 over Low power Wireless Personal Area Networks) compressions for IPsec payload headers [17]. Abdmeziem and Tandjaoui mention other proposed solutions like tailoring to Mikey-Ticket protocol for e-health applications in the context of IoT lightweight extensions to HIP DEX (Host Identity Protocol Diet Exchange). The framework could be mapped to DTLS and different delegation procedures of primitive of protocol can be commissioned to distribute the computational load to other avenues. However, they noticed that even these approaches may reduce the computational load of the devices under manifold constraints. They altered the end point principle including a different trusted party.

In addition to security solutions based on cryptography for e-health IoT environments [16, 17, 19–21] to control data access and authentication, some research works rely on adaptive approaches. Adaptive security solutions are in general based on risk analysis with rigorous identification of vulnerabilities. For e-health, the first vulnerability is related to the IoT device resulting from capacity limitation to implement complex security schemes. Additionally, we need a certain metric to quantify the risk and other parameters. Savola et al. [7] propose heuristics for the development of concerned security metrics, based on the risk-analysis results achieved through two view-points: the service provider's business perspective, and the end-user's perspective. Nevertheless, these analyzes don't focus on privacy and assume that data reside in a well-managed shared database on the service provider's premises. Authors, in [22], propose a risk-centric adaptive security framework for IoT in eHealth. They incorporated game theory based approach to analyze the monitored information and context awareness to measure and forecast dynamically for privacy risks and integrity towards potential benefits. The result of the analysis is used to make inferences and suitably adhere to post-event scenarios by adjusting different parameters (encryption parameters, security protocols and algorithms, security policies as well) or by keeping dynamic alterations in the paradigm of the security system. The work presented by the authors has been carried out in a research project ASSET (Adaptive Security for Smart Internet of Things e-health). In the same project, we can find in [23] references to adaptive security issues. In [24], the authors coined a state-of-the-art based on game theory models. Finally, a Markov game-theoretic model is developed for adaptive security in the IoT towards e-health applications. The test and evaluation are accomplished while simulating an adaptive security policy emphasizing on authentication policies. This approach delivers adaptive measures of security parameters with respect to the dynamic behavior of the environment. However, it is a reactive solution, therefore, it is necessary to test it under real conditions to validate the reactivity and efficiency. Finally, the solutions proposed in the literature for the safety of e-health environment are confronted principally with the IoT's security challenge that comes down to the difficulty of implementing effective security measures using heterogeneous technologies and within limited-resource devices (limitations in terms of energy, calculation and memory). This challenge is exacerbated by the dynamics of the environment induced by mobile devices. Therefore, substantial numbers of cryptographic solutions are not effective because they are static in nature, proposed for a dynamic environment. Furthermore, these solutions are not designed to detect a compromised IoT device or an abnormal behavior. Computational intelligence as ant colony is largely used in the literature in many fields like data retrieval in Cloud Computing [25], secure building [26], to control road traffic in emergency situations [27] or to propose a dynamic routing for IoT [28]. Ant colony algorithm is conceived through the social behavior of ants to reach towards the destination optimally. For example, it can be the instances to find the shortest path or finding and storing food. This is the collaboration of cooperative ants, that rely on their individual experience to determine a route based on deposition and evaporation of pheromone. Hence, using an algorithm which reproduces this model can solve many complex problems. Regarding security, ant colony approach is generally used to detect intrusion in networks or to enhance network security. The intrusion detection is based on a behavior analysis (resources use, access request, protocol, etc.) or on a pattern matching, which is less efficient to detect unknown threats. Authors of [29] proposed ant colony algorithm to find out vulnerabilities in networks. They deploy the algorithm on a network map obtained from network scanning, and remote OS/application detection tools. To improve existing solutions, they propose to detect vulnerabilities by traversing from one node to another, and by constructing a graph where ants move using a particular decision policy and a pheromone update. In [30], the authors propose to apply ant colony algorithm on a network model to analyze behaviours and to determine invasion route. This leads to identify and evaluate dynamically the system safety state, and to detect intrusion in this route in order to provide an appropriate response. Although, the ant colony algorithm resolves many problems, none of these solutions consider detecting threats in e-health with IoT environment in a strongly dynamic and constraint driven environment.

In addition, there are broader numbers of research initiatives accomplished on bio-inspired and quantum inspired computing, encryption based ECG hash code generation, watermarking approach for colour bio-medical images, telemedicine strategies towards diagnostic preservation and different secured registration approaches [31–38]. They all holistically contribute different computational intelligence techniques in bio medical and e-health driven applications.

2.1 Model, Parameters and Relevance: Bio-Inspired Algorithm and Pheromone Map

A real function q is assumed, with range [0, 1]. It is actually the preparedness of the system in terms of the suggested specifications. A low value, underestimated a given threshold, denotes that the system state is unacceptable, while a value close to 1 implies that most requirements are well defined and accomplished. The function q comprises of three parts:

- The agreement of security could be expressed in the function q_s;
- The degree of fulfilled QoS requirements, expressed in the function q_Q; and
- The costs that occur due to mitigation of threats.

The function q is then composed of a product of all partial functions of:

$$i \in \{S, Q, C\} : q = \prod_i q_i^{p_i} \quad (1)$$

where,

S represents: all reliable system states

Q: The acceptable states of the system under possible constraints

C: The cost to maintain essential security and quality of service.

Here, the p_i are the values of pheromone of ant colony agents as real numbers $o \leq p_i < \infty$ and express the importance of a single p_i, large values indicating more importance. Pheromone value $p_i = 1$ is considered as neutral. The importance of each parameter is defined by the evaluation system according to the nature of the requirement before assessing the q_i values.

Ant colony optimization is a nature-inspired meta-heuristic proposed by [6] Dorigo et al., which actually follows the social behavioral features of biological ants to explore relevant food sources. Each ant arbitrarily navigates to search without any prior information of food sources. They interact and communicate with each other by releasing a chemical known as pheromone in the traversed search trajectory. The density of pheromone on a relevant path implies the acceptability or assurance of the path in terms of obstacles. The density of pheromone for the given path will be evaporated gradually over time, if the path has not become acceptable or popular to the colony of ants. In other forms, the path will be reinforced accordingly. Higher pheromone concentration helps ants to establish a shortest yet optimal path between their nests and locations of food. The reinforcement strategy of the particular path also assists the follower to be nearer to the food source monitored and referred by the deposition of pheromone. The behavior of food foraging of ants has been implemented and modelled through an Ant colony algorithm. Finally, the foraging problem is interpreted as a classic optimization problem for food sources from the respective nests.

While incorporating terminologies in graph theory, it is assumed that the vertices and edges of any graph entity are the possible components of the solution, and each edge is adjunct with a pheromone value. A potential solution is constructed by an ant through the selection of components and features. The process is probabilistic, primarily depends on pheromone deposition. Following subsequent iterations, the solution is marked by an evaluation function and all the necessary constraints could be taken-care-off with the solution. It is evident that a higher pheromone concentration leads to a more effective solution. The follower ants can explore more feasible solution if the concentration of pheromone remains high and the level of constraints are maintained. Referring Table 1, it could be evident to position ants pheromone with e-health security contexts.

Let, i and j be two successive nodes on the traversal of an ant and $\tau_{ij}(t)$ be the pheromone concentration conceived by the ants at time t and related with the edge of the graph adjoining the nodes i and j.

Let $\rho > 0$ be the pheromone evaporation rate, and $\Delta\tau_{ij}^{k}(t)$ be the pheromone deposited by ant k at time t. Each ant k traverses through nodes i and j. Each ant constructs the possible optimal solution approach and deposits the pheromone for each edge of movement graph.

The ant colony optimization algorithm is pivoted on the concept of stochastic propagation of multiple moving agents (ants) while constructing a graph [3]. Categorically, the probabilistic value for the kth ant to move from node i to node

Table 1 Analogy of mobile objects with Ants

e-Health IoT	Ant colony and pheromone
Mobility of patients and their smart devices as phone, tablets	Exploits graph zone with minimum cost for health IoT
Presence of local memory device	Ant can refer, compare and evaluate from past experience
Initial position	Start state with transitions

j of the constructed graph is evaluated by *p* using Eq. (3). Moreover, at each step, the amount of pheromone is updated according to:

$$\tau_{ij}(t+1) = (1-\rho)\tau_{ij}(t)v\frac{Q}{L_k} \tag{2}$$

where, the parameter ρ describes the pheromone evaporation, $v = 1$ if the *(i, j)* edge was visited by the *k*th ant and zero otherwise, Q is a constant and L_k is the "cost" of the *k*-th path (typically its length).

In the original Ant Colony System, when building a traversing a graph, ant *k* at the current position of target graph *i* chooses the next location *j* to move according to pseudorandom proportional rule as stated:

$$p_{ij}^{k} = \frac{[\tau_{ij}]^{\alpha}[\eta_{ij}]^{\beta}}{\sum_{l \in N_i^k}[\tau_{il}]^{\alpha}[\eta_{il}]^{\beta}} \tag{3}$$

$j \in N_i^k$, where η_{ij} =1/d_{ij}, is a heuristic that is available a priori and α, β are the respective parameters to quantify the correlated influence of pheromone trail of sensing zone in real time, where τ_{il} and η_{il} represent the pheromone content and heuristic information on the edge connecting node i to node l respectively. The node l is included in N_i^k. N_i^k is the adequate neighbouring region of moving ant *k*, when being at locations, which is not still listed by the ant, i.e. that particular coordinate is un-traversed so far.

The contents of Table 1 have become significant to represent the analogical perspective of ants and mobile devices, which are being connected with e-health application and different relevant sensors. The concept of pheromone alert can be explained with a brief system set up of e-health application. The primary reason of choosing ant's pheromone is to combat with the uncertainty in threat detection. As chances of attack paths, the pattern of data leakage and tampering poses a significant uncertain problem to sensor and IoT interfaces, especially when facing a continuously environment like patients' different states, hence appropriate measures are required. To overcome uncertainty, social insects in the proposed application would continually gather information about their surroundings [5]. The foragers at certain central position of Graph of Things often have a well-developed memory [3]. In addition, social insects can share valuable information, such as safety, quality and authenticity of information flow towards a particular patient [4]. The proposed approach corresponds to the following salient points:

- The patient has been investigated with medical check up in different environments like home, clinic, dispensing room or from information on travel of the patient and he has to be monitored continuously through wireless sensors and IoT devices.
- Similar to device interaction of IoT, a GoT (Graph of Things) for different functions of q concerning different events can be formulated. GoT can be

expressed as a concept of fostering and monitoring extended data sources of IoT to provide a simple interface to proliferate, compound, enrich, and analyze the different patterns yielded through a graph. The graph can help to visualize the analytics of any business process in real time. It can detect emergency contexts, and automate immediate preventive measures [6].

- A pheromone alert is employed with a middleware framework of IoT and with the GoT orientation for the sensor framework. The patient positiones him at different places starting from home, travel, waiting in the clinic, and on the treatment phases. A group of ants can be positioned on any two random successive nodes of a linked graph of either IoT or GoT.
- The amount of pheromone deposition reinforces the possibility of data threats from sensors and IoT devices, the following broad outlines:
- Process of Replication: Each ant makes copies of itself. Replicated agents are placed on the node of GoT, where their parents are being attached. They inherit the parent's operational parameters as well as a constant amount of information flow across the Internet and Graph of Things. A mutation may occur at the probability of $1/n_b$ to randomly alter each of the inherited operational parameters. n_b denotes the number of operational parameters of each ant. Operational parameters can be mutated accordingly. Each child agent possesses the sensor data from its predecessors or parents during the traversal of GoT, and carries it to an initial or starting position. Different ants may choose different paths for initial position (where to traverse) depending on their operational and positional parameters.
- Swarming [39]: Each agent may converge with other agents at any intermediate node while going towards a terminal node. Positioning the intermediate node, it will be held for a particular period (t_w) as waiting state for other agents to arrive at the node. If it meets the ant agents, leading to the same terminal point, it merges with them and aggregates their sensor data. The operational parametric of swarming is evaluated through an objective function with respect to constraints. The swarming behavior is responsible for saving consumption of resources by aggregating multiple agents and reducing the number of data traversals across the distributed network. If a swarming behavior returns to any abnormal event, then the intrusion in aggregated and chained data sources needs to be monitored for possible occurrences of threats.
- Pheromone deployment and portability: On each intermediate node towards a starting point or node, the agent chooses the node of immediate hop in its portability by sensing three types of pheromones available on the local node: initial point, migratory and alarm pheromones. Each initial node sequentially reciprocates a heuristics rule to deposit pheromone to individual nodes. Their concentration reduces considerably on stochastic basis. All agents are exhausting on a node at the same time, arbitrarily selected one will survive for next hop. On each neighbouring nodes, agents can sense, where terminal points exist approximately with uncertain trends. It helps to move them by enhancing the appropriate concentration gradient of pheromone value of terminal point. At the time of migration to neighbouring nodes, agents disburse pheromones on their local nodes. Each portable pheromone marks the final node as an agent.

During the failure of migrations for a specific time-out period, migration pheromone also can be expressed. Migration failures may occur due to certain possible data integration issues or attacks, for example, node/link failures due to possible threats. A pheromone disappears, when its concentration deposition becomes gradually towards the least optimal value (could be zero). Each agent investigates Eq. (4) to determine, the next-hop node for a suitable migration.

- Mathematically, the representation will be similar to:

$$s_j = \sum_{t=1} wm_t \frac{p_{v,j} - p_{v_{\min}}}{p_{v_{\max}} - p_{v_{\min}}} \tag{4}$$

Here, weighted sum (s_j) against each neighbouring node j is expressed, and moves to a node of a highest weighted member sum. This could be a possible indication of alert and alarm as well. $\mathrm{wm_t}$ represents the weight of each node under t time iterations.

In this case, v denotes pheromone variations; $p_{1,j}$, $p_{2,j}$, $p_{3,j}$ represent the concentrations of leading point, portable and sensing pheromones on the node j respectively. $p_{v_{\max}}$ and $p_{v_{\min}}$ denote respectively the highest and the lowest concentrations of p_v among all adjoining nodes.

2.1.1 Properties and Validation of Pheromone Deposition on Internet of Things (IoT)

This work considers a few important concepts concerning the properties of ant colony and pheromone. The main logical assumption for dispersing pheromone across the IoT driven Graph of Things, is important to presume certain properties and to resolve the analogical model to identify the food sources of ant, nest and path where the ants are being traversed. The property foraging is the prime idea to be incorporated with ant movements across (foraging property, Refer appendix) IoT graph. In this model, food source are the pilot value(s) of any combination of sensors (specifically in terms of access control and time). Primarily, ants search for this pilot value through local pheromone deposition. if the pheromone deposition differs, then it can anticipate the possible reason or threats behind it. The proposed model is population based heuristics, it signifies that if there are larger dimensions of IoTs and GoTs, then a number of watch ants could be more to evoke alert signals. The primary parameters envisaged are:

- The density of ants (participated in foraging) in a particular space,
- The proportion of ants going back to the initial point with food,
- The concentration of pheromone,
- The concentration of food source,
- The specific rate of deposition of pheromone,
- The rate of evaporation of pheromone,
- The rate of removal of food sources through foraging ant.

Categorically, the diffusion process has not been included here, instead a constant deposition of pheromone on IoT graph is assumed (Refer Eq. (7)). However, the pheromone deposition and evaporation times are modelled by Poisson's distribution: each ant has a probability unit per unit of time to lay down a pheromone and each pheromone has a probability $1/T_p$ per unit of time to disappear or to evaporate. The pheromone deposition stimulates the interactions between the ants. This interaction is not pivoted to local space and time (as the ant with a pheromone value may have moved away substantially far before another ant interacts with it). More description can be referred in [40].

3 Proposed Algorithm: Pheromone Alert

The proposed algorithm pheromone alert is a specific algorithm (based on chemical from social insects e.g. pheromone) to be applied on undirected Graph of Things, yield from sensor networks. The network orientation keeps on changing for a specific patient on study, depending on his different physical positions and states. However, the protocol of all communications across the health sensors remains the same. The primary objective of the pheromone sense alert and alarm generation algorithm is to measure the possibility of threats, data leakage or attacks on the basis of deposition, duration and evaporation of pheromone across any random nodes of sensor graph yield through e-health application and interaction with a patient. The diffusion processes foster computational intelligence, so that the IoT driven paradigm of sensor networks can be monitored through the social insect's pheromone. The different phases are:

- The inclusion of pheromone defines the degree of rapidity of a particular pheromone to be released across the nodes of graph G,
- The evaporation rate, which determines how effectively and fast, the pheromone strength fades stochastically, if the particular path has not been referred again,
- The influence or impression, that characterizes, how much the pheromone influences the physical map of sensor organization. It means that the distribution of pheromone on GoT can also indicate critical points, which represent vulnerable attacks from which the e-health application may suffer.

While formulating the proposed algorithm, pheromone deposition and evaporation process are important. Formalization of the processes for deposition and evaporation across nodes of graph can be defined as follows.

3.1 *Formal Proposition: Pheromone Deposition*

Let $\rho > 0$ be the rate of evaporation of pheromone, and $\Delta\tau_{ij}^{k}(t)$ be the density of pheromone concentrated by ant k at time t:

$$\tau_{ij}(t) = (1-\rho)\tau_{ij}(t-1) + \sum_{k=1}^{m} \Delta\tau_{ij}^{k}(t) \tag{5}$$

From Eq. (5), the difference can be expressed as

$$\tau_{ij}(t) - \tau_{ij}(t-1) = -\rho\tau_{ij}(t-1) + \sum_{k=1}^{m} \Delta\tau_{ij}^{k}(t).$$

Conventionally, including differential operator $D \Rightarrow \frac{d\tau_{ij}}{dt}$ and finally the expression of pheromone deposition across the edge *(i, j)* is given as:

$$D = -\rho\tau_{ij}(t-1) + \sum_{k=1}^{m} \Delta\tau_{ij}^{k}(t) \tag{6}$$

$\Rightarrow (D+\rho)_{ij} = 0 \Rightarrow D = -\rho$ is the complementary form.

Considering the stable state of IoT protocol and the constant deposition of pheromone across IoT graph G, the complementary function and its particular integral is recombined at $\tau_{ij}(t) = C_k$. A stable state signifies a consistency and a stable standard for IoT protocol, after computing the particular integral for $\tau_{ij}(t) = C_k$.

Hence, the final deposition value of pheromone across the edge *(i, j)* is evaluated as:

$$\tau_{ij}(t) = \sum_{k=1}^{m} C_k/\rho \tag{7}$$

3.1.1 Formal Proposition: Pheromone Evaporation

Let the pheromone evaporation ρ at time t be ρ_t. The value of ρ_t, ranges in the closed interval of [0, 1]. Now, the relation is based on recurrence and thus for the evaporation of pheromone at time (t + 1) is given by [41]:

$$\rho_{t+1} = \alpha\rho_t + \beta(1-\rho_t) = z\,\rho_t + \beta \tag{8}$$

where α, β are two constants, such that $0 \le \alpha, \beta \le 1$ and $z = \alpha - \beta$.

3.2 Expected Output

Monitoring and stealing confidential information on patient Vital Signs

- Cost = Sensor jammed (level 1) possible attacks to information content on transit

- Damage = Deliberate collisions caused on GoT (level II)
- Selective forwarding: It is observed that in multi-iterative environment [15, 54, 56, 57], electronic actuator data centric components (i.e., comprising the health data or environmental data) are expected to be forwarded to the base station or a remote server through multi-referential routing protocol. The threat occurs in case the malicious nodes may be reluctant to send or to relay certain messages (e.g., ECG, body-temperature, etc.) and may simply relinquish them, so that they cannot be propagated further. The effect of this vulnerability could be more significant, if the attacker is included exclusively in the routing path and thereby impressing the effect of collision of packets, data items and the level of cost associated with it (level III).
- Sinkhole threat: In this specific malfunctioning, an attacker attempts to attract all adjoining nodes to establish paths through the already affected node: This will impress in the cost of traversal and the difference of time for traversal also could be important (level IV).
- Sybil Attack: This attack imposes multiple mis-guided identities for already infected and compromised nodes to other adjunct nodes in the homogeneous environment. With this broader expected output, the high level description of the algorithm is presented, however the algorithm can be extended for more pheromone mark ups and levels of authentication of e-health vulnerabilities.

The logical representation of the patients' states is given as the classification of sensor's paths under different states. In the Sect. 2.1 Eq. (1) describes brief about the objective function q for the entire IoT repositories. Referring the classical ant colony model as in Eqs. (2) and (3), the basic elements of the proposed solution is the induction of the classification rule on the basis of attribute terms, concerning e-health diagnostic and sensor based parameters. An Ant colony algorithm is used here for classification to quantify the logical level of vulnerability, path or attacks in the form of IF-THEN classification rules. The generic form is:

IF (conditions) THEN (class), where conditions adopts the form (term 1) AND (term 2) AND ... AND (term n).

Ideally, the consequent part and antecedent part of the rule can easily detect the classification rule. An instance that satisfies the IF part will be assigned the class predicted by the rule. Bursa and Lhotska (2007) in their work [42] described the clustering techniques used through ant colonies. Their study revealed two types of biological signals: Electrocardiograms (ECG) and Electroencephalogram (EEG). The recordings have been distinguished by a medical specialist into four pre-defined categories (wake, quiet sleep, active sleep and artefact for data movement). The sensors and IoT devices are incorporated. The recordings are validated in real time and any bi-furcation of recorded values could be sensed as alert for possible threats with initial pheromone values deposited on random nodes of Graph of Things (GoT).

Algorithm 1: High Level Description of the Proposed Algorithm Pheromone Alert

Input: Initialization of values S= 0; t = current time ; t[ ]=null; =100 initial alert pheromone value (say 100 is threshold value)
T= time stamp (consider 10 hrs of inspection) , Graph G , patient state q,
Constants : α, β , IoT $\in$ GoT $\in$ G , R = φ /*R: set of roots */

Output: Classification of threats or vulnerabilities **as Level 1, L II, L III or L IV**
/* Separate functions could be invoked*/

```
Begin
for each v ∈ S                    /* S : array of nodes in vulnerable area*/
        if v has no incoming edge
                R=R ∪ findR(v)
End for
findR (node u)          /* Function performs possibility of traversal on Graph*/
R'=ϕ
        if u is not yet traversed
                label u is traversed
        else return φ
        if u has no exiting edge return {u}
                for each e(u,v)
                        R'=R' ∪ findR(v)
                end for
                return R'
end findR      /* Identification of possibility*/
t[ ]= Recorded values of signal (pheromone) for patient initial state
while (each(t[ ]) matches with pilot _pheromone_value || actual
_pheromone_value)     /* Pheromone Measures*/
        Display as linked value to the recorded pheromone unit on graph G;
        Increment S value until end of signal and position value as per Eq. (1);
end while
Set of nodes that match for given signal on Graph G ={1,2,3,....,n}
do
        for all nodes of Graph G ={1,2,.....,n}
                Choose node i with random probability
        Repeat for relevant GoT
do pheromone updating and pheromone evaporation
        end for
Choose next immediate node j∈ s with probability until s = null
probation t[ ]= tokens (pheromone) while (each (t[ ]) matches with
 pilot_pheromone _value|| actual_pheromone value)
  /*  Performing Comparison of Pheromone value*/
Evaluate pheromone updating as per Eq. (3), (5) & (6)
        Calculate pheromone evaporation as per Eq. (8)
```

```
Detect Levels of Output
if actual pheromone_value > pilot _pheromone_value ≥ 100 units
        Pick Edge of Graph G as either of LI to L IV
end if
for all IoT∈ GoT
do pheromone updating and pheromone evaporation; // Eq. (5), (6) & (8)
end for
        Repeat until G is traversed
                End
```

Our proposed algorithm fits several use cases in eHealth with Internet of Things environment, by way of illustration; we can be inspired by Closed-Loop Insulin Delivery project or what may be called wearable artificial pancreas [43, 44]. This project involves implementing an insulin delivery closed loop system which consists of a sensor for real-time continuous glucose monitoring to record blood sugar continuously and transmits the values to a small laptop computer or a Smartphone that runs an algorithm to control a subcutaneous wireless insulin pump that delivers the required dose of insulin. Furthermore, we can allow to the Smartphone or the small laptop to transmit the patient data to a server for monitoring by the medical staff.

It is clear that the components of such a system are sensitive for threats that can compromise them. Thus, this use case is interesting and illustrative of the applicability of the proposed security solution. We have patients moving between connected objects (sensor, Smartphone, insulin pump) where at least one connected object (like a Smartphone) has a connection to a remote server.

4 Data and Implementation

The initial data source for instantiation of the proposal is the Machine Learning data Repository (UCI).[1] The standard raspberry Pi interface has been used and ACO-Pants 0.5.2 implementation of the ACO Meta-Heuristic also accomplished. Synthetic data set has been envisaged for pheromone trailing, intensity and direction across the nodes of graph G. Table 2 is the extraction of parameters being referred in the simulation model. The effect of all these parameters could be significant on the detection of vulnerability or raising the alert in terms of security system. If the number of ants and speed is increased from its present numerical values (at least 0.1 %), it indicates that the pheromone deposition rate also could be faster on a more secured path. Thus, the dissemination of information to the control

[1]http://archived.ics.uci.edu/ml/datasets/MHEALTH+Dataset.

Table 2 Numerical values of ants' parameters

Description	Value
No. of ants m	200
Speed of ant	2 cm/s
Pheromone deposition rate	0.2 s^{-1}
Pheromone lifetime	100 s
Threat detection radius	5 cm

panel must be faster and the pheromone life time is reduced with faster evaporation as well. The fine tuning of parameters can only be done with respect to e-health sensor set up of Ardunio and Raspberry Pi combination due to their compatibility.

In Fig. 3, a plot of experiments is presented. Reduced pheromone depositions are performed towards the initial traversal of ants across health sensors in different physical states (q) of patients. Definitely, the cycle could be completed once the ants compare the pilot values of pheromone and actual deposition value. The value could be different due to the possibility of intermediate data leakage and threats. Hence, on the reverse traversal, during the returning of ants to their initial position (swarming process, referred in Sect. 2.1), it has been observed that the deposition of pheromone gradient was bit lower and if the pheromone concentration was allowed to build up, it becomes higher (position B). Outwards ants deposited a reduced value of pheromone, if they would go on to c pertaining to a false alert decision. The traversed ants deposited more value of pheromone, if they had just performed

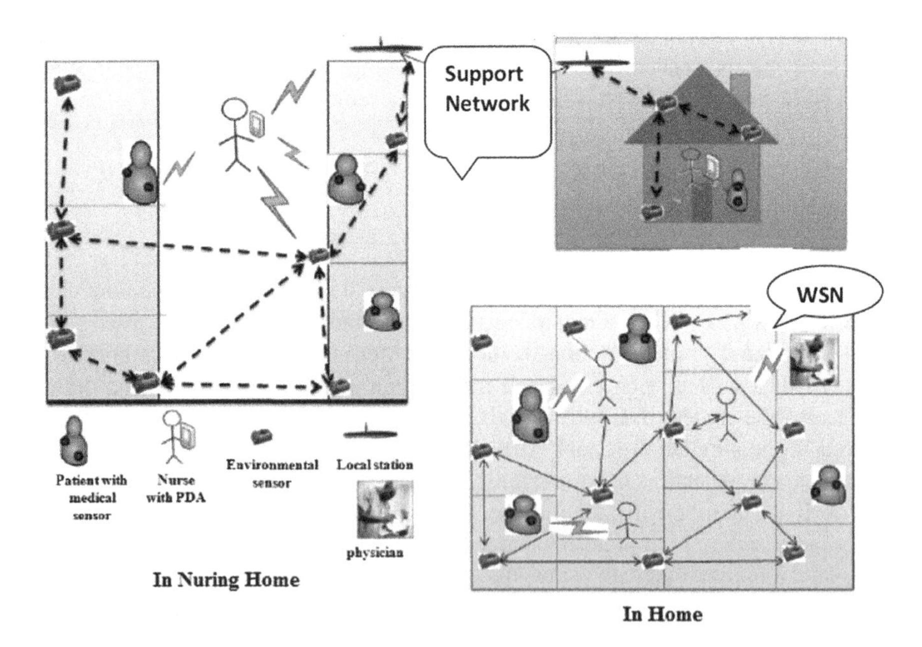

Fig. 3 Different dynamic physical locations of a patient

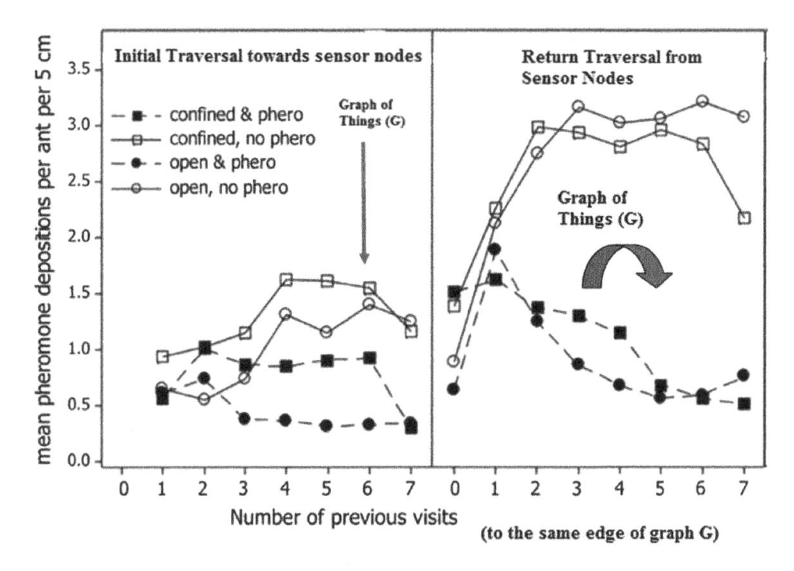

Fig. 4 Effect of pheromone deposition and traversal on IoT

an error value on the current traversal. The tendency of depositing pheromone could be maximum at this point. Data from both ants, which performed and did not perform the deposition pheromone, are merged in this figure. Data acquired from all open routes, and both types of bi-furcations of performing ants have been merged for effective representation of pheromone mapping. Not all the ants are positioned and deployed for pheromone deposition, as initially 2 random nodes were selected for movement on IoT graph (Fig. 4).

4.1 *Evaluation of Results*

The initial data set was referred from UCI, although for security level classification, data set was not directly available. Hence, synthetic data set was created in consultation of UCI. The distribution is known and the novelty of algorithm is tested. The initial dataset is two dimensional, comprising of four clusters. It is represented here as a square template of data. Ideally, a normal distribution expressed as $N(\vec{\mu}, \vec{\sigma})$ is followed to represent prior or posterior clusters of paths. The enumerated clusters, the capacity of clusters, the mean value of dispersion $\vec{\mu}$ and the vector of the standard deviation, statistically, $\vec{\sigma}$ for each normal distribution are deployed to yield the set. The dataset is initialized to 100 data elements. The idea can be referred from [45].

The set up of IoT and the yielded GoT can be formulated as a graph G and thereby considering the following parameters for initial statistical validation:

Table 3 Evaluation and post implementation parameters

Parameters	Primary	Mean	SD
Edge	5	8	1.4
Iterative step size	0.01	0.01	0
Operator on complement	1	4.95	3.48
Identification of threat as difference	1	1.5	0.5
Evaporation (%)	0.01	0.06	0.04
Remaining values	0	1.01	0.81

- Maximum Length of edge of selected path—the maximum number of steps associated on each edge;
- Size of steps—represented through standard deviation;
- Ant Complement—as a population based meta-heuristics, the number of ants present per node can be recorded;
- Range detection for statistical dimensions—The preferred value is better than a mean value (refer Eqs. (6)–(8));
- Quantity of Pheromone—A specific scaled value representing the quality aspect of pheromone deposition, good could represent higher density and quality of pheromone;
- Evaporation Rate—How much pheromone disappears over time component;
- Remaining Parameter—Portion of the sum of all pheromones deposited or concentrated across selected edges.

Table 3 snaps about the statistical measures of the parameters under consideration to demonstrate vulnerability pattern classification on IOT graph using pheromone alert algorithm.

However, the classification is compared (Refer Table 4) with standard precession, Recall and Jacquard coefficients for mean value and SD. For simple illustration, a primary deposition value is necessary which links two nodes when the pheromone concentration becomes stochastic and the distribution may evaporate, if the traversed path has not been acceptable to peer ants. Eventually, this is accomplished by the time required for the ant to traverse the deepest and extensive edge of yielded sensor graph path and still adequate pheromone on the first step is initiated assuming the deposition rate remains constant across the nodes at a random probability value. It is recommended that the aggregated edge lengths used are of approximately 8–10 steps, it signifies that an ant takes 8–10 time cycles an average to visit an edge. Hence, the pheromone layout on the edge must be sustained for the said time cycles. If the amount deposited is 30 units, assuming an evaporation rate of 10 %, then it is implied that after 8 steps, it will be nearly exhausted. The

Table 4 Statistical benchmarking of pheromone alert

Synthetic data set from UCI results	Mean	SD
Precession	0.98	0.01
Recall	0.94	0.021
Jacquard	0.92	0.02

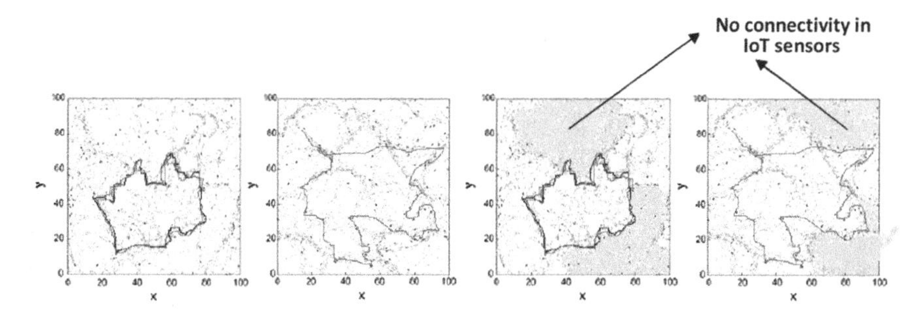

Fig. 5 Pheromone deposition and IoT interaction, at t = 500 s, 1000 s, 1500 s and 2000 s

evaporation parameter is important, as the classification of vulnerability or threat is irrelevant, where there is no pheromone. It denotes that either the connectivity of a sensor node is not being established or a Graph of Things (GoT) has not been produced.

As in the presented model, the approach of pheromone trail is an important parameter, hence an experimental simulation is made on IoT sensors to demonstrate with respect to different pheromone depositions sensor connectivity, considering changing physical locations of patients. Simulation parameters are chosen accordingly and the execution is accomplished with Python standard library. The ants are expressed in blue notation and the pheromones are denoted in green. Red mark up marks the IoT connectivity and where no pheromone is visible, it signifies no connectivity across IoT sensors (refer to numerical values of Table 2). These all possible positions are dynamically simulated with respect to the movement of patients.

At this present scenario, robustness of the solution has not been tested with different security test cases. The only emphasis of this solution is to initiate dashboard control of e-health and IoT devices including intelligent computaional agents. Even though all the sensor interfaces are not being addressed with the solution, the extension could be achieved, if more e-health library for IoT set up could be developed and included (Fig. 5).

4.2 *Limitations and Future Scope*

The present solution has been performed in a restricted simulation environment where all e-health sensor and their interfaces are not being considered. The genuine multi-objective optimization through ACO is not presented, the quality of service has only been investigated. Subsequently, the cost and energy efficiency of sensor devices can also be considered as the components of optimization effort. The optimization feature of ants could be deployed in a future solution as here the components of measuring pheromone strength are evaluated with respect to the medical data of intercepted sensing path of IoT devices. The inclusion of ant colony and the relevant libraries of agents can contribute significantly to monitor security threats through parallel programming. The optimization principle could also be satisfied and therefore the non-polynomial problem of searching and traversing the complex graph can be computationally mediated.

5 Conclusion

The presented chapter described a novel approach by utilizing a computational intelligence in security aspects of IoT (Internet of Things) primarily towards e-health applications. The prime objective of the contribution is to measure the degree of threats, vulnerabilities or attacks in case of dynamic data grabbing for a patient pertaining to different physical locations like from home to diagnostic centre. It is assumed that sensors of health centric paradigm are interconnected and in turn produce a connected graph. The intermediate protocol for exchanging information across the sensors remains homogeneous and thus intelligent agents like social insects could traverse across the interconnected graph and inspect the scope and tendency of the nodes. If the pilot standard value formulated for IoT sensors against time out and access point is found to be deviated, then ants can sense the scope of possible vulnerable conditions across the node of sensors and alert signals are initiated towards the main dash-board control. The entire functional unit is pivoted on the movement of pheromone, the chemical which can remotely communicate the connections across the sensor nodes under observation. The proposed model measured the pheromone deposition and evaporation amount to quantify the level and classification of e-health data exchange process. Several relevant parameters of ant colony, pheromone map and their analogical perspectives with IoT have been deployed. Experimentations are performed keeping the synthetic data set derived from public repository data source. At present, the security measures of IoT in e-health solicit conventional data integrity measures, instead of computational intelligence. The proposed model can justify such positioning of intelligent social insects to measure the degree of vulnerability and risk impact. Initially, the deposition of pheromone and no pheromone and the evaporation of pheromone in sensor connectivity graph are being considered to classify the possible risk level. The extended plug-in software can be compatible with Raspberry pi for more classification of risks. The autonomic control of application, after the detection of a possible vulnerability, can also be developed to control the inference and decision support level of data centre administrator. For higher precision, such applications will enhance e-health security in IoT context.

Appendix

Essential Definitions

- Internet of Things (IoT): The internet of things (IoT) is the linked relationship of devices, sensors, vehicles and all other eligible used components. The necessary concepts are co-adjured with software, embedded sensors, on-chip actuators, and broader network connectivity, which are being instrumental for the objects to collect and interact with data.
- e-health: e-health is an accomplished interface of medical and bio-medical informatics, a health enterprise framework, referring to service computing on health and information dispatched or extended through the web centric technologies.
- Computational Intelligence: Computational Intelligence (CI) is a vertical of artificial intelligence which highlights the heuristic algorithms such as fuzzy systems, neural networks and evolutionary computation.
- Ant colony Optimization: Ant colony optimization (ACO) is a population-based metaheuristic and it is basically used to find approximate solutions to difficult and hard optimization problems. In ACO, a set of software agents called artificial ants search for good solutions to a given optimization problem.
- Pheromone: A chemical substance that is usually yielded by social insects and serves especially as a stigmergy with a collective intelligence issue.
- Pheromone Evaporation and deposition: The process of accumulation and release of pheromone depending on the availability of an edge to reach the shortest path respectively.

References

1. SENSEI, EUFP7project, online at http://www.sensei-project.eu
2. IoT-A, EUFP7project, online at http://www.iot-a.eu
3. Harald Naumann, IOT/M2M COOKBOOK, Copyright © 2015 Harald Naumann, Neustadt, Germany
4. Gyrard, A., Patel, P., Datta, S., Ali, M.: Semantic web meets internet of things (IoT) and web of things (WoT). In: International Conference on Semantic Web, Kobe, Japan, October 2016 (2016)
5. Lake, D., Milito, R., Morrow, M., Vargheese, R.: Internet of things: architectural framework for eHealth security. J. ICT **3** & **4**, 301–328, River Publishers (2014)
6. Ant Colony Optimization Marco Dorigo Thomas Stutzle, A Bradford Book The MIT Press, Massachusetts (2004)
7. Savola, R.M., Savolainen, P., Evesti, A., Abie, H., Sihvonen, M.: Risk-driven security metrics development for an e-health IoT application. In: Information Security for South Africa (ISSA), 2015, pp. 1–6 (2015)
8. Beckers, R., Deneubourg, J.L., Goss, S.: Trail laying behavior during food recruitment in the antLasius niger (L.). Insects Soc. **39**(1), 59–72 (1992)

9. Lindh, W., Pooler, M., Tamparo, C., Dahl, B.: Delmar's Comprehensive Medical Assisting: Administrative and Clinical Competencies; Cengage Learning: Boston. MA, USA (2009)
10. Doukas, C., Pliakas, T., Maglogiannis, I.: Mobile healthcare information management utilizing Cloud Computing and Android OS. Conf. Proc. Annu. Int. Conf. IEEE Eng. Med. Biol. Soc. IEEE Eng. Med. Biol. Soc. Annu. Conf., vol. 2010, pp. 1037–1040 (2010)
11. Tang, W.T., Hu, C.M., Hsu, C.Y.: A mobile phone based homecare management system on the cloud. In: 2010 3rd International Conference on Biomedical Engineering and Informatics, vol. 6, pp. 2442–2445 (2010)
12. Karunarathne, M.S., Jones, S.A., Ekanayake, S.W., Pathirana, P.N.: Remote monitoring system enabling cloud technology upon smart phones and inertial sensors for human kinematics. In: 2014 IEEE Fourth International Conference on Big Data and Cloud Computing (BdCloud), pp. 137–142 (2014)
13. Tsoi, K.K.F., Kuo, Y.H., Meng, H.M.: A data capturing platform in the cloud for behavioral analysis among smokers: an application platform for public health research. In: 2015 IEEE International Congress on Big Data, pp. 737–740 (2015)
14. Gachet, D., de Buenaga, M., Aparicio, F., Padron, V.: Integrating internet of things and cloud computing for health services provisioning: the virtual cloud carer project. In: 2012 Sixth International Conference on Innovative Mobile and Internet Services in Ubiquitous Computing (IMIS), pp. 918–921 (2012)
15. O. for C. R. (OCR), Summary of the HIPAA Privacy Rule, HHS.gov, 07-May-2008. [Online]. Available: http://www.hhs.gov/hipaa/for-professionals/privacy/laws-regulations/index.html. Accessed 28 Jun 2016
16. Gope P, Hwang T.: BSN-Care: a secure IoT-based modern healthcare system using body sensor network. IEEE Sens. J. **16**(5), 1368–1376 (2016)
17. Abdmeziem, M.R., Tandjaoui, D.: An end-to-end secure key management protocol for e-health applications. Comput. Electr. Eng. **44**(C), 184–197 (2015)
18. Keoh, S.L., Kumar, S.S., Tschofenig, H.: Securing the internet of things: a standardization perspective. IEEE Internet Things J. **1**(3), 265–275 (2014)
19. Kocabas, O., Soyata, T., Aktas, M.K.: Emerging security mechanisms for medical cyber physical systems. IEEE ACM Trans. Comput. Biol. Bioinforma. IEEE ACM **13**(3), 401–416 (2016)
20. Gong, T., Huang, H., Li, P., Zhang, K., Jiang, H.: Medical healthcare system for privacy protection based on IoT. In: 2015 Seventh International Symposium on Parallel Architectures, Algorithms and Programming (PAAP), pp. 217–222 (2015)
21. Sharma, A., Goyal, T., Pilli, E.S., Mazumdar, A.P., Govil, M.C., Joshi, R.C.: A secure hybrid cloud enabled architecture for internet of things. In: 2015 IEEE 2nd World Forum on Internet of Things (WF-IoT), pp. 274–279 (2015)
22. Abie, H., Balasingham, I.: Risk-based adaptive security for smart IoT in eHealth. In: Proceedings of the 7th International Conference on Body Area Networks, ICST, Brussels, Belgium, Belgium, pp. 269–275 (2012)
23. Habib, K., Leister, W.: Threats identification for the smart internet of things in eHealth and adaptive security countermeasures. In: 2015 7th International Conference on New Technologies, Mobility and Security (NTMS), pp. 1–5 (2015)
24. Hamdi, M., Abie, H.: Game-based adaptive security in the internet of things for eHealth. In: 2014 IEEE International Conference on Communications (ICC), pp. 920–925 (2014)
25. Sriprasadh, K., Prakash Kumar, M.: Ant colony optimization technique for secure various data retrieval in cloud computing. Int. J. Comput. Sci. Inf. Technol. **5**(6) (2014)
26. Anita, Tyagi, S.S.: Providing security for the building using ant colony optimization technique. Int. J. Sci. Res. Publ. (IJSRP) (2013)
27. Peinado, A., Ortiz, A., Munilla, J.: Secure distributed system inspired by ant colonies for road traffic management in emergency situations. In: The Seventh International Conference on Emerging Security Information, Systems and Technologies Presented at the SECURWARE 2013, pp. 144–149 (2013)

28. Lu, Y., Hu, W.: Study on the application of ant colony algorithm in the route of internet of things. Int. J. Smart Home **7**(3), 365–374
29. Wang, Y., Wang, C.: Based on the ant colony algorithm is a distributed intrusion detection method. Int. J. Secur. Its Appl. **9**(4), 141–152
30. Chhikara, P., Patel, A.K.: Enhancing network security using ant colony optimization. Global J. Comput. Sci. Technol. Netw. Web Secur. **13**(4) Version 1.0, 201AD
31. Nandi, S., Roy, S., Dansana, J. et. al.: Cellular automata based encrypted ECG hash code generation: an application in inter human biometric authentication system. Int. J. Comput. Netw. Inf. Secur. (2014)
32. Biswas, S., Roy, A.B., et. al.: A bio-metric authentication based secured atm banking system. Int. J. Adv. Res. Comput. Sci. Softw. Eng. **2**(4), 172–182 (2012)
33. Samanta, S. et. al.: Quantum inspired evolutionary algorithm for scaling factors optimization during manifold medical information embedding. In: Bhattacharyya, S. et al (eds.) Quantum Inspired Computational intelligence: Research and Applications. Elsevier (2016)
34. Suri, J., et. al.: Diagnostic preservation of atherosclerotic ultrasound video for stroke telemedicine in watermarking framework. In: 2015 AIUM Annual Convention and Preconvention Program Hosting WFUMB Congress, Volume: Ultrasound in Medicine & Biology, vol. 41, Issue 4, Supplement, pp. S1-S188 (2015)
35. Santhi. V., Dey, N.: Intelligent techniques in signal processing for multimedia security. Intelligent Systems Reference Library series—Springer (2016)
36. Pal, A.K., et. al.: Hybrid reversible watermarking technique for color biomedical images. In: 2013 IEEE International Conference on Computational Intelligence and Computing Research Proceedings, pp. 1–6 (2013)
37. Chakraborty et al.: Firefly algorithm for optimized non-rigid demons registration. In: Yang, X. S., Papa, J.P. (eds.) Bio-Inspired Computation & Applications in Image Processing. Elsevier (2016)
38. Acharjee et al.: Watermarking in motion vector for security enhancement of medical videos. In: International Conference on Control, Instrumentation, Communication and Computational Technologies (ICCICCT), pp. 532–537 (2014)
39. Hecker, J.P., Letendre, K., Stolleis, K., Washington, D., Moses, M.E.: Formica ex Machina: ant swarm foraging from physical to virtual and back again. In: Proceedings of the Eighth International Conference on Swarm Intelligence (2012)
40. Diestel, R.: Graph Theory, electronic edn. Springer, Heidelberg, Germany (2005)
41. Kumar, P., Raghavendra, G.S.: On the evaporation mechanism in the ant colony optimization algorithms. Ann. Comp. Sci. Ser. **9**, 51–56 (2011)
42. Bursa, M., Lhotska, L.: Ant colony cooperative strategy in electrocardiogram and electroencephalogram data clustering. In: Nature Inspired Cooperative Strategies for Optimization (NICSO 2007), pp. 323–333 (2007)
43. Leelarathna, L., Dellweg, S., Mader, J.K., Allen, J.M., Benesch, C., Doll, W., Ellmerer, M., Hartnell, S., Heinemann, L., Kojzar, H., Michalewski, L., Nodale, M., Thabit, H., Wilinska, M.E., Pieber, T.R., Arnolds, S., Evans, M.L., Hovorka, R.: Day and night home closed-loop insulin delivery in adults with type 1 diabetes: three-center randomized crossover study. Diabetes Care **37**(7), 1931–1937 (2014)
44. Renard, E., Farret, A., Kropff, J., Bruttomesso, D., Messori, M., Place, J., Visentin, R., Calore, R., Toffanin, C., Di Palma, F., Lanzola, G., Magni, P., Boscari, F., Galasso, S., Avogaro, A., Keith-Hynes, P., Kovatchev, B., Del Favero, S., Cobelli, C., Magni, L., DeVries, J. H., AP@home Consortium: Day-and-night closed-loop glucose control in patients with type 1 diabetes under free-living conditions: results of a single-arm 1-month experience compared with a previously reported feasibility study of evening and night at home. Diabetes Care **39**(7), 1151–1160 (2016)
45. Handl, J., Knowles, J., Dorigo, M.: Ant-based clustering: a comparative study of its relative performance with respect to k-means, average link and 1d-som. In: Proceedings of the Third International Conference on Hybrid Intelligent Systems, IOS Press (2003)

46. Atay, F., Stojmenovic, I., Yanikomeroglu, H.: Generating random graphs for the simulation of wireless ad hoc, actuator, sensor, and internet networks. In: Proceedings 8th IEEE Symposium on a World of Wireless, Mobile and Multimedia Networks WoWMoM, Helsinki, Finland, June 2007 (2007)
47. Bonabeau, E., Dorigo, M., Theraulaz, G.: Inspiration for optimization from social insect behaviour. Nature **406**, 39–42 (2000)
48. Brambilla, M., Ferrante, E., Birattari, M., Dorigo, M.: Swarm robotics: a review from the swarm engineering perspective. In: IRIDIA Technical Report (2012)
49. Le-Phuoc, D., Nguyen-Mau, H.Q., Parreira, J.X., Hauswirth, M.: A middleware framework for scalable management of linked streams. Web Semant. Sci. Serv. Agents World Wide Web **0**(0) (2012)
50. Amorim, P.: A continuous model of ant foraging with pheromones and trail formation. Proc. Ser. Braz. Soc. Appl. Comput. Math. **3**(1), 2015 (2015). doi:10.5540/03.2015.003.01.0323

Vitality of Robotics in Healthcare Industry: An Internet of Things (IoT) Perspective

Ankit R. Patel, Rajesh S. Patel, Navdeep M. Singh and Faruk S. Kazi

Abstract Since last two decade robotics is one of the emerging, challenging, developing and innovative fields of research among researchers, industries universities. It is very difficult to distinguish robots from other machines; robots can be defined as machines that are capable of perform variety of task with more autonomy and degree of freedom (DoF) than humans. Nowadays healthcare services and systems become very complex and encompass a vast number of entities that are characterized by shared, distributed, and heterogeneous devices, sensors, and information and communication technology. With the advent of Internet of Things (IoT), robots are integrated as a 'thing' and establish connections with other things over the Internet. This chapter clearly indicates the long term benefits of human being in healthcare sector, medical emergencies, e-health, etc. using robotics and IoT. Also, the phase of adoption, interaction, challenges for future is to be discussed.

Keywords Robotics · Internet of Things (IoT) · Surgical robotics · Medical technology · Medical robots · Robot operating system (ROS)

A.R. Patel (✉)
Department of Electrical & Computer Engineering, Faculty of Engineering, University of Jeddah, Jeddah, Kingdom of Saudi Arabia
e-mail: majorankit@gmail.com

R.S. Patel
Department of Mechanical Engineering, School of Technology, Pandit Deendayal Petroleum University (PDPU), Gandhinagar, Gujarat, India
e-mail: rajesh.patel@sot.pdpu.ac.in

N.M. Singh · F.S. Kazi
Department of Electrical Engineering, Veermata Jijabai Technological Institute (VJTI), Mumbai, India
e-mail: nmsingh@vjti.org.in

F.S. Kazi
e-mail: fskazi@vjti.org.in

C. Bhatt et al. (eds.), *Internet of Things and Big Data Technologies for Next Generation Healthcare*, Studies in Big Data 23,
DOI 10.1007/978-3-319-49736-5_5

1 Introduction

Today, a good percentage of world population is aging rapidly and co-morbidities will continue to rise largely as a result of lifestyles associated with economic development such as smoking, obesity, harmful consumption of alcohol, unhealthy diet and sedentary lifestyle. According to World Health Organization (WHO) report, the healthcare Internet of Things (IoT) market segment is poised to hit USD 117 billion by 2020. Increasingly, Internet of Things start-ups are finding new applications within healthcare and leveraging connected sensors to better diagnosis, monitor, and manage patients and treatment. Many are focused on clinical-grade wearable to more robustly track patient data, while others see opportunity for sensor networks within hospitals and practices to optimize healthcare delivery and monitor patient adherence [1].

As IoT having features of reconnect with different entities like apps, devices and people interaction, which gives the better solution for healthcare and medical industry. Thus, it is clear that IoT offering new promises with great efficiency to ensure safety and care of patients, cost reduction, value of treatment as a future healthcare and medical systems. The major advantage of the IoT driven healthcare units include the following:

- Decreased costs of medical treatment
- Improved outcomes of treatment
- Improved diseases management
- Reduced errors
- Enhanced patient experience
- Enhanced management of drugs

With the rapid development in the field of robotics, machine learning and IoT, we have all the pieces of technology to make this happen and it's just a matter of time when this technology pieces will be integrated to transform our way of living. Robotics deals with programmed machines designed to do labour intensive work. Machine Learning is the science of getting computers and machines to function without being programmed to do so. The combination of Robotics and Machine Learning results in Robots with the capability to do the jobs on their own. Machine Learning tasks can start with supervised learning, then moving to a semi-supervised state and then unsupervised learning. It basically contains the essence of statistical pattern recognition, parametric/non-parametric algorithms, neural networks, recommender systems, etc. Machine Learning is and advanced state of intelligence—With Internet of Things (IoT), multiple robots can get interconnected. IoT platform provide unique facility to interconnection between objects or people, transfer data between the two without human to computer or humans interaction. IoT can be applied to monitoring and capturing data from anything and everything connected to a network—e.g. media, environment monitoring, infrastructure management, manufacturing, energy management, building and home automation or transportation, medical and healthcare systems.

The organization of chapter as follow: Sect. 2 presents the field of robotics with its applications, growth, demands, and future challenges. In Sect. 3, we discuss about Internet of Things (IoT) probable architecture (or structure), applications and challenges for implementation. In Sect. 4, the main topic is to be presented that how robotics plays a vital role in IoT based healthcare applications. The last part of the chapter includes future open research problems and conclusion.

2 Robotics

2.1 History and Definition

In 1921, Czech writer Karel Capek introduced the word "Robot" in his play R.U.R. (Rossuum's Universal Robots). "Robot" in Czech comes from the word "Robota", meaning "compulsory labour". The word robot was defined by the Robotic Institute of America as 'a machine in the form of a human being that performs the mechanical functions of a human being but lacks sensitivity'. As per Issac Asimov's series of robots in 1940s story, there are basically three main laws of robots are as under:

a. A robot may not injure a human being, or, through inaction, allow a human being to come to harm.
b. A robot must obey the orders given it by human beings except where such orders would conflict with the First Law.
c. A robot must protect its own existence as long as such protection does not conflict with the First or Second Law.

A prime application or intense behind the invention of robots was to work like humans, but as it was developed step by step and adding features it shows that it can do more than it was developed. Till today applications of robotics in many areas to be developed but there are still new scope are available in this area. A simple definition of a robot is: 'any machine programmed to do work'. However, basic machine automation is now so commonplace that this classic definition is being replaced with a more apt phrase—'a machine with intelligence'. The field of robotics comprise by telemanipulators and numerical control systems.

2.2 Medical Robotics

For healthcare and medical industries robots are performed integrated duties using the field of mechanical and electronics, like force or movement measurement or domain, sensor system technology, etc. The concern duties done by robots are total care of patients, rehabilitation, artificial prosthetics, medical interventions if needed, e-health, monitoring [2].

According to that definition, medical robotics is considered to have a huge value in healthcare in terms of health, societal, and economical benefits. Robotics can offer solutions for a significant proportion, especially for patient groups with certain needs such as amputees, strokes suffers, or cognitive or mental disability patients. Depending upon applications, and market analysis, there are six areas of medical robotics:

- Smart medical capsules
- Surgical robotics
- Prosthetics using Surgical robots
- Motor co-ordination analysis and treatment by robots
- Robot assisted mental and social therapy
- Robotized patient monitoring systems [3].

2.3 *Applications of Robotics in Healthcare Paradigm*

In surgery, medical robotics proved that with it both timing and risks are reduced. Due to its widespread, today prostate and cardiac procedures performed by robots in many countries. Robots also proved its ability in rehabilitation and in intelligent prostheses. Nowadays, social robotics is a challenging branch being developed having a capabilities of monitoring and motivating the patients. The market growth of medical and healthcare robotics is about USD 17.9 from 2014 to 2020, this is due to presence of medical robotics in healthcare industry [4].

The growing demand of information technology in healthcare and medical sector leads to robotics into it. In addition, robotics having advanced applications in healthcare domain boosts market growth in upcoming years. As the world population increases the use of minimally invasive robotic surgeries increases which will provides sustainability to the disorders such as neurological, orthopaedics and others. Countries like India, Brazil and China having lots of possibilities in this sector, will boost new opportunities to researchers and scientists to do more effort and adopt new technologies [4]. A market growth for robotics applications shown in Fig. 1.

It is obvious that the ability of computer integrated systems (CIS) provide more accuracy for surgeon's technical capability in term of current procedures or by making it possible in any abnormal environment. In such a cases the advantages by humans or by robot describes in Table 1.

Other advantages by CIS for surgical use are as:

- It gives technical solution in different procedures.
- By help of this, it is easy to monitor online all information which requires for surgery.
- Its working in delicate anatomical to dangerous proximity environments.

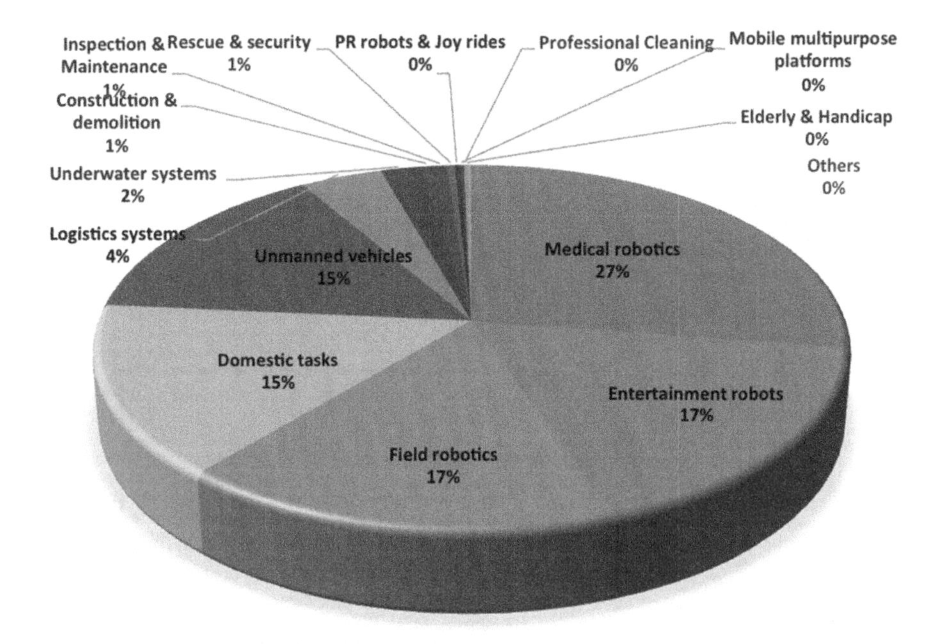

Fig. 1 Growth of robotics in different sectors [4]

Table 1 Strengths and limitations of robots and humans [6]

	Strengths	Limitations
Humans	Judgment is excellent	Prone to fatigue and interaction
	Excellent hand-eye coordination	Tremor limits fine motion
	Dexterity is excellent	Outside natural scale it has limited ability and dexterity
	Having capability of integration of multiple information sources	Not possible to see by tissue
	Trained by easily	Bulky end effectors, hence accuracy decreases
	Able and versatile to improvise	Geometrically less accurate
		Sterility is not easy
		Quickly infected and not protest against radiation
Robots	Higher geometric accuracy	Poor decision
	Untiring and stable	Adoption is not fast
	Fight against radiation	Limited dexterity
	Having many degree of freedom in motion analysis	Problems in hand-eye coordination
	Able to integrate multiple sources of numerical and sensor data	Not up to mark haptic sense
		Problem occurs when complexity

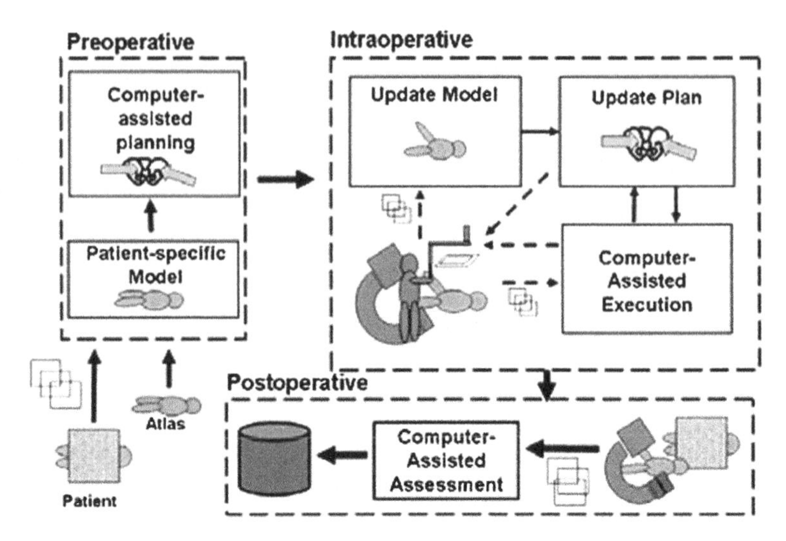

Fig. 2 The flow of information for computer integrated surgery systems

The different research domain in medical robotics shown in Fig. 3.

The nature of robotics systems is to connection between the real world data and physical world. The field of robotics is being always interdisciplinary having not only engineering but also includes biomechanics, computational science, neurology, cognitive science, sports science, biomedical, etc. Main challenge is to facing with medical robotics is that how to interface sensor, motor and human-adoption abilities in different environments.

Figure 2 works with humans to data of information with the physical world to perform a given task [5].

When we are talking about medical robotics, there are certain factors are to be kept in mind, like motion, autonomy, intelligence, etc. *Motion* includes actuated mechanism programmable in more than one axis and moving within its environment. *Autonomy* tells us level of human involvement in overseeing the operation of the robot or robotic device both in normal operation and particularly when there is a problem or fault in the system.

Intelligence indicates built in expert knowledge or skill to allow an operator (or perhaps no operator at all) to perform tasks with less skill/knowledge than would be required of a human performing the same task on their own [7].

It is very difficult to say that by which criteria robotics will helpful to medical and healthcare sector. There are so many methods to describing it, but apart from all here taking by its application.

Accordingly to Medical Treatment: There are total five different groups defined in [8].

(a) The first is *Prevention*, in which there is targeted that no further treatment required. If it is found something abnormal then go to next step, known as *diagnosis*, done by robotic systems (Fig. 3).

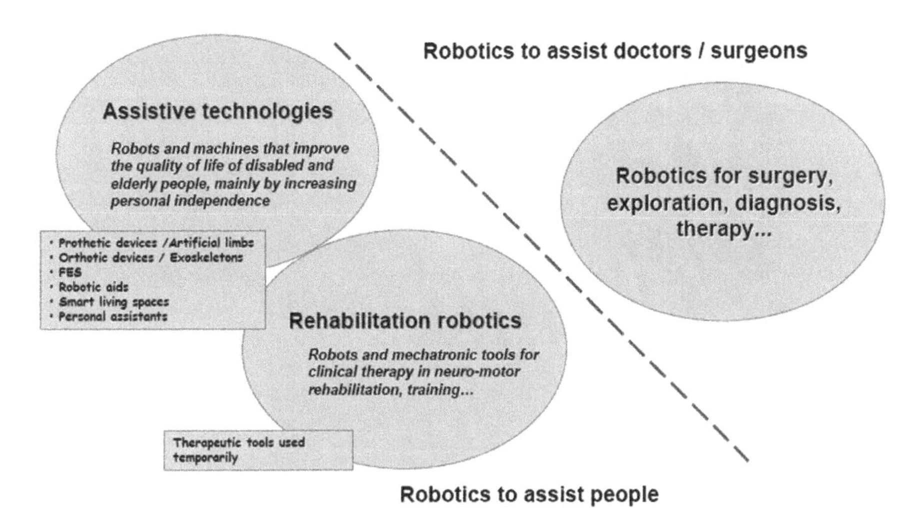

Fig. 3 Medical robotics research areas

Toyota developed the "Balance Training Assist" as in Fig. 4, in which two wheel robots used to balance. A patient moves his/her weight depending upon the information given by the machine shows different games displays on monitor [9].

(b) A *surgery (robotic systems for medical interventions)*: The option of surgery opens when physicians not able to perform a given task because of precision, repeatability and endurance. Furthermore, with a very small space robots can perform well inside the human body. Due to above advantages nowadays robots are become popular in the following fields:

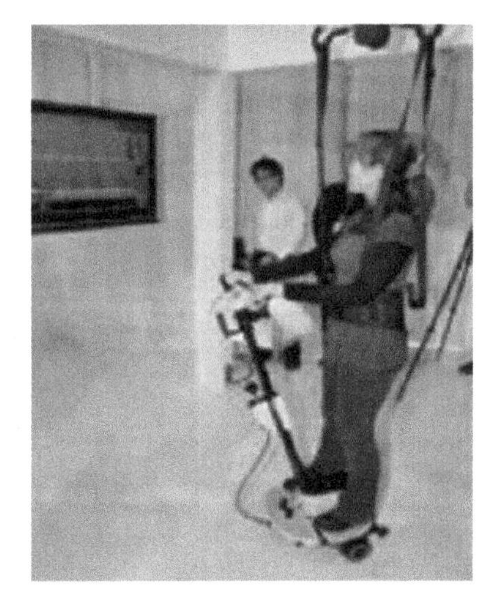

Fig. 4 Balance training assist from Toyota Corporation Ltd. [10]

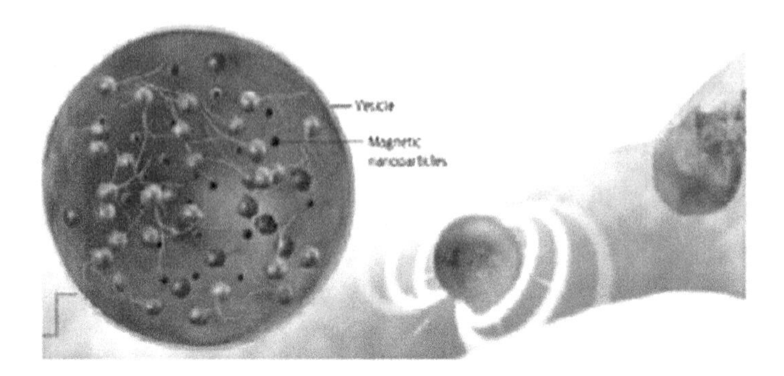

Fig. 5 The Nanobot [11]

- Precision and Micro surgery
- Minimal invasive surgery by robots [12]
- Nanobots
- Remote surgery via Internet or IoT based platforms
- In some cases, medical interventions by robots
- Surgery assistance by robots [13]

For drug therapy and ocular diseases *Nanobots* are used. It is made of flat nickel parts, sometimes known as "*Steerable Surgeons*" as shown in Fig. 5. The working of Nanobot is by external electromagnetic coils which produces magnetic fields inside it.

(c) *Professional care (robotic systems for professional care)* in hospitals: This category of robotic care is used for generally ageing people only. It includes monitoring, aid for nurses and physical activities in terms of care provision [14] and paramedic task [15].

Cody is a 'human-scale' mobile manipulator as in Fig. 6. By using "*Direct Physical Interface*" (DPI) in healthcare robotics systems, a nurse have capability to direct control of movement of the robot. DPI provides direct assist to nurse that

Fig. 6 Working of Cody Robot [16]

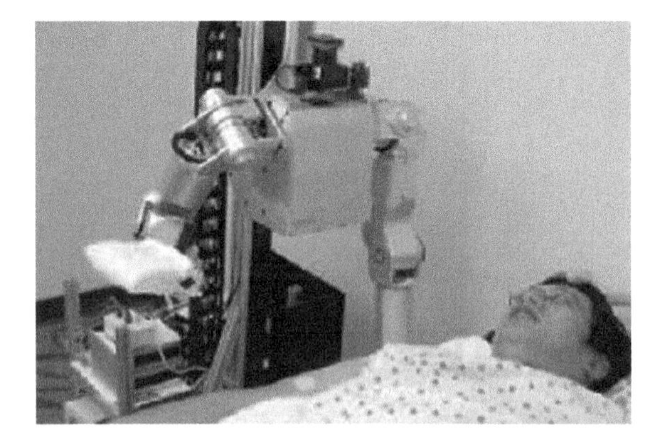

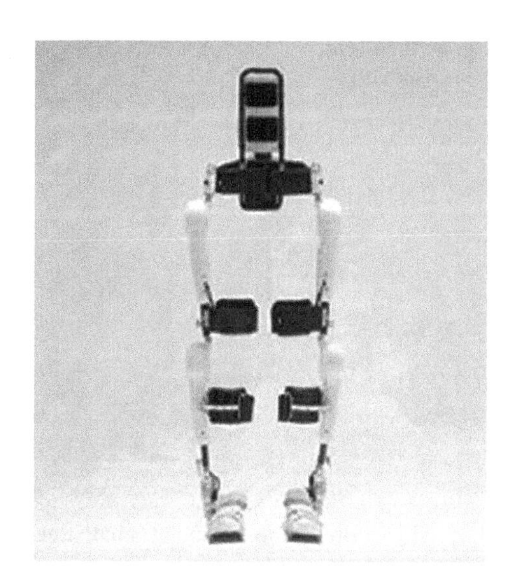

Fig. 7 Hybrid assistive limb

Cody is making direct contact with body. When the patient tries to getting any movement, Cody responds accordingly.

(d) *Rehabilitation treatment*: This kind of treatment is given at hospitals or at home. It can be divided into: (a) Motor coordination therapy, and (b) Sustaining muscle therapy. Behaviour of patient plays an important role in cognitive and mental problems.

'Hybrid Assistive Limb' (HAL) in Fig. 7 is a 'cyborg-type robot'. The main features of HAL that it provides support for wearer's bodily and enhanced [17]. Due to disorders of the cerebral and nervous muscular system, the lower limb disabilities occur in human body. In such a cases brain does not work properly. HAL provide support for lower limb to move accordingly to patient's intention [18]. It gives command/signal to brain that how to move the legs.

(e) *Daily Living Activities*: This is known as assistance of life. It has basically three main functions: (i) To assist users for doing daily activities. (ii) Provide mobility to disabled people, and (iii) Replace organs by intelligent prosthetics [20].

The electric wheelchair '*Friend*' (Fig. 8) having basic components like robot arm, computer and sensors. A Joysticks is also given for operate robotic system. With this facility provision it is possible to read book pages and also turns it.

2.4 Advantage and Disadvantage of Robotic Surgery

Today, it is estimated that only 5 % of the general surgery market has been penetrated by robotic procedures, leaving 95 % of the opportunity unmet. As robotic surgery continues to gain acceptance in many surgical specialities, thousands of hospitals are expressing interest in the next generation of robotic surgical platforms

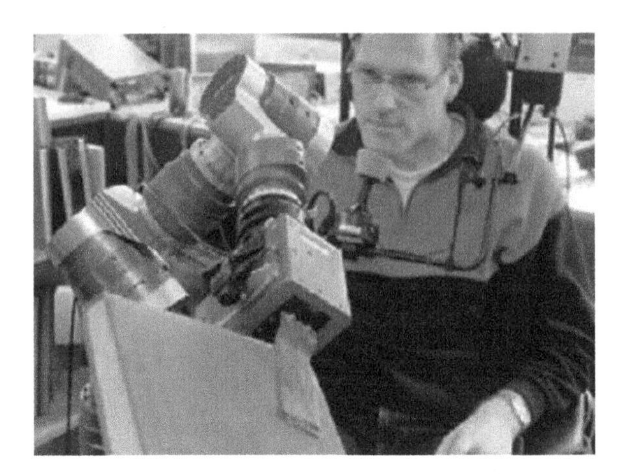

Fig. 8 The electric wheelchair [19]

that will address the financial challenges and operational inefficiencies being experienced with the current robotic platforms. According to Wintergreen Research, the robotic surgery market is growing USD 20 billion by 2021 [21]. In this context, here we are going to compare the advantage and disadvantage of the same (Table 2).

Table 2 Advantage and disadvantage of robotic surgery [22]

	Robotic equipment based surgery	Conventional surgery by doctors
Advantages		
	Filtration of tremor	Affordable, ubiquitous
	Stereoscopic visualization	Some haptic feedback
	7 DOF	Well developed, established technology
	Dexterity improvement	
	Elimination of Fulcrum effect	
	Motion scaling	
	Ergonomic positioning	
	Tele-surgery	
	Hand-eye coordination is better	
Disadvantages	Minimal haptic feedback	2-D visualization available
	Expensive	Compromised dexterity
	Longer set-up times	Limited degree of freedom
	Footprint is large	Hand-instrument motion reversal
	Emerging technology	

3 Internet of Things (IoT)

3.1 Definition

Currently, the definition of Internet of Things (IoT) is varying depending upon applications, persons, or domain areas. According to [23], the 'things' defined by three main areas: information, machine (it includes sensors, actuators, embedded systems, etc.) and people.

Figure 9 defines three basic environment of IoT: Things oriented, Internet oriented, and Semantic oriented. The Things oriented IoT will be defined as: 'Things having identities and virtual personalities operating in smart spaces using intelligent interfaces to connect and communicate within social, environmental, and user contexts' [25]. The Internet oriented IoT will be defined as: 'In future Internet, the interconnected objects plays an important role'. The Semantic oriented IoT will be defined as: 'A world-wide network of interconnected objects uniquely addressable based on standard communication protocols' [26]. In fact, IoT is simply shifting of paradigm using different technologies. It gives anytime, anyplace connectivity for anything [27].

It is very difficult to give a definition of IoT, but the following common things are includes in all [28]:

- The nature of connectivity is ubiquitous.
- The everything is to be connected.
- Data exchange through Internet or by the private network.

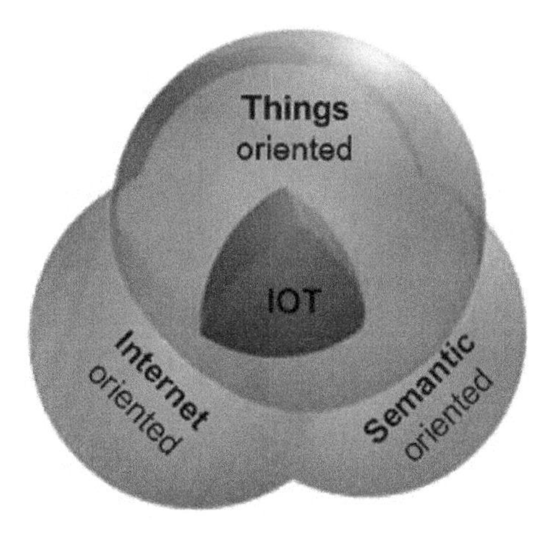

Fig. 9 IoT define in various environments [24]

3.2 Architecture of IoT

The Internet will enable the robot's real world to be connected to the virtual world.

If taken into account, with the emerging robot operating system framework, communication with the internet via Bluetooth requires only a set of application programming interface (API) calls shown in Fig. 10 [29].

Future robots will become part of the IoT and capable of seamlessly communicate with the cloud. These robots will have the potential to the smart mobility and context-aware computing to internet relevantly with their surrounding physical environment. Using cloud orchestration and messaging, a robot can also interact with any service, business process or device connected to the cloud. Communicate with the cloud can be either asynchronous or synchronous (a robot waits for the response before proceeding with the next action), based on the exposed web services invoked on the cloud.

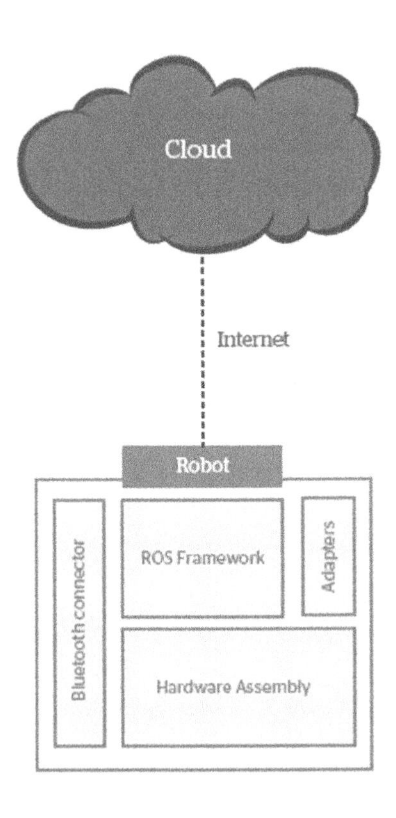

Fig. 10 Architecture of robot to Internet connectivity

3.3 IoT Platforms

The IoT platforms provide connection between real to virtual world environment. *Pachube* [30] is IoT platform for real time infrastructure having capability of manage millions of data points from millions of organizations, companies and individuals. *SenseTele* [31] is an IoT application which gathers data from various sources like embedded systems, sensors, physical objects, etc. Whatever the line data coming, it is used or shared via social networking platforms. *Nimbits* [32] provide cloud based service for people, sensors and devices. It is also open source platform. With this kind of tools anyone can define points and feed various information into it. This data points have the capabilities to perform various operations like statistics, generate alarms, connect to social networks, calculations, etc. *ThingSpeak* [33] gives freedom to users to store and retrieve data from things by exploitation of HTTP protocol over the Internet or via LAN. Using ThingSpeak, location tracking and sensor logging applications created. A continuous status updates kind of social network is also create by ThingSpeak. Further, it allows storing data and doing calculations through cloud. The integration of data into applications done by JSON, XML and CSV type data representations.

The standardization of IoThNet is explained in [34]. As shown in Fig. 11, there are basically three main categories of standardization interface.

(a) Interfacing of hardware and software.
(b) Health related data information (e.g. e-health records, etc.).
(c) Security schemes.

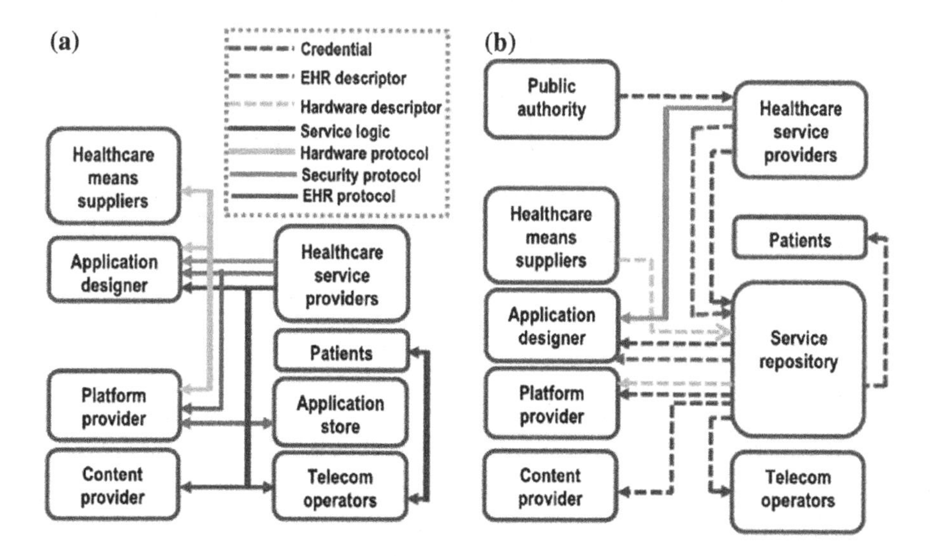

Fig. 11 IoThNet platform interfaces **a** without standardization **b** with standardization

A clear idea about rehabilitation process is discussed in [35], using IoThNet platform.

3.4 IoT Impact in Healthcare Sector

The healthcare system defined by IoT platform based on various factors like supervision of chronic diseases, care for elderly patients, health management systems, among others. For better understand it is also categories into two parts: (a) Application based, and (b) Service based. Further application based is divided

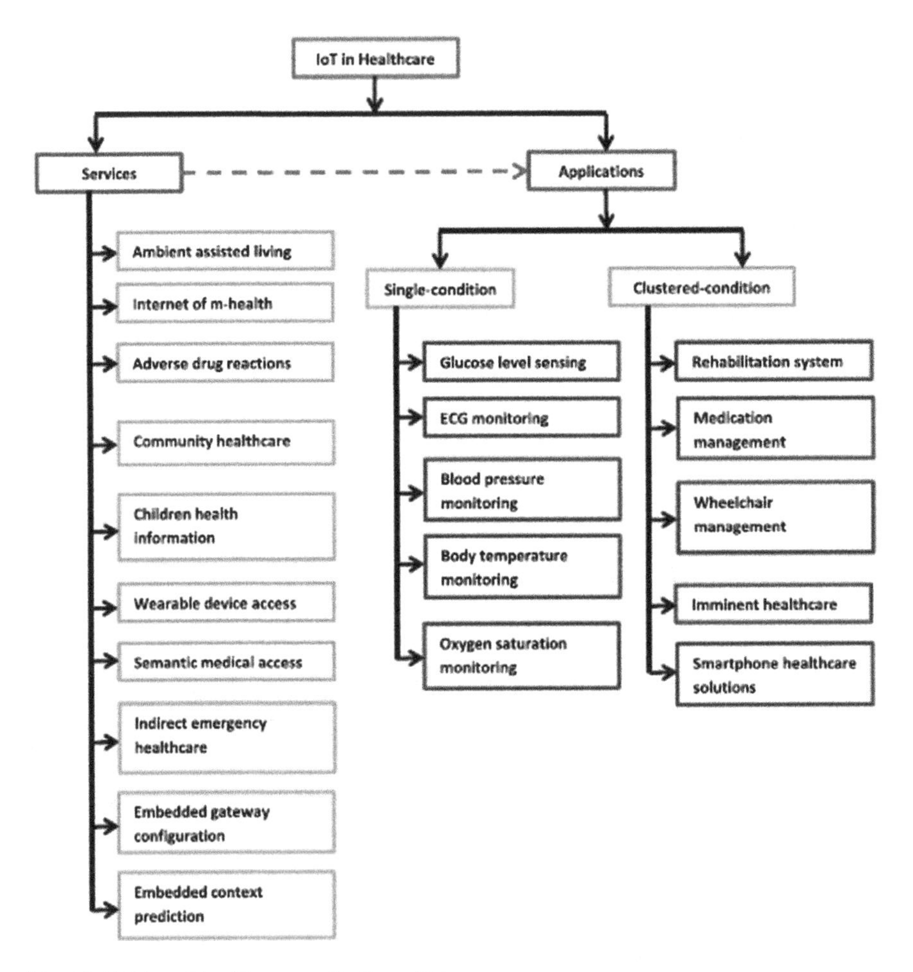

Fig. 12 IoT based healthcare applications [36]

into: Single condition based and Cluster condition based. A single condition refers to specific diseases, while cluster condition refers with multiple diseases as shown in Fig. 12. This is based on today's IoT healthcare systems, having dynamic nature to add more single or cluster condition based disease in future.

4 Connectivity: Robotics and IoT in Healthcare Domain

Figure 13 gives detail scope of robotic interaction with both the physical and virtual worlds. It considers a range of inputs (both active control and perception driven) and shows examples of the numerous possible outputs, actions or roles that can arise. Using this kind of model, the role of Information Technology (IT) services as an enabling and necessary part of the robotic interaction ecosystem begins to emerge. A robot may have a direct physical manifestation that allows it to mechanically act and react in the real world, but it may also operate in the virtual world using underlying information technologies as a conduit for eventual real-world interaction (e.g. communicate contextual information to remote observers). A robot can also have perception, i.e. it has an ability to assimilate real-world inputs, make 'contextual sense' of them and act according to its programming and what it has learned. This view of perception, control and interaction serves well, but misses one point that can often be found in the world of science fiction, whether or not a robot can be truly sentient [29].

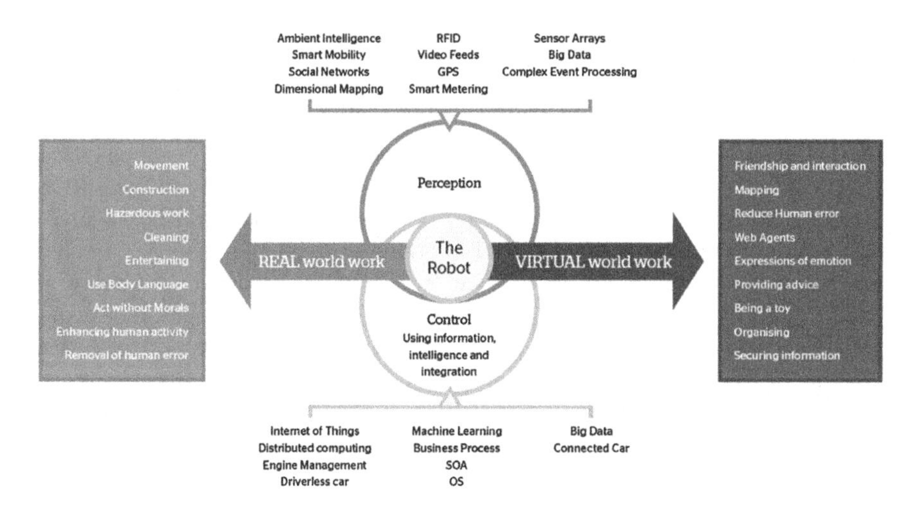

Fig. 13 Robot interactions to IoT

4.1 Robot Operating System (ROS)

In the coming days, interest of development of IoT will be increasing rapidly as per the different surveys. It will be necessary that to provide easier development tool to connect physical world to IoT based networks. As IoT is a new developing technology hence tools for the different solutions in IoT platform not fully/trustworthy developed yet. In this regards, ROS provide attractive opportunity for the IoT platform for infrastructure connectivity. ROS having its own features like high abstraction level to access any hardware attracts researchers and scientific organizations. Additional functionalities includes that it can be easily incorporated to the platform due to modular implementation [37].

The Internet Engineering Task Force (IETF) created the IPv6.0 to standardize the low power wireless personal group and network in 2005 [38]. In [39] shows that how two categories build for classification of IoT elements. According to [39], firstly reduced functionality devices, which not provide any packet routing due to their processing and memory limitations. Secondly, complex functionalities devices, having more capacity that the later one and hence it is acting as router and will be provide service to simple device and/or other external elements which is not a part of network. The more information about it is given in [40].

A common solution for the robotic field or area being provide by ROS platform. Depending upon the different components used, robot works accordingly [41, 42]. The uniformity of components makes the process of software development difficult, which is finally connect to hardware. The making of complex system dependent on knowledge of hardware specific and its interfacing. This leads to ROS to implement in robotic domain easier than any other platform [43].

While applying ROS platform to robotic systems, it is to be noted that it uses Peer to Peer (P2P) communication not centralized communication. A main advantage of this communication is when multiple nodes propagate, information collected by sensors to processing nodes. Even though maximum communication on ROS is works on P2P platform, but ROS naming service is centralized. ROS node communication system shown in Fig. 14. A 'scan' service offer by 'hokuyo' node, later it connects to master node for informing entry point of service. Another node 'viewer' used to access the service 'scan'. ROS gives more flexibility to system developer compare to other programming or scripting languages. It provides modular development which allows small modules to perform big work. Due to this feasibility of ROS, the developers can reuse the same coding for different projects. Still there are some difficulties to adopt ROS as a complete solution for robotic based IoT platform as: (a) Interoperability [44] (b) Open Standards (c) Scalability (d) Conflict Resolution [45] (e) Dynamic Infrastructure (f) Quality of Service (g) Privacy and Security.

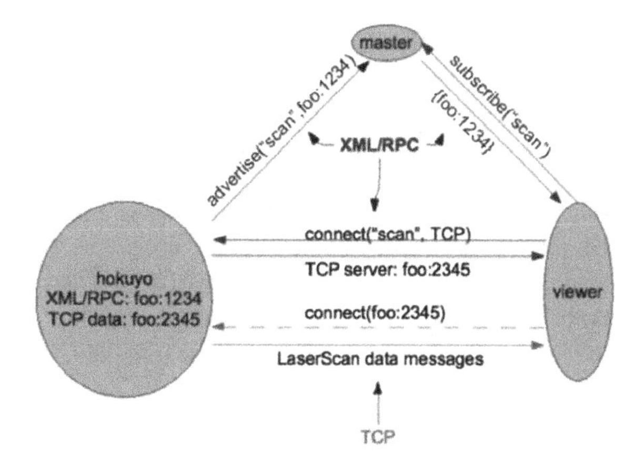

Fig. 14 Communication in ROS

5 Future Challenges

Robotic system plays a vital role in all surgical medical fields in past few years. Scientists are trying to overcome the electromechanical limitations of actual robotic systems. In the future robotic systems with smaller instruments, lower overall costs, shorter set-up time with the help of a very well trained team and remote telementoring will become available.

Although its popularity and affectness of IoT in healthcare and medical sector is being rapidly increases there are issues for adoption of it, includes sophisticated health monitoring system, expensive medical equipment used onsite, robots, etc.

The rapid development of healthcare sectors at hospitals and homes requires latest remote sensing devices of all kinds connected to healthcare providers and care takers fulfill the broad objective of IoT driven robotic applications [46]. According to [47], total cost of IoT based devices will be 19 trillion dollars in next decade. However, there are many issues and challenges related to smarter health is to be addressed including the quality of service during care, user engagements, data privacy and security, medical Big Data, and ethics of physician or/and system developer [48].

Whenever discussion between robots and objects going on, it is obvious to know the issues related to them: security, consensus theory, communication technology for short range, semantic based services and information centric networking are still open challenges. Finally, when more number of traffic in IoT driven environments added, the more requirements are difficult to be accomplished. It is noted down that The Netherlands becomes world's first nation having IoT based network with 1.5 million connections in July 2016.

6 Conclusions

I think that in the next coming years, there will be more advanced and cheaper technology in the field of healthcare and medical sector is available. This will be provides a solution to IoT based Robotics systems, which will be worked smoothly even in different functionality, environment and having more complexity. It means that robotics will play a vital role even in the fourth industrial revolutionary technology, namely Internet of Things (IoT). There are many organizations and researchers involve fulfilling IoT challenges, its adoption issues, infrastructure improvement and standardization; this is in progress and getting some good results worldwide in near future.

Acknowledgments The authors are very much thankful to Dr. Ali Zahrani, Chairman, Department of Electrical and Computer Engineering, Faculty of Engineering, University of Jeddah, Kingdom of Saudi Arabia for his moral support thought the journey.

References

1. World Health Organization (WHO): The world health report 2016, Geneva, Switzerland, pp. 8–9 (2016)
2. Butter, M., Rensma, A., van Boxsel, J., Kalisingh, S., Schoone, M., et al.: Robotics for healthcare—final report, p. 12. European Commission, DG Information Society, Brussels (2008)
3. Report of TNO Quality of Life. Robotics for healthcare (2008)
4. Report on Medical Robotic Systems Market to 2020—Industry Size, Growth Prospects. Grand View Research Inc., pp. 4–9 (2015)
5. Taylor, Russell H.: A perspective on medical robotics. IEEE Proc. **94**, 1652–1664 (2006)
6. Cleary, K.: Workshop Report: Technical requirements for image-guided spine procedures. Georgetown University Medical Center, Washington D.C., 113 pp. (1999)
7. Myklebust, J.B.: Robotics in healthcare: what the future holds in standards. In: 20th Annual AAMI/FDA International Conference on Medical Device Standards & Regulations, March 9–10, 2010, Reston, VA, USA (2010)
8. Butter, M., et. al.: Robotics for Healthcare, pp. 36–38 (2008)
9. Butter, M., et. al.: See also: Toyota Deutschland (Ed.) Toyota entwickelt Roboter fur Pflege-und Gesundheitswesen. 20 pp. (2011)
10. McNickle, M.: 10 Medical Robots that could change Healthcare, 11 pp. (2012)
11. McNickle, M.: 10 Medical Robots that could change Healthcare, 8 pp. (2012)
12. Scutti, S.: Medical robots are not just the future of healthcare, but part of the present, 2 pp. (2015)
13. Butter, M., et. al.: Robotics for Healthcare, 55 pp. (2008)
14. Pluta, W.: Cody wascht bettlagerige Patienten, Online (2010)
15. Steeves, R.: Robots invade your pharmacy, Online (2013)
16. McNickle, M.: 10 Medical Robots that could change Healthcare, 6 pp. (2012)
17. Cyberdyne Inc.: What's HAL. The world's first Cyborg Robot HAL, Online (2015)
18. Cyberdyne Inc.: HAL for Medical Use, Online (2015)
19. DPA (ed.): Roboter hilft Behinderten beim Arbeiten, Online (2012)
20. Steeves, R.: Robotic wheelchair can smoothly traverse even the bumpiest terrain, Online (2012)

21. Titan Medical Letters, pp. 1–8 (2016)
22. Wall, J., Chandra, V., Krummel, T.: Robotics in General Surgery, Medical Robotics. In Tech Publications, pp. 491–506 (2008)
23. Lee, G.M.: The Internet of Things—Concept and Problem Statement. Institute TELECOM, Online (2012)
24. Atzori, L., Iera, A., Morabito, G.: The Internet of Things—a survey. Comput. Netw. **54** (2010), 2787–2805 (2010)
25. Botterman, M.: Internet of Things: an early reality of the future Internet. In: Meeting at EU, Prague. Online (2009)
26. European Union Report. Internet of Things in 2020—a roadmap for the future, Online (2008)
27. ITU Internet Reports. The Internet of Things, November 2005
28. Advantech: The Internet of Things, The Future is Connected—Riding the wave of IoT growth, Technical White Paper. Online (2011)
29. Elliott, S., Hall, J., Smith, M., Wechalekar, P.: Connected robots, Atos ascent white papers, November 2012, pp. 4–10 (2012)
30. http://www.pachube.com
31. http://www.sensetele.com/teaser.htm
32. http://www.nimbits.com
33. http://www.thingspeak.com
34. Pang, Z., Chen, Q., Tian, J., Zheng, L., Dubrova, E.: Ecosystem analysis in the design of open platform-based in home healthcare terminals towards the Internet of Things. In: Proceeding of International Conference on Advanced Communication Technology, January 2013, pp 529–534 (2013)
35. Fan, Y.J., Yin, Y.H., Xu, L.D., Zeng, Y., Wu, F.: IoT based smart rehabilitations systems. IEEE Trans. Indus. Inform. **10**(2), 1568–1577 (2014)
36. Riazul Islam, S.M., et al.: The Internet of Things for Healthcare—A Comprehensive Survey, IEEE Access, The Journal for Rapid open access publishing, vol. 3, pp 678–708 (2015)
37. Hax, V.A., et al.: ROS as a middleware to Internet of Things. J. Appl. Comput. Res. **2**(2), 91–97 (2012)
38. Arkko, J., Devarapalli, V., Dupont, F.: Using IPSec to protect mobile IPv6 signaling between mobile nodes and home agents, Online (2005)
39. Kosmatos, E., Tselikas, N., Boucouvales, A.: Integrating RFIDs and Smart Objects into a unified Internet of Things Architecture. Adv. Internet Things **1**(1), 5–12 (2011)
40. Sachs, K., Petrov, L., Guerrero, P.: From Active Data Management to Event-Based Systems and More, pp. 242–259. Springer, Berlin (2010)
41. Marder-Eppstein, E., Berger, E., Foote, T., Gerkey, B., Konolige, K.: The office marathon: robust navigation in an indoor office environment. In: IEEE International Conference on Robotics and Automation (ICRA), Anchorage, 2010, pp. 300–307 (2010)
42. Achtelik, M., Weiss, S., Siewart, R.: Onboard IMU and monocular vision based control for MAVs in unknown in-and outdoor environments. In: IEEE International Conference on Robotics and Automation (ICRA), Shangay, 2011, pp. 3056–3063 (2011)
43. Quigley, M., Conley, K., et al.: ROS: An Open Source Robot Operating System. In: ICRA Workshop on Open Source Software, Kobe, Japan (2009)
44. Sundmaeker, H., Guillemin, P., Friess, P., Woelffle, S.: Vision and Challenges for Realizing the Internet of Things, p. 229. Publications Office of the European Union, Luxembourg (2010)
45. Vincent, H., Issamy, V., Georgantas, N., et al.: Choreos: scaling choreographies for the internet of future. In: Middleware '10, Bangalore, India, 10 pp. (2010)
46. Chui, M., Loffler, M., Roberts, R.: The Internet of Things. McKinsey Q. **2**, 2010 (2010)
47. Evans, D.: The Internet of Things: how the next evolution of the Internet is changing everything, April 2011 (2011)
48. Geissbuhler, A., et al.: ICOST. Springer Lecture Notes in Computer Science, vol. 9102, pp. 373–378 (2015)

Internet of Things Meets Mobile Health Systems in Smart Spaces: An Overview

D.G. Korzun

Abstract A mobile health (mHealth) system is responsible to support and provision of healthcare services using mobile communication devices, such as mobile phones and tablet computers. Although mHealth system development for Internet of Things (IoT) environments is still in the early stage, the existing research shows the essential potential impact on the healthcare service industry. This chapter overviews important IoT use cases in healthcare focusing on the proposed IoT solutions for smart services provided by an mHealth system. The study discusses recent experience on development of smart space based mHealth systems. IoT-aware opportunities and properties of healthcare services are considered, including our vision on service intelligence in the mHealth case. Smart spaces based methods are described for mHealth system development, including multi-agent architectures, semantics-oriented information sharing, and operation with multisource heterogeneous data.

Keywords Mobile healthcare · mHealth · Internet of Things · Smart space · Service-oriented information system · Service intelligence

1 Introduction

The traditional style of health monitoring and healthcare by visiting a hospital or clinic to meet a doctor is still the most popular, especially in developing countries. Although a medical information system (MIS) can provide effective digital service support, this form of medical operation is expensive. To make healthcare more effective, continuous health monitoring and use personal analysis of the critical health parameters can be established for the remote patients. This demand drives the development of new approach to healthcare called mobile health or mHealth [1–3].

D.G. Korzun (✉)
Department of Computer Science, Petrozavodsk State University, Lenin Ave., 33, Petrozavodsk, Republic of Karelia 185910, Russia
e-mail: dkorzun@cs.karelia.ru

C. Bhatt et al. (eds.), *Internet of Things and Big Data Technologies for Next Generation Healthcare*, Studies in Big Data 23,
DOI 10.1007/978-3-319-49736-5_6

An mHealth system is responsible to support and provision of healthcare services using mobile communication devices, such as smartphones and tablets [3, 4]. Mobile devices are primarily responsible for collecting various health parameters data, delivery of healthcare information to medical personnel and patients, online monitoring of patient vital signs, and direct provision of healthcare services. In fact, an mHealth system makes remote users virtually closer to healthcare backend services (located in an existing MIS), e.g., as if the user is located in the hospital.

Internet of Things (IoT) is making a rapid progress in the Internet by providing connectivity of "things" in the physical surroundings of our everyday life. Now IoT provides fusion of real (physical) and virtual (information) worlds, and the IoT concept evolves to service-oriented information interconnection and convergence [5, 6]. The emerging case of Internet of Things (IoT) environments is considered [7, 8]. An IoT environment is associated with a physical spatial-restricted place equipped with and consisting of a variety of devices. In addition to local networking, the environment has access to the global Internet with its diversity of services and resources. Evolving from the world of embedded electronic devices, an IoT environment includes many mobile participants; each acts as an autonomous decision-making entity [6, 9].

Smart spaces form a programming paradigm with software engineering methods for creating a wide class of ubiquitous computing environments. Nowadays smart spaces become more and more closely integrated with IoT [9, 10]. More precisely, a smart space enables information sharing in a given IoT environment, supporting construction of advanced digital services by the participants themselves. Such services are often referred as "smart", emphasizing the new level of service recognition (detection of user needs), construction (automated preprocessing of large data amounts), perception (derived information provision to the user for decision-making). This chapter focuses on the Smart-M3 platform as a promising open source solution for smart spaces based systems in IoT environments [10, 11]. The M3 architecture (multidevice, multivendor, multidomain) for smart spaces enables concept development of intelligent service-oriented applications based on information sharing by software agents that run on various devices and act as knowledge processors in the IoT environment.

Although mHealth systems development for IoT environments is still in the early stage, the existing research prototypes show the essential potential impact on the healthcare service industry [12]. This chapter overviews IoT use cases in healthcare focusing on proposed IoT solutions for smart services provided by an mHealth system. As summary of the recent experience on development of smart space based mHealth systems is presented. The IoT-aware opportunities and properties of healthcare services are systemized, including a vision on service intelligence in the mHealth case. Smart spaces based methods are described for mHealth system development, including multi-agent architectures, semantics-oriented information sharing, and operation with multisource data. The key contribution of this study is a concept model of the semantic layer that is responsible for connecting the mobile user and her/his surrounding equipment with healthcare backend services in the hospital facilities and powerful processing entities in the global Internet.

The rest of the chapter is organized as follows. Section 2 introduces the IoT concept for use in healthcare. Section 3 overviews several mHealth use cases that show how IoT can be used to create an effective and cheap way to construct healthcare services and to deliver them to remote users. Section 4 discusses our vision on the new generation of healthcare services when the traditional services are enhanced to support their adaptation, ubiquitous assistance, emergency treatment, personalization, proactive delivery, and some other properties. Section 5 reviews and systematizes existing smart spaces based solutions for mHealth systems. The focus is on a new semantic layer that connects the user (in a personalized manner) with healthcare services and powerful processing entities. Finally, Sect. 6 concludes the chapter.

2 IoT-Enabled mHealth

The IoT concept defines ubiquitous connectivity of a multitude of "things" in the physical surroundings of our everyday life [6]. Basically, the IoT technology provides a way (an infrastructure and supporting mechanisms) to uniquely identify and link objects from out physical surrounding to their virtual (information) representations in the global Internet. Some of these objects can represent medical equipment such as sensors in the user's personal and body area networks [12]. Actions on physical objects and their resources can be replaced by operations on the virtual reflections, leading to a new approach to development of healthcare services. This section introduces the IoT opportunities for developing mHealth applications, following works [2, 5, 13].

The classic style of healthcare is limited by the time and space barriers [3], and a patient always has to visit a doctor in hospital or clinic. Information and communication technologies (ICT) provide a powerful tool to break these barriers. Traditional healthcare systems provide backend services located in medical facility. Such a system is enhanced with information services consumed remotely by mobile patients and medical personnel. Consider the following existing application concepts for the use of ICT in healthcare and well-being services provision.

- *eHealth* (electronic health): healthcare is supported by digital services that are constructed using electronic processes and communication.
- *Telemedicine*: a form of eHealth to provide clinical healthcare at a distance, including physical and psychological diagnosis based on telemonitoring of patients functions.
- *mHealth* (mobile health): Personal mobile devices are used for continuous collecting, aggregating and analysis of patient-level health data. On the one hand, services provide healthcare information to medical personnel as well as to the patients. On the other hand, direct provision of healthcare services can be performed using mobile telemedicine.

- *Cybermedicine*: the Internet is used to deliver healthcare services, such as medical consultations, diagnosis, and prescriptions. Services allow patients online access to consultations and treatment with medical professional.

As in many other application domains, IoT can enable healthcare using fusion of real (physical) and virtual (information) worlds [14]. This fusion supports a new level of interconnection and convergence of service-oriented information coming from both worlds. Healthcare services are constructed within IoT environments. Such an environment is associated with a physical spatial-restricted place equipped with and consisting of a variety of devices. In addition to local networking, the environment has access to the global Internet with its diversity of services and resources, including traditional medical information systems.

Evolving from the world of embedded electronic devices, an IoT environment includes many mobile participants; each acts as an autonomous decision-making entity [1, 6]. Furthermore, an IoT environment can be non-fixed: the environment is formed ad hoc or occasionally (e.g., when some users appear) in a spatial area or the environment is mobile (e.g., around the user) to make a user-centric system accompanying the user [7].

The classes of advanced eHealth/Cybermedicine applications are summarized in Table 1, following survey work [15]. The IoT technology supports their realization

Table 1 Advanced eHealth/cybermedicine applications

Class of application	Healthcare function	IoT enabler objects
Health monitoring	Continuous monitoring of individual health/physiological parameters using wearable and implantable medical sensors (ECG, blood pressure, EMG, etc.)	Medical sensor network (MSN) around the user
Behavioral monitoring	Continuous monitoring of human behavior (watching TV, sleeping, location, etc.)	Personal mobile sensors of physical state (e.g., on smartphone) as well as surrounding environmental sensors
Emergency detection	Continuous monitoring of individual patient status, possibly in respect to defined health risks (hazards, falls, etc.)	Advanced personal mobile computers such as smartphones of patients and medical personnel
Assisted living	Creating a smart environment for supporting patients and elderly people during their daily activities	Embedded devices and consumer electronics
Therapy and rehabilitation	Supporting patients who require rehabilitation healthcare in their common everyday living settings	Mobile medical devices (wearable, implantable) as well as home-use medical equipment
Well-being	Assisting people for motivation of them to follow a healthier life style. Analyzing emotions and improving well-being based on neurological and psychological insights	Portable personal mobile computers such as smartphones and recommendation services in the internet
Smart hospital	Improving communication and responsiveness within a hospital between patients, medical personnel and other stakeholders	Industrial IoT devices for medical domain

using the ubiquitous connectivity (anywhere, anytime, any device) and the opportunity to involve into the computation not only traditional computers but also appropriate digital objects from physical and information worlds.

An mHealth system can be characterized with the following properties.

1. A personal mobile device such as smartphone is a local server of the personal part of the system [16].
2. Local devices of the patient are interconnected on the personal part to make local continuous data collection, analysis, and response [17, 18].
3. Remote healthcare resources from MIS are introduced using the Internet connectivity [8, 19] and appropriate decision-making [15, 20, 21].
4. Provided services are smart, i.e., they are constructed based on analysis of local and global information [4, 7].
5. The access to personal part is secured. In particular, biometric authentication is used [22] and cryptographic mechanisms are applied to prevent malicious adversary from gaining the control over local devices [18].
6. The transfer of private data between the personal part of patient and the entire healthcare system is secured [1, 23].

The focus of this chapter in on the service intelligence property, which is achieved primarily by the first four properties above. An interested reader can study mobile communication and security properties in works [6, 1, 18, 22, 23, 19] and references therein.

Since mobile IoT devices, including smartphones and wireless sensors, become covering the essential share in IoT-enabled healthcare services, the role of mHealth is growing in the general concept of eHealth and its evolution to cybermedicine. Many already proposed mHealth scenarios employ the known approach of personal mobile gateway [16]. A generic IoT-enabled architectural model for inclusion of a personal mHealth system into existing healthcare and medical information systems is shown in Fig. 1 (derived from our previous work [18]).

A personal m-Health system of the patient is organized over the sensor network. The personal system can access the existing healthcare system (backend services) using the patient's personal gateway attached to the global Internet. The healthcare system collects all data coming from many patients. In the other direction, the healthcare system provides its services (e.g., MIS services in hospital) to remote patients and medical personnel. This way, certain medical facilities are made open for remote participants, including remote patients (in their everyday life) and remote medical personnel (nearby the patient).

The sensing devices create a personal information space, which is local to the patient. This space covers data sensed by devices of Body Area Network (BAN) and Personal Area Network (PAN). BAN includes various medical wearable and implantable devices such as ECG or glucose sensors, insulin pumps, accelerometers, and RFID tags. PAN includes environmental sensors deployed around or mobile devices of the patient. For example, temperature and humidity

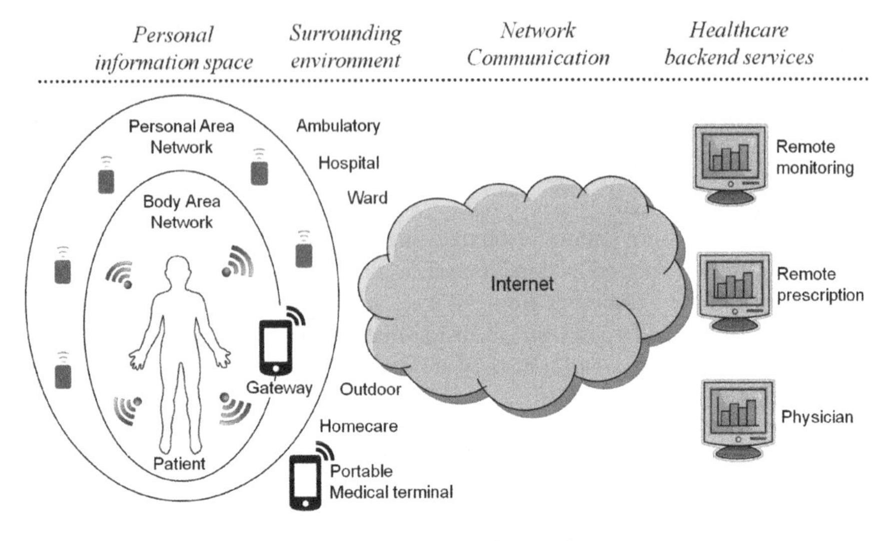

Fig. 1 Generic view on personal m-Health system of the patient

sensors, RFID readers, and smartphones. Such devices are rich sources of personal and environmental data, which can be effectively used in healthcare.

Each personal mHealth system has a gateway. The latter is responsible for communication with the outside world, i.e., using the global Internet. The gateway collects, aggregates, processes, and transfers information to the healthcare system with its existing healthcare services running on backend servers. They are physically located on the hospital side, in medical facility.

Although the gateway becomes a control point for decision-making, complex processing can be delegated to clouds or other Internet resources. Basically, healthcare backed services need input data from the patient and her/his surrounding physical environment. The input can be a result of preprocessing performed on the patient's side or somewhere else. Moreover, backend services can be composed with services in the Internet such that the patient receives a new service. For example, remote monitoring of patient's well-being can benefit on diet planning services.

A personal mHealth system also supports Portable Medical Terminal (PMT) for medical personnel on the patient side. This solution ensures dependability. In fact, PMT is similar to the gateway. The aim is to allow nearby medical personnel to directly access patient's mHealth system. If the system is in normal operation mode, then PMT communicates directly with the gateway. In abnormal situations (e.g., if the gateway is unavailable), PMT replaces the gateway and directly communicates with devices of the mHealth system. An example situation is when the patient cannot function due to emergency, and nearby medical personnel have to take control. Another example is when the gateway device is broken or lost.

In summary, the considered architectural model exploits the IoT support for creating various mobile information services that combine sensor data coming from the personal information space and processing power of local mobile devices and remote healthcare services. The patient's personal mobile device becomes a single window both to locally monitored data and to healthcare backend services. Importantly that new services can be constructed combining resources from these two sides: the local side of patient and the remote side of medical facility.

3 IoT Use Cases for mHealth

The considered architectural model of personal mHealth systems opens the opportunity for developing essentially advanced service scenarios in healthcare. Based on the recent research literature this section overviews several use cases that demonstrates IoT benefits for creating an effective and cheap way to construct mHealth systems and to deliver their information services to mobile users.

The overviewed use cases are summarized in Table 2. One of the primary IoT application goals is to improve the quality and content of human everyday life. This goal is achieved by automating some tasks and activity that humans need to perform [8]. This automation concerns mainly monitoring and decision making, and makes the key benefit of all the considered use cases. Note that the automation is not replace humans, as it happens in many traditional automation systems. Data collection, information production, and hidden facts discovery is subject to the automation. Human are still responsible for final decision making, based on the provided information.

Table 2 Example IoT use cases for mHealth

Use case	Mobility	Personalization
Ambient Assisted Living (AAL) for elderly people	Indoor mobility is supported at home environment equipped with consumer electronics	The assistance is for current situation which the patient gets in
First aid assistance for patients	Mobile users are patients with chronic deceases	Emergency situation detection is based on monitoring of individual health parameters and human behavior
Personalized healthcare assistance and advisory	Mobile users perform their daily activity	Recommendations are constructed based on individual health parameters and human behavior
Professional services for medical personnel	Doctors serve patients remotely	The personalization property of a doctor-to-patient serving is preserved despite of the spatial distance
Personal well-being applications	Mobile user is provided with recommendation on healthy and active way of life	The service fits personal user's interest in her/his recent situation anywhere and anytime

Ambient assisted living (AAL): the use case provides assistance for people at their home environment [14, 24], particularly to elderly people. Sensors are used as health monitoring equipment. The information collected by these sensors is made available to medical personnel in hospital, to family members, and to other interested parties. As a result, the services improve treatment and responsiveness for the monitored patients. Importantly that personal IoT devices can be used now to monitor a patient's current medicines. A possible option is the risk evaluation for new medications (e.g., allergic reactions). AAL primarily aims at extending the time that elderly people live independently in their home environment using information and communication technology to advance personal healthcare [5]. Aging is an important factor for new healthcare practice problems. In particular, the proportion of elderly people is growing fast, even faster than the total population.

The AAL use case can be extended to other parts of human population. In particular, active people are busy with their work duties and different social activities. This part of world population cannot spend time for regular monitoring of the health since it requires much individual resources from the person. Such people typically contact a doctor only when some extraordinary health problem has appeared. The case happens when the disease is on its middle or even further phase.

The AAL style reduces the cost of health monitoring and diagnostics. In many cases there is no need to visit a doctor in the hospital. Applying the IoT technology leads to a new generation of hospitals (e-hospitals or smart hospitals). The patients are equipped with a set of IoT-enabled devices for monitoring many health parameters and activity. As a result, the patients receives more detailed monitoring comparing with the traditional healthcare style in a hospital. More precise information is measured when the patient is at home since the home environment is more comfortable and closer to real-life. Indeed, in emergency situations, hospitalization is still mandatory, since treatment at home can be too risky or even impossible.

First aid assistance: the use case aims at detection and assistance in various emergency situations for mobile patients. A typical example is chronic cardiovascular deceases when emergency situations are rare but can happen during everyday activity [2, 13]. The sudden cardiac death is considered as a crucial public health problem. Much efforts are now directed to increase survival rates after cardiac arrest. In city areas, the ambulance response time may vary over a wide range. The first pre-doctor aid in an emergency situation can be provided even by some people nearby. First aid is a set of simple actions that any person can take regardless of education level or a special training. In many countries, people have the right to provide first aid even without medical training in case of trauma and emergencies directly at the place of the accident before arrival of medical personnel.

A patient is equipped with such medical devices as electrocardiograph sensors. Vital signs of the patient are continuously monitored. Preliminary analysis is made by the smartphone trying to detect the emergency symptoms as fast as possible. Whenever an emergency situation is detected the assistance service needs to notify all interested parties (physicians and doctors, ambulance staff, attracted people nearby), to make recommendation for the first aid (in the form of instructions), to help in transportation to the hospital (e.g., accompany support) as well as to support preparation in selected hospital before the arrival. Then the patient receives clinical treatment in the hospital. The goal is making the medical and other pertinent care as soon as possible, applying all situation-aware knowledge and resources.

A lot of research is now focused on various variants of personalized healthcare assistance, not only for emergency situations. In particular, work [25] introduced a smartphone sensor-based system. The system aims at facilitating the life of bipolar disorder patients. Also, support of their treatment is provided based on the smartphone as a primary control tool. The system covers different medical aspects of the human activity and behavior, providing an important information source to healthcare professionals. Another example of health parameters monitoring is mobile application CardiaCare [26]. The application runs on a smartphone communicating with a heart activity monitor used by the patient. The assistant service is pure local: arrhythmias detection for the heart function is performed directly on the smartphone.

4 Healthcare Service Intelligence

The term "smart service" is in the very widespread use today, including the mHealth application domain. IoT environment operates with multiple data sources from information world and physical world. In fact, the aim is make service construction solving a puzzle over such local and global information. This section discusses several properties of service intelligence for this type of service construction and delivery, focusing on the personalized mHealth systems in healthcare.

Modern data processing systems and particularly the Internet provide huge amounts of information, and the amounts continue to grow fast. The users cannot efficiently utilize these resources, which are often now considered as Big Data. An important research problem for these data is how to make their services intelligent and sensitive to users, e.g., see [15, 27]. The mobile users as patients need in context-aware and personalized services, which can be proactively identified, constructed, and delivered depending on the recent situation. The key challenge, which is observed now, is the high fragmentation in existing Internet services due to the lack of mechanisms for information exchange between services.

As a result, information produced by one service is not easily accessible and usable by other services [5]. The bridge is typically constructed manually by the user when she/he solves a problem using several existing services. The challenge is intelligent use of all available information appropriate for the situation. In this case, service provision chains become lengthy and, in addition to Internet resources, involve a multitude of heterogeneous devices, services, and users localized in the physical surrounding: various embedded and consumer electronics devices as well as personal equipment that accompanies human.

In the IoT concept, entities of the physical world are transformed into smart objects [6]. The term "smart" emphasizes individual intelligence attributes: each object acts autonomously, makes continuous sensing the environment, communicates with other nearby and faraway objects, applies available resources of the global Internet, and visually interacts with the end-users. A smart object can make own decisions when processing the data and communicating. As a result, IoT environment is formed by many heterogeneous digital objects. Importantly that computationally advanced personal mobile devices (e.g., smartphones) and various digital gadgets (including medical and well-being wireless devices) cover a very growing class of such smart IoT objects.

A computing environment is made smart or intelligent by its information services [28]. They acquire and apply knowledge about the whole environment as well as about its users. The goal is to achieve high user experience of service consumption. The term "smart" goes beyond the individual intelligence attributes. Cooperative activity of participating objects creates the intelligence and enables construction of advanced services in the environment. That is, many objects become data processing entities, trying to overcome the Big Data and service fragmentation challenges.

Therefore, many smart objects, which are individually smart, create a smart environment, which provides advanced services [9]. The users perceive the intelligence via these information services. Nevertheless, each smart object acts autonomously: it reasons about, controls, and adapts to conditions of the physical environment and observable user context. A typical cycle of this activity is the following: (i) perceiving the state of the current environment base on all available information, (ii) reasoning about this state to understand the role in service construction, and (iii) making actions in order to cover the part of service construction.

In the simplest case, a smart object constructs services based on own direct observations, i.e., acting as a provider of one or more services. More advanced case is when service construction is cooperative activity. Multiple smart objects process information about available resources of the environment and about semantics of ongoing processes. For instance, in healthcare the continuous mobile monitoring of recent correlation between different health parameters can provide valuable knowledge on the patient's current health status.

Both individual and cooperative activity of smart objects aims at automating many basic tasks that humans must perform in their daily activities. This kind of automation is different from classical automated systems where the intelligence power targets computational issues [7]. Let us introduce the following properties for the service intelligence, which have general value and can be considered beyond the architectural model of personal mHealth systems.

Knowledge adaptation: Information in the environment is regularly changed due to dynamics of the involved participants and their processes. This information and derived knowledge is accessible for service construction in such a way that allows service adaptation to the situation and user's status. For example, in health monitoring, the service can analyze online motional activity of the user and provide appropriate recommendations when the activity indicates a risk.

Situational context-awareness: Mobile users are rich sources of contextual data, including geolocation and status. An example is an emergency service when in emergency situations the patient becomes associated with mobile medical personnel that are nearby and have appropriate medical resources (e.g., qualification and equipment).

Service personalization: Each user has own personal information representation in the smart environment. The environment applies this knowledge in order to customize and personalize the service construction. For example, medicine and well-being recommendations should consider the known signs and instances of patient's allergy. Furthermore, the personal mobile device (smartphone) should be able for making own interpretation of the information. The service applies this interpretation for selecting the most appropriate visualization on the end-user side.

Proactive service delivery: The environment provides knowledge on the situations when a service is needed. This knowledge is explicitly represented and shared. The representation is detected to start construction of appropriate services. For example, a mobile user can be notified about nearby hospitals when the need to visit a doctor is detected.

In an IoT environment, the conventional input and output no longer exist in a fixed form. Instead, the sensors and processing devices are integrated into everyday equipment and personal gadgets to work together in cooperation. Services are constructed within this distributed cooperative activity. Many possibilities become available on each construction step, in contrast to traditional services with the fixed request–response scheme. This freedom enables the service intelligence: a smart service can flexibly sense, understand, and adapt to the user needs, as the properties above defined. In the architectural model of personal mHealth systems, the service intelligence supports enhancing health and social care provision in a way to complement existing healthcare backend services.

Let us discuss certain "intelligence attributes" to form a generic vision on a smart mHealth service. The most essential attributes are summarized in Table 3. As we will see in the subsequent section the attributes can be received based on the IoT technology and smart spaces methods.

Table 3 mHealth service intelligence attributes

Use case	Mobility
Service ubiquity	Services are available for their patients anywhere and anytime, independently on the location and situation
Multisource data	Services exploit multiple data sources, either medical or nonmedical, personal or collectively created
Context-awareness	Services apply contextual and situational information, which is sensed by many medical and physical sensors
Knowledge reasoning	Services derive new knowledge from big data corpuses, which can be online accesses, dynamically evolved, and fragmented
Service construction	A service is constructed for the current need to best fit the situation of the remote user. The simplest form of pure transfer of a healthcare backend service to a remote user is extended with available service discovery and their composition to the required service

The possibility to provide a "mobile" healthcare service, outside of hospital, is a clear result of the emerging IoT technology, including the use of wireless sensors and personal mobile devices [19]. Continuous monitoring and data processing on the side of patient is performed. Network interaction with backend healthcare services is established when needed. mHealth services become "ubiquitous" or, in other words, they persistently accompany and surround their patients.

mHealth services are not limited with such conventional medical information as electronic health records (EHR). The latter typically provide short and highly fragmented history. The IoT technology enables accessing and sharing various data sources. The information is made available to medical personnel and other interested parties, aiming at improving the healthcare quality. Some information can be non-medical, e.g., geolocation (of a patient) or community opinions (from social networks). These data naturally become sources of contextual and situational information, which can be shared and further used in service adaptability, self-learning, personalization, and proactive delivery.

When a lot of data appears then knowledge reasoning over these data collections becomes inevitable part of a smart service. Based on deduced knowledge, recommendations to assist a patient can be constructed. A special form is prediction, which is important for early detection of patient state changes. In particular, machine learning methods are used for examining the activities of daily living in terms of start time, duration and frequency. If changes in human behavior are detected, then situations that require further health evaluation can be identified.

5 Smart Spaces Based Methods for mHealth System Development

Smart spaces provide an approach to creating service-oriented information systems with high intelligence support in IoT environments. The approach provides methods for semantic information sharing in the IoT environment, operation over the collected information, and cooperative service construction by all participants themselves. This section shows application of the principal smart spaces methods to mHealth system development.

A smart space establishes an information-centric intelligent environment (e.g., on the top of IoT environment) for service construction and delivery. The participants act as service providers and consumers. They are represented by software agents. Available digital devices and systems can be used to run the agents, either surrounding or remote. To support cooperation the key idea is to collect and semantically relate the information coming from all available sources [7, 28]. The collection is in shared use by all participants. The semantic relation supports the intelligent use. The established environment has the layered structure shown in Fig. 2. Importantly that human users receive, consume, and experience information

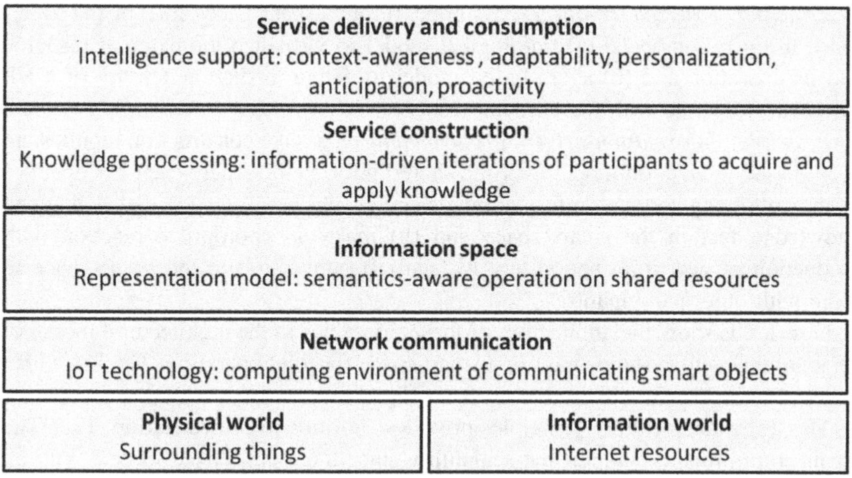

Service delivery and consumption
Intelligence support: context-awareness, adaptability, personalization, anticipation, proactivity

Service construction
Knowledge processing: information-driven iterations of participants to acquire and apply knowledge

Information space
Representation model: semantics-aware operation on shared resources

Network communication
IoT technology: computing environment of communicating smart objects

Physical world Surrounding things	**Information world** Internet resources

Fig. 2 Layers of a smart space deployed in IoT environment

services based on cooperative activity of participating objects in acquiring and applying common knowledge about the environment, its resources and users.

A promising software development platform for smart spaces is Smart-M3 [10, 11]. It provides an open source technology, which can be used in many application domains. Semantic information broker (SIB) is a central element of the platform architecture. An appropriate SIB is deployed running on a dedicated host machine of the IoT environment. To collect information content the SIB provides an RDF-based knowledge base, which implements an RDF triplestore with support for information search and processing extensions. The RDF representation leads to interoperable information sharing. Agents directly communicates with their SIB to access the content. In the simples case, read and write operations allows collecting and sharing the content (RDF triples are basic data unit). The subscription operation enables advance information-driven cooperation of agents when one agent can detect changes in the shared content. The Smart-M3 term "knowledge processor" (KP) makes distinguishing for this class of software agents from the general term from multi-agent systems and agent-based communication. That is, KPs target asynchronous collective knowledge generation and utilization via information sharing and semantic relations.

The smart space approach provides software engineering methods, which can be successfully applied for creating and deploying mHealth systems. In particular, personalized m-Health systems can be made by smart space participants, as it is discussed in proposals [4, 13, 14, 17, 21]. The smart spaces based methods follow the design principles listed below.

Principle: *Information hub*. An IoT environment has a knowledge base to create the smart space with ontological models to describe semantic representation of involved participants, service construction processes, and available resources.

Principle: External resources. External resources are accessible in the smart space using two models: (a) ontological model to virtualize the external resource and its operation and (b) agent-based model to define mediation activity of a KP assigned to operate with the external resource.

Principle: Information-driven programming. Service construction applies an agent-based interaction model over the shared information where each KP operates in the following loop of information detection and reaction: (a) detect a given knowledge fact in the smart space and (b) make an appropriate reaction with production of new information and its (partial) publication in the smart space to share with other participants.

Now let us show the application of these principles in the architectural model of personal mHealth systems that use a smart space for joint operation. The basic idea is depicted in Fig. 3, which evolves from Fig. 1.

The information hub principle provides information localization [7]. The localization property support the scalability since there is no need to deal with all available data in one giant storage. Data from the whole world are not duplicated in the smart space. Instead, they are represented as related locally problem-aware fragments from multiple sources. Regular data are typically too big, and they should be kept in appropriate external databases (e.g., on backend servers). Service construction is cooperative agent-based activity of several KPs. Instead of direct agent-to-agent communication, each KP accesses the shared semantic information hub. This indirect KPs interaction exploits the publish/subscribe coordination model to detect information changes in the shared content.

The semantics are kept in the smart space in the form of relations (e.g., named links) between information fragments. Ontology modeling provides a way to represent concepts of the application domain and their instances, thus forming

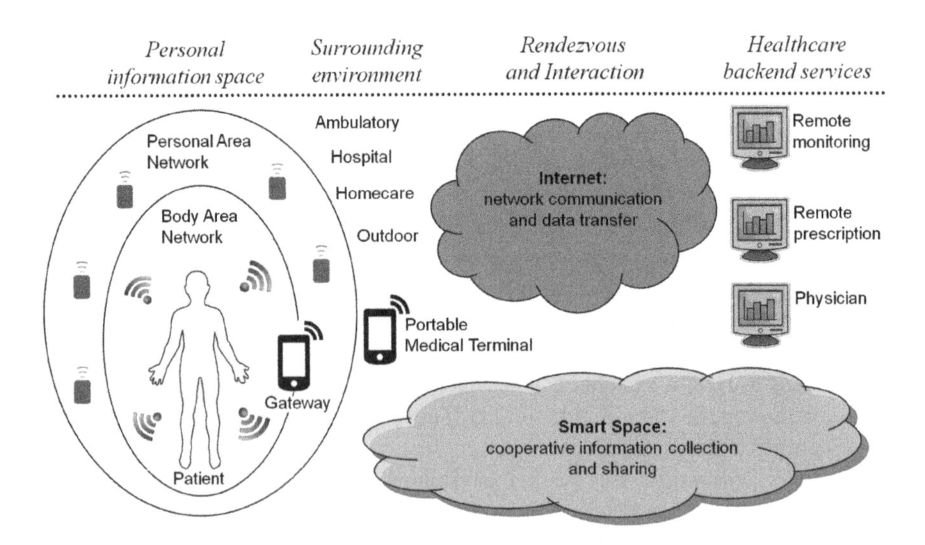

Fig. 3 Smart spaces based personal mHealth system

information fragments (objects) in the smart space. In mHealth scenarios, these objects are patients, medical personnel, medical supplies, recommendations, etc. Semantic relations suit well for representing such knowledge as a patient has pneumonia or as correspondence of medicines to concrete patients (e.g., taking personal allergy reaction into account).

Ontology provides an effective model to describe this kind of knowledge. In particular, the efficiency is shown for context modeling in IoT environments with a multitude of sensors generating big data [29]. In work [30], an ontological model is applied to support the management of chronically ill patients at home and in the personalized manner. The ontology describes general medical knowledge as well as medical knowledge about the patients. Work [31] considered senior homecare assistance to show the advantage of use of ontology in knowledge representation for integrating medical, social, and familiar resources.

The use of ontology for localized semantic representation of collected and shared knowledge in a smart space has the following important goal. The smart space should enable the integral healthcare of the mobile patient in her/his current environment (hospital or home, outdoor or in a building). The relevance of this way of ontology use in person-centric healthcare systems was demonstrated in [21]. The proposal is to link the following three information layers.

- User plane: local continuous health monitoring and feedback provision for the patient. The plane is for interactions by and with the patients.
- Medical plane: expertise assessment and decision-making. The operation is based on sensed medical and clinical data. Services support diagnosis, treatment (planning and execution), and recommendation (feedback) to the patient. The plane is for interactions by and with the doctors.
- Statistical plane: Summarized expertise work. The operation involves external knowledge management. The plane is for interactions with medical researchers.

The important activity of KPs is derivation of new knowledge [17, 21]. This property is achieved using the ontology model. It allows any KP to understand the semantics currently represented in the smart space. Based on this knowledge a KP rationally participates in service construction and delivery. Such a KP becomes able to recognize and react on various situations, for instance:

- a new patient joins the smart space,
- the need of an assistance service appears for a doctor,
- to make a recommendation an advanced information search in several medical information systems is needed,
- the recommendation is constructed and the information is ready for delivering to the end-user.

The external resources principle allows operation with many external data sources, thus semantically integrating them into a smart space. The IoT technology enables accessing and sharing various data sources. In particular, work [32] described an approach to database schema design for continuously monitored health parameters that form a highly diverse medical data collection with multidimensional and sparse structure.

The use of external resources also means construction of composed services [7]. Existing healthcare backend services are not straightforwardly delivered to the users using the IoT communication. These services can be enhanced by augmentation with other available data. In particular, it can be used for adaptation and personalization.

Following the information-driven principle, the coordination in a smart space is based on reacting on observations in the shared, semantically-linked, and cooperatively-generated information. The steps are as follows.

1. Read access to the smart space content: information is accessible by instant queries and subscriptions, including advanced search features.
2. Information-driven analysis: making own interpretations and decisions based on (a) shared information in the smart space and (b) private local knowledge on the KP side.
3. Cooperation activity: reaction of each KP is a part of service construction. KP actions addresses the environment as well as new content is published in the smart space.

Consequently, the smart spaces approach evolves the generic IoT vision on smart objects. They are not just augmented with basic functions such as sensing, actuation, processing, and networking. More importantly that each object acts autonomously. It can make its own decisions based on sensed environment, communications with other objects, access to Internet systems, and interactions with end-users. For mHealth systems this IoT potential has already indicated in [1, 33].

The discussed smart spaces based approach makes many opportunities for advancing services of mHealth systems. First, the smart space makes semantic-oriented integration of data from one or more patients. This information is enhanced with semantic links to other informational pieces and external sources. The representation of this information and its interpretation is based on ontology. Second, healthcare service construction is personalized, oriented to a concrete person. This smart space support allows proactive service delivery, which is uttermost important in healthcare applications with detection of personal needs for the service provision to the patient.

6 Conclusions

This chapter overviewed the IoT concept and its possible use cases for mHealth. Our study shows how IoT can be used to create an effective and cheap way to construct healthcare services and to deliver them to remote users. Our vision on the new generation of healthcare services is discussed: the traditional services are enhanced to support their adaptation, ubiquitous assistance, emergency treatment, personalization, proactive delivery, and some other properties. The smart spaces approach is applied to mHealth system development for IoT environments and systematized existing smart spaces principles. The key contribution is the concept model of a semantic layer that connects the user (in a personalized manner) and her/his surrounding equipment with healthcare backend services and powerful processing entities in the global Internet.

Acknowledgments This work is financially supported by the Ministry of Education and Science of Russia within project # 14.574.21.0060 (RFMEFI57414X0060) of Federal Target Program "Research and development on priority directions of scientific-technological complex of Russia for 2014–2020".

References

1. Jara, A.J., Zamora-Izquierdo, M.A., Skarmeta, A.F.: Interconnection framework for mHealth and remote monitoring based on the internet of things. IEEE J. Sel. Areas Commun. **31**(9), 47–65 (2013)
2. Korzun, D., Borodin, A., Paramonov, I., Vasyliev, A., Balandin, S.: Smart spaces enabled mobile healthcare services in internet of things environments. Int. J. Embed. Real-Time Commun. Syst. (IJERTCS) **6**(1), 1–27 (2015)
3. Tachakra, S., Wang, X., Istepanian, R.S., Song, Y.: Mobile e-health: the unwired evolution of telemedicine. Telemed. J. e-Health **9**(3), 247–257 (2003)
4. Korzun, D., Nikolaevskiy, I., Gurtov, A.: Service intelligence support for medical sensor networks in personalized mobile health systems. In: Proceedings of the 8th conference on Internet of Things and Smart Spaces (ruSMART 2015). LNCS 9247, pp. 116–127, Springer International Publishing (2015)
5. Balandina, E., Balandin, S.I., Koucheryavy, Y.A., Mouromtsev, D.: IoT use cases in healthcare and tourism. In: Proceedings of the 17th IEEE Conference on Business Informatics (CBI 2015), vol. 2, pp. 37–44 (2015)
6. Kortuem, G., Kawsar, F., Sundramoorthy, V., Fitton, D.: Smart objects as building blocks for the internet of things. IEEE Int. Comput. **14**(1), 44–51 (2010)
7. Korzun, D.: On the smart spaces approach to semantic-driven design of service-oriented information systems. In: Proceedings of the 12th Int'l Baltic Conference on Databases and Information Systems (DB&IS 2016), pp. 181–195. Springer International Publishing (2016)
8. Whitmore, A., Agarwal, A., Xu, L.: The internet of things—a survey of topics and trends. Inform. Syst. Front. **17**(2), 261–274 (2015)
9. Korzun, D., Balandin, S., Gurtov, A.: Deployment of smart spaces in internet of things: overview of the design challenges. In: Proceedings of the 13th Int'l Conference Next Generation Wired/Wireless Networking (NEW2AN 2013) and 6th Conference Internet of Things and Smart Spaces (ruSMART 2013). LNCS 8121, pp. 48–59, Springer International Publishing (2013)
10. Korzun, D., Kashevnik, A., Balandin, S., Smirnov, A.: The Smart-M3 platform: experience of smart space application development for internet of things. In: Proceedings of the 15th Int'l Conf. Next Generation Wired/Wireless Networking and 8th Conference on Internet of Things and Smart Spaces (NEW2AN/ruSMART 2015). LNCS 9247, pp. 56–67, Springer International Publishing (2015)
11. Honkola, J., Laine, H., Brown, R., Tyrkkö, O.: Smart-M3 information sharing platform. In: Proceedings of the IEEE Symposium on Computers and Communications (ISCC'10), pp. 1041–1046. IEEE Computer Society (2010)

12. Islam, S.M.R., Kwak, D., Kabir, M.H., Hossain, M., Kwak, K.S.: The internet of things for health care: a comprehensive survey. IEEE Access **3**, 678–708 (2015)
13. Korzun, D., Borodin, A., Timofeev, I., Paramonov, I., Balandin, S.: Digital assistance services for emergency situations in personalized mobile healthcare: smart space based approach. In: Proceedings of the SIBIRCON-2015. pp. 62–67. IEEE (2015)
14. Korzun, D., Nikolaevskiy, I., Gurtov, A.: Service intelligence and communication security for ambient assisted living. Int. J. Embed. Real-Time Commun. Syst. (IJERTCS) **6**(1), 76–99 (2015)
15. Acampora, G., Cook, D.J., Rashidi, P., Vasilakos, A.V.: A survey on ambient intelligence in healthcare. Proc. IEEE **101**, 2470–2494 (2013)
16. Silva, B.M.C., et al.: Mobile-health: a review of current state in 2015. J. Biomed. Inform. **56**, 265–272 (2015)
17. Borodin, A., Zavyalova, Y., Zaharov, A., Yamushev, I.: Architectural approach to the multisource health monitoring application design. In: Proceeding of the 17th Conference of Open Innovations Association FRUCT, pp. 36–43 (2015)
18. Nikolaevskiy, I., Korzun, D., Gurtov, A.: Security for medical sensor networks in mobile health systems. In: IEEE 15th Int'l Symposium on A World of Wireless, Mobile and Multimedia Networks (WoWMoM), pp. 1–6. IEEE (2014)
19. Pal, A.K., Dey, N., Samanta, S., Das, A., Chaudhuri, S.S.: A hybrid reversible watermarking technique for color biomedical images. In: IEEE Int'l Conference on Computational Intelligence and Computing Research (ICCIC), pp. 1–6 (2013)
20. Demirkan, H.: A smart healthcare systems framework. IT Prof. **15**(5), 38–45 (2013)
21. Vergari, F., Cinotti, T.S., D'Elia, A., Roffia, L., Zamagni, G., Lamberti, C.: An integrated framework to achieve interoperability in person-centric health management. Int. J. Telemed. Appl. (2011)
22. Nandi, S., Roy, S., Dansana, J., Ben, W., Karaa, A., Ray, R., Chowdhury, S.R., Chakraborty, S., Dey, N.: Cellular automata based encrypted ECG-hash code generation: an application in inter human biometric authentication system. Int. J. Comp. Netw. Inform. Secur. **6**(11), 1–12 (2014)
23. Bose, S., Madhulika, A.S., Chowdhury, S.R., Chakraborty, S., Dey, N.: Effect of watermarking in vector quantization based image compression. In: Int'l Conference on Control, Instrumentation, Communication and Computational Technologies (ICCICCT), pp. 503–508 (2014)
24. Memon, M., Wagner, S.R., Pedersen, C.F., Beevi, F.H.A., Hansen, F.O.: Ambient assisted living healthcare frameworks, platforms, standards, and quality attributes. Sensors **14**(3), 4312–4341 (2014)
25. Grunerbl, A., Muaremi, A., Osmani, V., Bahle, G., Ohler, S., Troster, G., Mayora, O., Haring, C., Lukowicz, P.: Smartphone-based recognition of states and state changes in bipolar disorder patients. IEEE J. Biomed. Health Inform. **19**(1), 140–148 (2015)
26. Borodin, A., Pogorelov, A., Zavyalova, Y.: The cross-platform application for arrhythmia detection. In: Proceedings of the 12th Conference of Open Innovations Association FRUCT and Seminar on e-Tourism, pp. 26–30 (2012)
27. Evers, C., Kniewel, R., Geihs, K., Schmidt, L.: The user in the loop: enabling user participation for self-adaptive applications. Future Gener. Comput. Syst. **34**, 110–123 (2014)
28. Augusto, J., Callaghan, V., Cook, D., Kameas, A., Satoh, I.: Intelligent environments: a manifesto. Hum.-Centric Comput. Inf. Sci. **3**, 12 (2013)
29. Perera, C., Zaslavsky, A., Christen, P., Georgakopoulos, D.: Context aware computing for the internet of things: A survey. IEEE Commun. Surv. Tutorials, **16**, 411–454 (IEEE) (2014)
30. Riano, D., Real, F., Lopez-Vallverdu, J.A., Campana, F., Ercolani, S., Mecocci, P., Annicchiarico, R., Caltagirone, C.: An ontology-based personalization of health-care knowledge to support clinical decisions for chronically ill patients. J. Biomed. Inform. **45** (3), 429–446 (2012)
31. Valls, A., Gibert, K., Sánchez, D., Batet, M.: Using ontologies for structuring organizational knowledge in home care assistance. Int. J. Med. Inform. **79**(5), 370–387 (2010)

32. Borodin, A., Zavyalova, Y.: On an EAV based approach to designing of medical data model for mobile healthcare service. In: Proceedings of the 9th Int'l Conference on Mobile Ubiquitous Computing, Systems, Services and Technologies (UBICOMM 2015), pp. 20–23. IARIA XPS Press (2015)
33. Nee, O., Hein, A., Gorath, T., Hulsmann, N., Laleci, G.B., Yuksel, M., Olduz, M., Tasyurt, I., Orhan, U., Dogac, A., Fruntelata, A., Ghiorghe, S., Ludwig, R.: SAPHIRE: intelligent healthcare monitoring based on semantic interoperability platform: pilot applications. IET Commun. **2**(2), 192–201 (2008)

Part II
Big Data in Healthcare

Big Data Knowledge System in Healthcare

Gunasekaran Manogaran, Chandu Thota, Daphne Lopez, V. Vijayakumar, Kaja M. Abbas and Revathi Sundarsekar

Abstract The health care systems are rapidly adopting large amounts of data, driven by record keeping, compliance and regulatory requirements, and patient care. The advances in healthcare system will rapidly enlarge the size of the health records that are accessible electronically. Concurrently, fast progress has been made in clinical analytics. For example, new techniques for analyzing large size of data and gleaning new business insights from that analysis is part of what is known as big data. Big data also hold the promise of supporting a wide range of medical and healthcare functions, including among others disease surveillance, clinical decision support and population health management. Hence, effective big data based knowledge management system is needed for monitoring of patients and identify the clinical decisions to the doctor. The chapter proposes a big data based knowledge management system to develop the clinical decisions. The proposed knowledge system is developed based on variety of databases such as Electronic Health Record (EHR), Medical Imaging Data, Unstructured Clinical Notes and Genetic Data. The proposed methodology asynchronously communicates with different data sources and produces many alternative decisions to the doctor.

G. Manogaran (✉) · D. Lopez
VIT University, School of Information Technology and Engineering,
Vellore, Tamil Nadu, India
e-mail: gunavit@gmail.com

C. Thota
Albert Einstein Lab, Infosys Ltd, Hyderabad, India

V. Vijayakumar
VIT University, School of Computing Science and Engineering, Chennai,
Tamil Nadu, India

K.M. Abbas
Department of Population Health Sciences, Virginia Tech, Blacksburg, USA

R. Sundarsekar
Priyadarshini Engineering College, Vellore, Tamil Nadu, India

C. Bhatt et al. (eds.), *Internet of Things and Big Data Technologies for Next Generation Healthcare*, Studies in Big Data 23,
DOI 10.1007/978-3-319-49736-5_7

Keywords Big data · Knowledge system · Health care system · Electronic Health Record (EHR) · Medical Imaging Data · Unstructured Clinical Notes · Genetic Data

1 Introduction

"Big Data" initially meant the volume, velocity and variety of data that becomes tricky to analyze by using conventional data processing platforms and techniques [1]. Nowadays, data production sources are improved rapidly, such as telescopes, sensor networks, high throughput instruments, streaming machines and these environments generate massive amount of data. Nowadays, big data has been playing a crucial role in a variety of environments such as healthcare, business organization, industry, scientific research, natural resource management, social networking and public administration. Big data can be categorized by 10V's as follows (Fig. 1). *Volume*: The big volume indeed represents Big Data. Recently, the data generation sources are augmented and it causes diversity of data such as text, video, audio and large size images. In order to process the enormous amount of data, our conventional data processing platforms and techniques has to be enhanced [2]. *Velocity*: The rate of the incoming data has increased dramatically this velocity indeed represents Big Data. The phrase velocity represents the data generation speed. The data explosion of the social media has changed and causes variety in data. Nowadays, people are not concerned in old post (a tweet, status updates etc.) and notice to most hot updates [2]. *Variety*: The variety of the data indeed represents Big Data. Nowadays, the collection of data types is also increased. For example, most organizations use the following type of data formats such as database, excel, CSV, which can be stored in a plain text file. Nevertheless, sometimes the data may not be in the anticipated format and it causes difficulties to process. In order to defeat this issue the organization has to be identified the data storage system which can analyze variety of data [2]. *Value*: The value of data indeed represents Big Data. Having continuous amounts of data is not helpful until it can be turned into value. It is essential to understand that does not always mean there is value in Big Data. The benefits and costs of analyzing and collecting the big data is more impartment thing when doing big data analytics. *Veracity*: This veracity of data indeed represents Big Data. Veracity represents the data understandability; it doesn't represent data quality. It is significant that the association should perform data processing to prevent 'dirty data' from accumulating in the systems. *Validity*: It is essential to ensure whether the data is precise and accurate for the future use. In order to take the right decisions in future the organizations should valid the data noticeably. *Variability*: Variablity refers to the data consistent and data value. *Viscosity*: Viscosity is an element of Velocity and it represents the latency or lag time in data transmit between the source and destination. *Virality*: Virality represents the speed of the data send and receives from various sources. *Visualization*: Visualization is used symbolize the Big Data in a complete view and determine the

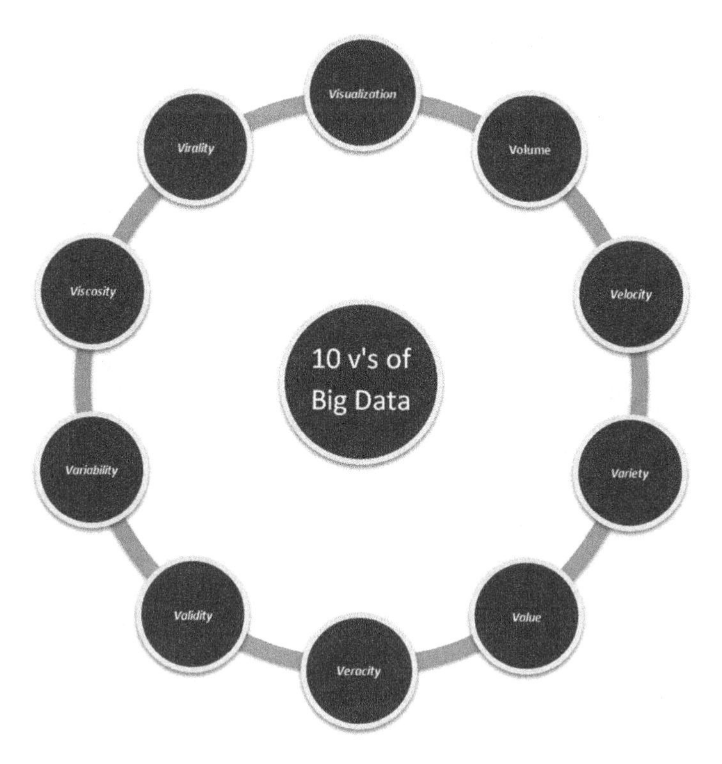

Fig. 1 10V's of Big Data

hidden values. Visualization is an essential key to making big data an integral part of decision making.

Big Data also impact more in healthcare. Nowadays, health care systems are rapidly adopting clinical data, which will rapidly enlarge the size of the health records that are accessible, electronically [3, 4]. A recent study expounds, six use cases of big data to decrease the cost of patients, triage and readmissions [5]. In yet another study, big data use cases in healthcare have been divided into number of categories such as clinical decision support, administration and delivery, user behavior, and maintain services. Jee et al. described that how to reform the healthcare system based on big data analytics to choose appropriate treatment path, improvement of healthcare systems, and so on [6]. The above use cases have utilized the following big data in health care implementation. (1) Patient-centered framework produced based on the big data framework to approximate the amount of healthcare (cost), patient impact (outcomes), and dropping re-admission rates [7]. (2) Virtual physiological human analysis combined with big data analytics to create robust and valuable solutions in silico medicine [8].

Table 1 Comparison of various databases for Big Data

Name	Spark SQL	HBase	Hive
Description	Spark SQL is a component on top of 'Spark Core' for structured data processing	Apache HBase is a scalable and distributed database is used to store the data on top of the HDFS	Apache Hive is a SQL interface and relational model for querying, analyzing and summarizing large size of datasets stored in HDFS
Database model	Relational DBMS	Wide column store	RDBMS
Technical documentation	spark.apache.org/-docs/-latest/-sql-programming-guide.html	hbase.apache.org	cwiki.apache.org/-confluence/-display/-Hive/Home
Developer	Apache software foundation	Apache software foundation	Apache software foundation
Initial release	2014	2008	2012
Current release	v2.0.0, July 2016	1.2.2, July 2016	2.0.0, February 2016
MapReduce	N/A	Yes	Yes
Database as a Service (DBaaS)	No	No	No
Implementation language	Scala, Java, Python, R	Java	Java
Supported programming languages	Java, Python, R, Scala	C, C#, C++, Groovy, Java, PHP, Python, Scala	C++, Java, PHP, Python
Data scheme	Yes	Schema-free	Yes
Typing	Yes	No	Yes
XML support	No	No	N/A
Secondary indexes	No	No	Yes
SQL	No	No	No
APIs and other access methods	JDBC, ODBC	Java API RESTful HTTP API Thrift	JDBC, ODBC, Thrift
Server-side scripts	No	Yes	Yes
Triggers	No	Yes	No
Transaction concepts, concurrency	No	No	No
Concurrency and durability	Yes	Yes	Yes
In-memory capabilities	No	No	N/A

Table 2 Comparison of various platforms for Big Data

Name	MapReduce	Strom	Spark streaming
Description	Hadoop MapReduce is a type of programming model used for processing huge size of data sets across a Hadoop cluster	Storm on YARN is powerful for scenarios requiring real-time analytics, machine learning and continuous monitoring of operations	Apache Spark follows in-memory database so that it can generate one hundred times quicker output for user queries on stream of data
Website	https://hadoop.apache.org/docs/r1.2.1/mapred_tutorial.html	strom.apache.org	spark.apache.org/streaming/
Developer	Apache software foundation	Apache software foundation	Apache software foundation
Execution model	Batch	Streaming	Batch, streaming
Supported language	Java	Any language	Java, Python, R, Scala
Associated ML tools	Mahout	SAMOA	MLlib, Mahout, H2O
In-memory capabilities	No	Yes	Yes
Low latency	No	Yes	Yes
Fault tolerance	Yes	Yes	Yes
Enterprise support	No	No	Yes

2 Overview of Big Data Tools and Technologies

This section describes various tools and technologies for big data. The comparison of various databases and various platforms for big data are depicted in Tables 1 and 2 respectively.

2.1 Hadoop Architecture

Apache Hadoop consists of master/slave architecture that uses namenode and datanode to process the huge data. The namenode performs as the master and datanodes act as slaves. The namenode manages the access of all datanodes. The main accountability of datanodes is to administrate and store the huge data across multiple nodes. User configures the number of block replication in Hadoop architecture (Fig. 2).

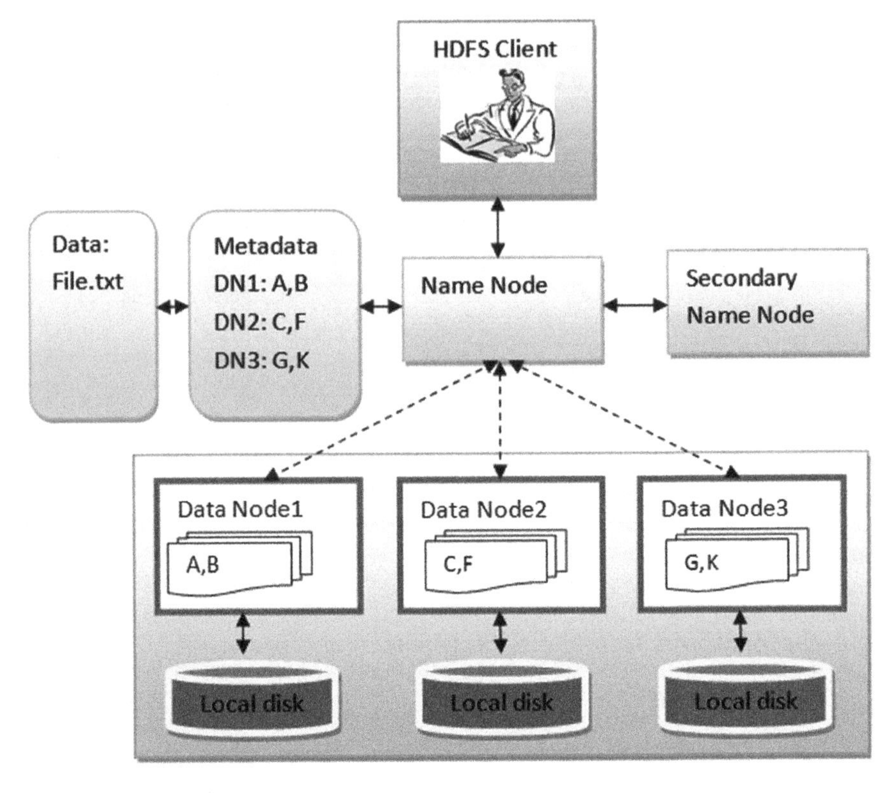

Fig. 2 HDFS architecture

2.2 Hadoop Components

Hadoop Distributed File System (HDFS): The HDFS is initially intended to process on cluster of nodes. HDFS stores data in distributed manner and used for many applications those have large data. The typical HDFS architecture is depicted in Fig. 1.

HDFS architecture does the following tasks:

- Distributed File System (DFS) always makes getting new data as simple as adding a new file to the folder, which contains the master dataset
- Distributed file system distributes the huge size of data across a cluster of commodity hardware. As more number of computers is added, the storage space and I/O throughput increase
- Distributed file system uses MapReduce framework to process the huge data in parallel manner
- Distributed file system restricts the users to delete or modify files in the master dataset folder. This feature protects the master data against human mistakes or bugs.

Namenodes: The namenode is always serves as the master server and it does the following tasks:

- Controls the file system namespace
- Periodically stores information about the metadata of the data blocks
- Data blocks' location is stored on the data node
- Name also perform following functions such as opening files and directories, renaming and closing, Once the namenode of the system crashes, then the entire Hadoop system goes down.

Datanode: In general, every node in the Hadoop cluster maintains at least one datanode. These nodes focus on managing the data storage of their system and are accountable of the following tasks:

- Performs write/read functions on the Hadoop file systems based on the client's request
- According to the instructions of the namenode it perform operations such as block creation, deletion, and replication
- Periodically send the blocks information to the namenode.

Secondary Namenode: This node is used to make a copy of name node. In other words, this makes a secondary copy of namenode.

JobTracker: This node used to track all the data nodes. It includes scheduling, monitoring of all task.

TaskTracker: TaskTracker is always runs on the datanodes of the hadoop cluster to run map task and reduce task. This node does the following tasks:

- Performs write/read functions on the Hadoop file systems based on the client's request
- According to the instructions of the namenode it perform operations such as block creation, deletion, and replication
- Periodically send the blocks information to the namenode.

2.3 Hadoop MapReduce

Hadoop MapReduce is a type of programming model used for processing huge size of data sets across a Hadoop cluster. Hadoop framework also provides the scheduling, distribution, and parallelization services to process the big data. Hadoop MapReduce programming consists of following features:

- MapReduce programming languages C++, Java or Python can be chosen by programmers developers
- MapReduce programming model is an ability to process petabytes of data, stored in Hadoop cluster

- MapReduce Parallel processing is an ability to process the huge size of data in minutes
- MapReduce manages node failure on its own, hence, if any one machine fails, an additional machine is take care of the node failure
- MapReduce model is also used to increase the processing speed and reduce the network I/O patterns.

2.4 Apache Sqoop

Apache Sqoop can extract data from Hadoop Distributed File System (HDFS) and export it into external structured data stores (relational databases). Apache Sqoop consists of the following functions to incorporate bulk data transfer between Hadoop and relational databases:

- Performs transformation of huge data between Hadoop Distributed File System and relational databases
- It consists of improved compression and light-weight indexing technique for efficient query performance
- Used to transfer data from EDWs and external storage into Hadoop file system for cost-effectiveness of combined data processing and storage
- Faster performance and better resource utilization
- Transferring huge data from external storage into Hadoop system
- Schema-on-read data lake is used in the Sqoop to merge structured data with unstructured data, so that effectiveness of the data analysis is enhanced
- Provide excessive storage to other systems and load processing.

2.5 Apache Flume

Apache Flume is used for transferring batch files, log files and high-volume streaming data into HDFS for storage. Flume consists of the following functions:

- Enables stream data from numerous sources into Hadoop system for analysis and storage
- It follows channel-based transactions to assure reliable data delivery. For example, when a message is transferred from one machine to another, two transactions are happening concurrently, one is represented on the destination side and the other one is on the source side
- It follows horizontal scaling to consume most recent data streams and additional storage.

2.6 *Apache Pig*

Apache Pig maintains the generation of batch views. This query approach consists of numerous functions together in a single pipeline; so it decreases the number of data scanning. Apache Pig also supports the traditional data functions like joins, filters, ordering, etc. and nested data types like tuples, maps, and bags on structured, semi-structured, or unstructured data. In general, Apache Pig often used while joining new incremental data with the previous data results.

2.7 *Apache Hive*

Apache Hive is a SQL interface and relational model for querying, analyzing and summarizing large size of datasets stored in HDFS. HiveQL is a type of query language for hive, which converts normal SQL-like queries into MapReduce jobs executed on Hadoop Distributed File System (HDFS).

2.8 *Cloudera Impala*

Cloudera Impala is used to provide fast response to the user queries, instead of long batch jobs previously related to SQL-on-Hadoop methodologies. Impala has incorporation with Apache Hive metastore database so that user can distribute the databases and tables between both components.

2.9 *Apache Mahout*

Apache Mahout is used to provide more accurate result for the user queries. In general, machine learning is an artificial intelligence that allows computers to learn based on data alone; it provides better performance as more data is analyzed. It provides several scalable data mining techniques such as clustering, classification, filtering, dimensionality reduction, pattern mining and so on.

2.10 *Apache Hadoop Yarn*

Apache Hadoop Yarn is used to distribute the big data analytics jobs by Map Reduce and HDFS. YARN consists of following features for Hadoop framework such as security, resource management and data governance tools. As its architectural center, YARN improves Hadoop compute cluster in the following ways:

- It provides open-source or proprietary tools to use Hadoop system for real time and batch processing
- Apache YARN follows dynamic allocation of system resources that increases resource utilization compared to static MapReduce model rules used in previous Hadoop versions
- Apache YARN is capable handling petabytes of data across hundreds of nodes in the Hadoop cluster
- Apache YARN also process existing MapReduce applications without any disruption.

2.11 Apache Parquest

Apache Parquest supports master data management when user needs columnar storage. In addition, Apache Parquest doesn't store the complete data into the memory; as an alternative it stores those data which are actually required, thus dropping the required space in the memory as well as raising the speed.

2.12 Apache Spark Streaming

Apache Spark is fundamentally works based on cluster computing framework. Unlike Hadoop's MapReduce paradigm, Apache Spark follows in-memory database so that it can generate one hundred times quicker output for user queries on stream of data. Spark streaming has been provided as a part of Spark, which finds its application in real-time for example to monitor, control the access of end users on a website and fraud detection in real time.

2.13 Apache HBase

Apache HBase is a scalable and distributed database is used to store the data on top of the HDFS. It has been identified after the Google's BigTable was developed and can store millions of rows and columns. In view of the fact that HBase maintains Master/Slave architecture, it is extremely accessible to all nodes in the cluster.

3 Proposed Big Data Knowledge System in Healthcare

3.1 Role of Knowledge System in Healthcare

Knowledge is the combination of information, data, and experience. It is developed based on the trainings, analysis and various work experience. This knowledge is used to develop decisions at emergency situations and complex problems. Nowadays, knowledge developed from various experience are often used in critical healthcare problems and disease diagnosis. In addition, clinical management, surgical environment and drug recommendation are also used knowledge system to get desired output. In addition, more knowledge is developed from past issues and mistakes. In general, knowledge is classified into two type's namely tacit and explicit knowledge based on the generation sources. Explicit knowledge is easy to collect, format, and distribute with various persons. Hospital and medical procedures and disease diagnosis are considered as some of the example for explicit knowledge [9]. Alternatively, tacit knowledge is developed based on the individuals' experience [10]. Because of the difficulty, subjectivity, and objectivity, tacit knowledge is very complex to collect, format, and distribute to other individuals.

3.2 Types of Knowledge in Healthcare

Knowledge can be further classified in the three types [11].

Provider Knowledge: Medical experts have both tacit and explicit knowledge. In general, every doctor is required to identify typical medical diagnosis or details from various available sources. Years of experience in medical diagnosis is used to take better decisions.

Patient Knowledge: Tacit knowledge is developed from the patients and it is considered "health status". Generally speaking, practitioners and doctors may not know about the current and past medical conditions of the patients.

Organizational Knowledge: Organizational Knowledge is also a vital role in patient treatments and diagnoses for preventative maintenance and illnesses. Most medical organizations have other familiar resources that are available for doctors and patients to contact. Organizational Knowledge is developed from text-based materials, medical diagnostic systems, and other sources.

3.3 Sources of Big Data in Healthcare

The most familiar big data sources in medical environments include Electronic Health Record (EHR), Medical Imaging Data, Unstructured Clinical Notes and Genetic Data.

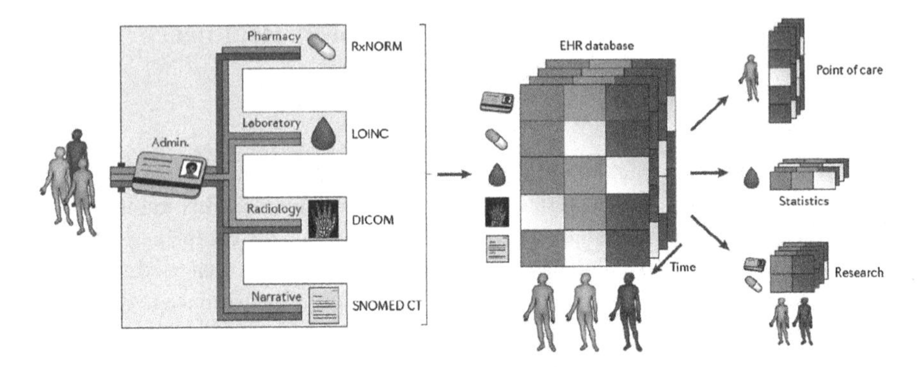

Fig. 3 Various types of Electronic Health Records (EHRs)

Electronic Health Records (EHRs): The following information is generally available in all EHRs are: laboratory results, billing data, medication records, and test details [12]. In most of the cases laboratory results and billing data are in the structured "name-value pair" data. Recently, more number of researchers is trying to develop big data based electronic phenotype algorithms to identify diseases from the EHR. Figure 3 represents the various types of Electronic Health Records (EHRs) [13].

(a) *Billing data*: Billing data are uses various codes to document the patients' symptoms, clinical records and lab results. International Classification of Diseases (ICD) and Current Procedural Terminology (CPT) are often used to document the billing data. This codes and data derived from ICD is most often used for research purposes. Summary of the ICD and CPT are depicted in Tables 3 and 4 respectively.
(b) *Laboratory data*: Laboratory data and vital signs are mostly in the structured format. It follows coding scheme to store the huge amount of lab related data.

Table 3 Summary of ICD

	ICD
Ease of use	• High
Format	• Structured
Advantages	• Simple to work and good prediction
Disadvantages	• Disease codes frequently used for all cases • Less accuracy

Table 4 Summary of CPT

	CPT
Ease of use	• High
Format	• Structured
Advantages	• Easy to work and high precision
Disadvantages	• Data is not accurate

Table 5 Summary of laboratory data

	Laboratory data
Ease of use	• High
Format	• Mostly structured
Advantages	• Data validity is high
Disadvantages	• May require to calculate cumulative dissimilar variations

Nowadays, many dictionaries and various algorithms are developed to reduce the complexity if laboratory data [9–11]. Summary of laboratory data are depicted in Table 5.

(c) *Medication records*: Medication records are used to identify accurate phenotype characterization. In addition, medication records also used to improve the disease diagnosis and drug recommendation in healthcare industry. This record is also used to avoid unwanted lab test and clinical care for individuals who are not actually affected by the disease. In addition, medical records are also used to identify the significance and importance of various drugs for number of diseases. Nowadays, format and variety of the medication records are increasing noticeably, it would helps to identify the number of hospital stays and reduce fault diagnosis rate [14]. Summary of medication records are depicted in Table 6.

Table 6 Summary of medication records

	Medication records
Ease of use	• Medium
Format	• Structured and unstructured
Advantages	• High data validity
Disadvantages	• Need to develop communication platform between inpatient and outpatient data
Summary	• Useful for disease diagnosis and clinical care

Table 7 Summary of clinical notes

	Clinical notes
Ease of use	• Medium
Format	• Unstructured
Advantages	• More details about doctors' judgment
Disadvantages	• Difficult to process without human intervention • Precision is fully depends on processing method • Cut, copy and paste are often affect the quality of the data
Summary	• Clinical documents are often used to identify common and well known diseases

Unstructured Clinical Note: Clinical documentation is often in the form of unstructured and it is widely used to improve the disease diagnosis [15]. Clinical notes are also considered as big data and scalable algorithms are used to process such huge size of data. For example, natural language processing and text search algorithms are widely used to process such huge size of clinical notes. Normally, clinical notes are created with the help of dictated and transcribed or computer-based documentation (CBD) systems. Summary of the clinical notes are depicted in Table 7.

Medical Imaging Data: Medical images are most often used for diagnosis, planning and therapy assessment [16, 17]. Recently, imaging techniques are increased such as Computed Tomography (CT), X-ray, molecular imaging, Magnetic Resonance Imaging (MRI), ultrasound, photoacoustic imaging, fluoroscopy and mammography. Nowadays, size of the medical videos and CT scans are also increased rapidly [18, 19, 20]. Such data requires huge storage space and fast algorithms to process and disease diagnosis [21, 22]. Medical imaging consists of different image acquisition methodologies generally utilized for various clinical applications. For example, visualizing blood vessel structure can be done using CT, MRI, photoacoustic imaging, and ultrasound. The main challenge with the image data is that it is not only large size, but also complex and multi dimensional [15].

Documentation from Reports and Tests: Nowadays, the cost to sequence the human genome (encompassing 30,000–35,000 genes) is quickly decreasing with the improvement of high-throughput sequencing tools and methods. Nowadays, it is difficult to process huge size of genome data and compute results. This would require advance scalable algorithms to process such huge size of clinical records. In order to overcome this issue, researchers are developed P4 medicine paradigm (i.e. predictive, preventive, participatory, and personalized health) with omics outline [15].

(d) *Wearable Sensor Devices*: Nowadays, more wearable medical devices are developed for patients' continuous health monitoring [23, 24]. These devices generate huge amount of health data continually. The typical communication among wearable things is depicted in Fig. 4. More familiar used wearable sensors and it functionalities is depicted in the Table 8. Security requirements and solutions in wearable medical devices are depicted in Table 9.

4 Big Data Genomics and Its Requirements

4.1 Acquisition for Big Genomics Data

The huge growth in genomic data is creates an opportunities decrease the overall prices, increase throughput and accuracy. The advancement in big data analytics is used in genomes sequencing to progress the accuracy and decrease the time taken

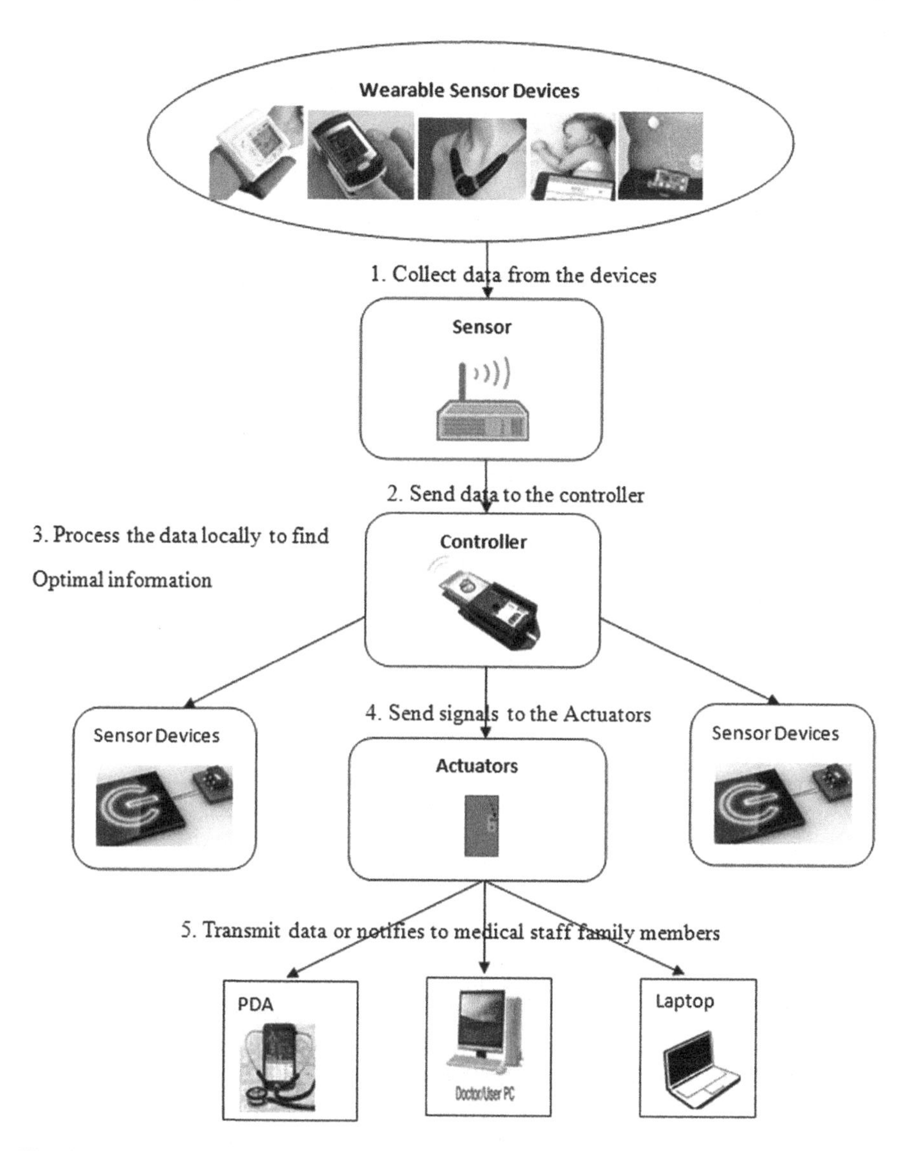

Fig. 4 Communication among wearable things in healthcare

for rapid diagnosis. Huge big genomics data provides high value insights and meaningful results for better prediction in healthcare.

Table 8 Sensors in human body

SNO	Name of the sensor	Sensor use	Sensor placement
1	Accelerometer	Measuring the human energy expenditure	Wearable
2	CO_2	Measuring the carbon dioxide level from mixed gas	Wearable
3	Electrocardiogram sensor	Measuring the electrocardiograph signal	Wearable
4	Accelerometer	Measuring the angular velocity with respect to the body axis	Wearable
5	Moisture sensor	Measuring the sweating rate	Wearable
6	Blood monitoring sensor	Measuring the percentage of oxygen saturation in blood	Wearable
7	Stress sensor	Measuring the pressure changes of the underside of foot	Wearable/ surrounding
8	Breath monitoring sensor	Measuring the rate of breathing	Wearable
9	Heat sensor	Measuring the rate of body temperature	Wearable
10	Image sensor	Capturing the motion, length, location, and area	Wearable/ surrounding
11	Blood pressure monitoring sensor	Measuring the systolic and diastolic pressure	Wearable
12	Heart rate monitoring sensor	Measuring the heart rate	Wearable
13	Blood sugar monitoring sensor	Sensors record glucose levels continuously around the clock	Wearable

4.2 *Storage for Big Genomics Data*

In healthcare industry there is a need to develop the storage system for large size of genomics data. Recently, 3-D memory and scalable methodologies are invented to increase the scalability and computing features of genomes and omics data. The above mention technologies are five time faster than the traditional optical switching technologies. Nowadays, compression and indexing systems are rapidly increased to store big genomes and omics data. For example, scalable MapReduce based algorithmic technologies are used to compare one genome to many others in an efficient way. In addition, many of the researchers are developing streaming methods to make on-the-fly comparisons for genome sequencing applications.

Table 9 Various security requirements and solutions in components of wearable healthcare system

Components in the wearable healthcare system	Vulnerabilities	Types of threats and attacks	Available security requirements and solutions
Physical objects	• Physical layer devices have limited communication, calculation and storage resources • Physical objects are distributed in various regions. Hence, unauthorized user can accesses the devices and performs damages and illegal actions such as reprogram the device, extract security keys and information.	• DoS/DDoS attacks • Physical attacks • Integrating WSNs • Integrating RFID • Unauthorized access control and data access	• Encryption/Cryptographic techniques • Continuously evaluates the suspicious nodes' behaviour can reduce the influence of malicious user access • Authentication • Authorization • Access control • Identification
Communication technologies	• IoT is a dynamic network infrastructure • Power issues • Network issues • Selection of security technique and its challenges	• Wireless WAN communications • Wireless LAN/PAN communications • Secure IoT communication protocols in constrained resources environment • Secure transmitted data	• Encryption/decryption is used to provide confidentiality service • Strong authentication also used to provide security solutions • Backup solution is used when network fails • Authorized access and availability

(continued)

Table 9 (continued)

Components in the wearable healthcare system	Vulnerabilities	Types of threats and attacks	Available security requirements and solutions
Applications	• Data coverage • Cloud computing • Security issues in web application • Secure communication	• DoS • XSS attack • CSRF attack • SQL injection • Data protection • Data access • PHRs attacks • Malicious user attacks • Sharing data in different environments • Real-time information processing • Sharing the same sensed data by several applications	• Encryption/decryption mechanisms • Secure data access • Scheduling techniques • Assuring identification • Assuring authentication • Firewall and antivirus • Intrusion detection

4.3 *Distribution for Big Genomics Data*

Cloud computing technologies are most often used for distributing genome sequences at a population scale. These technologies reduce the data movement and increases code federation. For example, Google, Amazon, and Facebook uses distributed computing framework to store large amount of data in distributed manner. Nowadays, cloud computing technologies are used for large scale genomic data querying and sequencing. For example, TCGA and BGI-cloud are uses cloud computing based platforms to store huge genomes and omics data in distributed manner. Though, efficient storage and processing methodologies are available to process such huge amount of genome data. There is a need to provide authentication, encryption, and other security frameworks to make certain that genomic data remain private.

4.4 *Analysis for Big Genomics Data*

The vital role of genome sequencing is to measure and observe the changes of DNA mutations and find the other molecular measurements relate to various diseases. In order to achieve the above task, there is a need to develop the scalable computing methodologies for processing such huge amount of genomics data. R, Mahout, and Hadoop machine learning algorithms are most often used to process such huge size of genome data.

5 Big Data in Descriptive Epidemiology

The Global Burden of Disease, Injuries and Risk Factors (GBD) study exemplifies an ongoing project on big data in descriptive epidemiology. The GBD studies generate estimates and trends of epidemiological metrics—morbidity, mortality and risk factor rates by age, sex, cause, year and geography [25]. A suite of analytical and statistical methods are used in the estimation process, and Disability Adjusted-Life Year (DALY) is used as an objective comparative metric for 310 diseases and injuries, and 79 behavioral and risk factors for 188 countries from 1990 to 2015. DALYs combine the morbidity metric of Years of Life lost due to Disability (YLD) and mortality metric of Years of Life Lost due to premature mortality (YLL); that is, DALY = YLD + YLL.

The GBD studies are led by the Institute of Health Metrics and Evaluation [26], in collaboration with more than 1700 collaborators from 125 countries. Dynamic data visualizations enable user-specific analysis and derive new insights [27], and data is publicly accessible through the Global Health Data Exchange [28]. Figure 5

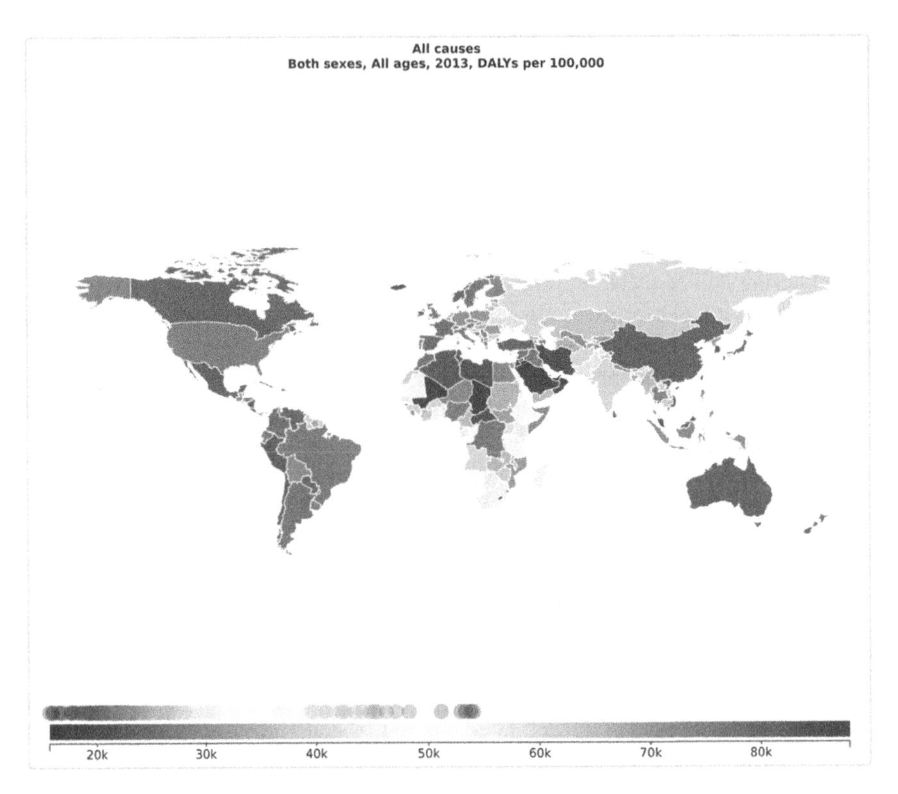

Fig. 5 Global burden of disease in 2013. Global burden of disease (DALYs per 100,000 people) due to all causes for both sexes and all ages in 2013

illustrates the global burden of disease due to all causes for both sexes and all ages in 2013, expressed through the metric of DALYs per 100,000 people.

The GBD studies follow the Guidelines for Accurate and Transparent Health Estimates Reporting (GATHER), which is a checklist and standard of 18 best practices for health estimates to improve transparency, accuracy and reliability [29, 30]. The GBD studies compile data from multiple health databases and epidemiological studies across different countries, and analyze over a billion data points. The GBD analytic method enables regular updates with data from new epidemiological studies. Policymakers of different countries, including China, India, Mexico, United Kingdom, and other countries are adopting the GBD approach to measure and analyze the population health of their respective countries.

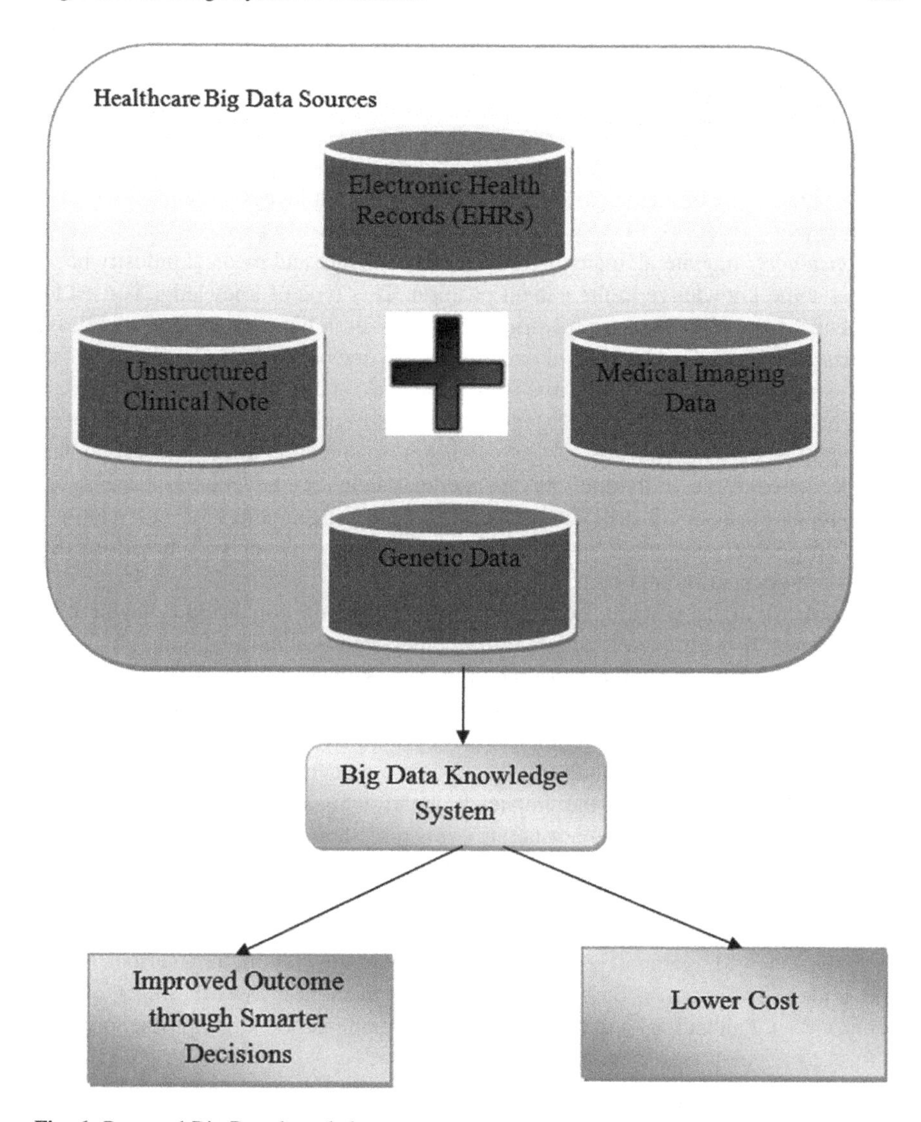

Fig. 6 Proposed Big Data knowledge system

6 Functionalities of Proposed Knowledge System

Big Data base knowledge system is shown in the Fig. 6. It consists of variety of databases such as EHR, Medical Imaging Data, Unstructured Clinical Notes and Genetic Data.

6.1 Identifying Different Decisions Using Levels of Healthcare System

The Healthcare Leadership Alliance (HLA) organized the healthcare system into four general levels or themes of analysis: consumers, employees, organizations, and environment [31].

Consumers: In general, many organizers in healthcare and medical industry have at least some knowledge in the patient position. This type of knowledge is used to enable the manager with a helpful structure of indication but also generate sightless. In general, users frequently tend to over generalize one patient's experience to those of others and in the procedure miss individual differences. In order to develop an efficient knowledge system the organization should understand the patient's need.

Employees: The employees of the healthcare organization are considered as the well knowledgeable individuals in the medical industry; nevertheless, the environment of proficient instruction creates for composite tapestry of interrelationships. In general, the goals, income and organizational power vary based on the healthcare occupation and spot.

Organization: In general, healthcare services directly connected with the end users. Hence, it is completely different from other organizations and industries. This creates "receiving it right the first time" for various business organizations; due to this reason the healthcare organization is one of the most regulated of all the organizations in the globe. In general, it is very important to understand the systems context for professionals joining into healthcare organization from other trade. For example, individuals from the financial departments are normally adapted to working under significant authoritarian oversight; though, those individuals feel difficult to face with various work forces. In addition, Individuals from production environments are familiar with skill set for increasing the operational efficiency, but they may not expertise in developing a healthy product.

Environment: In general, healthcare organizations are classified by various levels and trades. The changes in the economy and awareness toward fitness of the country would affect the healthcare delivery. More interaction among these forces is helpful to develop better knowledge in healthcare.

6.2 Developing Knowledge in the Healthcare System

Developing knowledge in the healthcare system consists of following ways [31]:

Knowledge Development in Consumers:

- Conduct interview with patient families
- Contribute in meetings and/or society outreach procedures and programs.

Knowledge Development in Employees:

- Monitoring the healthcare providers activities
- Participate staff meetings from other professions/departments
- Study applicable professional information and publications sources.

Knowledge Development in Organization:

- Increase mentoring relationships with head of the departments (e.g., finance/billing, legal affairs, community affairs, public health department)
- Contribute in community relations events and groups.

Knowledge Development in Environment:

- Study the healthcare division of business and common interest periodicals
- Examine relevant scholarly and employment journals (e.g., Health Affairs, Healthcare Executive)
- Participate seminars and workshops provided by special interest groups
- Volunteer in community activities.

7 Limitations and Future Work

This chapter discusses only about Electronic Health Record (EHR), Medical Imaging Data, Unstructured Clinical Notes and Genetic Data. The other sources of big data in healthcare are not discussed. The future work of this chapter is to combine the various other sources of big data in healthcare such as social media, web searches and mobile devices and developing the knowledge system.

8 Conclusion

Nowadays, health care systems are rapidly adopting clinical data, which will rapidly enlarge the size of the health records that are accessible, electronically. This chapter studies the characteristics and challenges for big data in healthcare, and proposes a big data based knowledge system. The proposed knowledge system is developed based on variety of databases such as EHR, Medical Imaging Data, Unstructured Clinical Notes and Genetic Data.

References

1. Manogaran, G., Thota, C., Kumar, M.: MetaCloudDataStorage architecture for Big Data security in cloud computing. Procedia Comput. Sci. **87**, 128–133 (2016)
2. Victor, N., Lopez, D., Abawajy, J.: Privacy models for big data: a survey. Int. J. Big Data Intell. **3**, 61 (2016)

3. Lopez, D., Sekaran, G.: Climate change and disease dynamics—a Big Data perspective. Int. J. Infect. Dis. **45**, 23–24 (2016)
4. Lopez, D., Gunasekaran, M., Murugan, B.S., Kaur, H., Abbas, K.M.: Spatial Big Data analytics of influenza epidemic in Vellore, India. In: IEEE International Conference on Big Data, pp. 19–24, Oct 2014
5. Bates, D., Saria, S., Ohno-Machado, L., Shah, A., Escobar, G.: Big Data in health care: using analytics to identify and manage high-risk and high-cost patients. Health Aff. **33**, 1123–1131 (2014)
6. Jee Kim, G.: Potentiality of Big Data in the medical sector: focus on how to reshape the healthcare system. Healthc. Inform. Res. **19**, 79 (2013)
7. Chawla, N., Davis, D.: Bringing Big Data to personalized healthcare: a patient-centered framework. J Gen. Intern. Med. **28**, 660–665 (2013)
8. Viceconti, M., Hunter, P., Hose, R.: Big Data, big knowledge: Big Data for personalized healthcare. IEEE J. Biomed. Health Inform. **19**, 1209–1215 (2015)
9. Lopez, D., Gunasekaran, M.: Assessment of vaccination strategies using fuzzy multicriteria decision making. In: Proceedings of the Fifth International Conference on Fuzzy and Neuro Computing (FANCCO-2015), pp. 195–208. Springer International (2015)
10. Kothari, A., Hovanec, N., Hastie, R., Sibbald, S.: Lessons from the business sector for successful knowledge management in health care: a systematic review. BMC Health Serv. Res. **11**, 173 (2011)
11. Chen, E.T.: An observation of healthcare knowledge management. Commun. IIMA **13**, 95–106 (2013)
12. Denny, J.: Chapter 13: mining electronic health records in the genomics era. PLoS Comput. Biol. **8**, e1002823 (2012)
13. Jensen, P., Jensen, L., Brunak, S.: Mining electronic health records: towards better research applications and clinical care. Nat. Rev. Genet. **13**, 395–405 (2012)
14. Poon, E., Keohane, C., Yoon, C., et al.: Effect of bar-code technology on the safety of medication administration. Obstet. Gynecol. Surv. **65**, 629–630 (2010)
15. Belle, A., Thiagarajan, R., Soroushmehr, S.M., Navidi, F., Beard, D.A., Najarian, K.: Big data analytics in healthcare. BioMed. Res. Int. **10**, 1–16 (2015)
16. Virmani, J., Dey, N., Kumar, V.: PCA-PNN and PCA-SVM based CAD systems for breast density classification. In: Applications of Intelligent Optimization in Biology and Medicine, pp. 159–180. Springer International Publishing (2016)
17. Bhattacherjee, A., Roy, S., Paul, S., Roy, P., Kausar, N., Dey, N.: Classification approach for breast cancer detection using back propagation neural network: a study. In: Biomedical Image Analysis and Mining Techniques for Improved Health Outcomes, p. 210 (2015)
18. Suri, J., Dey, N., Bose, S., Das, A., Chaudhuri, S.S., Saba, L., Shafique, S., Nicolaides, A.: 2084743 Diagnostic preservation of atherosclerotic ultrasound video for stroke telemedicine in watermarking framework. Ultrasound Med. Biol. **41**(4), S133 (2015)
19. Dey, N., Mukhopadhyay, S., Das, A., Chaudhuri, S.S.: Analysis of P-QRS-T components modified by blind watermarking technique within the electrocardiogram signal for authentication in wireless telecardiology using DWT. Int. J. Image, Graph. Sign. Process. **4**(7), 33 (2012)
20. Acharjee, S., Ray, R., Chakraborty, S., Nath, S., Dey, N.: Watermarking in motion vector for security enhancement of medical videos. In: IEEE International Conference on Control, Instrumentation, Communication and Computational Technologies (ICCICCT), pp. 532–537, July 2014
21. Bose, S., Acharjee, S., Chowdhury, S.R., Chakraborty, S., Dey, N.: Effect of watermarking in vector quantization based image compression. In: IEEE International Conference on Control, Instrumentation, Communication and Computational Technologies (ICCICCT), pp. 503–508, July 2014
22. Pal, A.K., Dey, N., Samanta, S., Das, A., Chaudhuri, S.S.: A hybrid reversible watermarking technique for color biomedical images. In: IEEE International Conference on Computational Intelligence and Computing Research (ICCIC), pp. 1–6, Dec 2013

23. Nandi, S., Roy, S., Dansana, J., Karaa, W.B.A., Ray, R., Chowdhury, S.R., Chakraborty, S., Dey, N.: Cellular automata based encrypted ECG-hash Code generation: an application in inter human biometric authentication system. Int. J. Comput. Netw. Inf. Secur. **6**(11), 1 (2014)
24. Biswas, S., Roy, A.B., Ghosh, K. and Dey, N.: A biometric authentication based secured ATM Banking System. Int. J. Adv. Res. Comput. Sci. Softw. Eng. ISSN, 2277
25. Murray, C.J., Barber, R.M., Foreman, K.J., Ozgoren, A.A., Abd-Allah, F., Abera, S.F., Aboyans, V., Abraham, J.P., Abubakar, I., Abu-Raddad, L.J., Abu-Rmeileh, N.M.: Global, regional, and national disability-adjusted life years (DALYs) for 306 diseases and injuries and healthy life expectancy (HALE) for 188 countries, 1990–2013: quantifying the epidemiological transition. The Lancet **386**(10009), 2145–2191 (2015)
26. Healthdata.org: Global Burden of Disease (GBD)| Institute for Health Metrics and Evaluation. http://www.healthdata.org/gbd (2016). Accessed 8 Aug 2016
27. Healthdata.org: GBD Data Visualizations| Institute for Health Metrics and Evaluation. http://www.healthdata.org/gbd/data-visualizations (2016) Accessed 8 Aug 2016
28. Healthdata.org.: Global Health Data Exchange (GHDx)| Institute for Health Metrics and Evaluation. http://www.healthdata.org/about/ghdx (2016) Accessed 8 Aug 2016
29. Stevens, G., Alkema, L., Black, R., Boerma, J., Collins, G., Ezzati, M., Grove, J., Hogan, D., Hogan, M., Horton, R., Lawn, J., Marušić, A., Mathers, C., Murray, C., Rudan, I., Salomon, J., Simpson, P., Vos, T., Welch, V.: Guidelines for accurate and transparent health estimates reporting: the GATHER statement. PLoS Med. **13**(6), e1002056 (2016)
30. Stevens, G., Alkema, L., Black, R., Boerma, J., Collins, G., Ezzati, M., Grove, J., Hogan, D., Hogan, M., Horton, R., Lawn, J., Marušić, A., Mathers, C., Murray, C., Rudan, I., Salomon, J., Simpson, P., Vos, T., Welch, V.: Guidelines for accurate and transparent health estimates reporting: the GATHER statement. The Lancet (2016)
31. Garman, A.N., Tran, L.: Knowledge of the healthcare environment. J. Healthc. Manag. **51**, 152–155 (2006)

Big-Data Analytics, Machine Learning Algorithms and Scalable/Parallel/Distributed Algorithms

Anindita Desarkar and Ajanta Das

Abstract Smart data analysis has become a challenging task in today's environment where disparate data set is generated across the globe with enormous volume. So there is an absolute need of parallel and distributed framework along with appropriate algorithms which can handle these challenges. Various machine learning algorithms can be deployed effectively in this environment as they can work with minimal manual intervention. The objective of this chapter is first to present various issues faced in storing and processing big data and available tools, technologies and algorithms to deal with those problems along with one case study which describes an application in healthcare analytics. In the subsequent section it discusses few distributed algorithms which are widely used in the data mining domain. Finally it focuses on various machine learning algorithms and their roles in the big data analytics world.

Keywords Big data analytics · Machine learning · Distributed algorithms · Parallel algorithms

1 Introduction

Big data analytics is the methodology of processing and finding hidden patterns, unknown correlations, market trends and other useful business information from large volume of data sets consisting of heterogeneous data types, coming from various sources across the globe. Based on this analytical findings, more business

A. Desarkar · A. Das (✉)
Department of Computer Science & Engineering, Birla Institute of Technology, Mesra, Ranchi, 1582 Rajdanga Main Road, 4th Floor, Kolkata Campus, Kolkata 700107, India
e-mail: ajantadas@bitmesra.ac.in

A. Desarkar
e-mail: aninditadesarkar@gmail.com

C. Bhatt et al. (eds.), *Internet of Things and Big Data Technologies for Next Generation Healthcare*, Studies in Big Data 23,
DOI 10.1007/978-3-319-49736-5_8

growth can be achieved within a short period of time. Basic analytical methods and reporting tools which are working on calculating sums, counts, averages, execution of SQL queries depending on human intervention for the performed activities. This type of human dependency is a great challenge in the domain of big data where velocity, variety and volume are major concerns.

On the other hand, Internet of Things (IoT) which will be the next technological revolution is basically the other side of the coin where big data resides in one side. Basically IoT is the concept where every object or devices should have built in sensors to capture data across a network. So managing this huge amount of data, heterogeneous in nature is a huge challenge facing by all organizations. A proper analytics platform or framework is highly required for this data management and taking actions on it. These actions include event co-relation, metric calculation, and statistics preparation along with analytics and can vary depending on scenario.

Machine Learning comes into the picture which is perfect for exploiting the hidden knowledge within this large volume of distinct dataset with little reliance on human direction. It learns based on available data inputs and/or outputs, basically data driven and runs at machine scale, capable of handling huge variety of variables as well as data complexity which is quite essential in today's big data world. Machine learning consists various data analysis disciplines, starting from predictive analytics and data mining to pattern recognition and various algorithms are used for these purposes.

Big data analytics gained the momentum over traditional business intelligence program for its unique capability to deploy ideas into solutions, adapt with the changed environment along with its flexible nature. As a result, newer class of technologies that includes Hadoop and related tools such as YARN, MapReduce, Spark, Hive and Pig as well as NoSQL databases have been introduced. The current trend is using Hadoop as distributed data management system which has a flexible data storage mechanism for storing heterogeneous voluminous data coming across various sources. MapReduce is used as a parallel programming model in Hadoop for large scale data processing using commodity clusters.

Centralised healthcare monitoring and clinical analysis for caregiver or medical practitioner becoming a challengning issue. Healthcare monitoring system is based on lots of wearable body sensors, convenient handheld devices and broadband wireless services [1]. Electronic health records (EHR) includes various signal processing and time series data. So these different types of sources generate huge data, which turns into big data. Thus big data machine learning approaches need to be applied to provide clinical care. In this arena high performance computing or parallel/distributed algorithms ensures efficient storage and data retrieval for heterogeneous medical images or data [2].

The primary goal of this chapter is to discuss various machine learning algorithms along with their implementation roadmap in the analytics domain. As a first step, it discusses various challenges faced to handle big data and the mitigation techniques to overcome the same which includes common tools and technologies available in the market. It also includes various existing applications along with a proposed one in the healthcare domain which describes the importance of analytics in our day to day life. There are various data mining algorithms which are basically machine learning algorithms, briefly described in the next section. The next section presents various types of machine learning methodologies includes supervised learning, unsupervised learning and reinforcement learning and few algorithms under each bucket. It also gives the brief description of the application where these algorithms are implemented successfully.

The structure of the chapter is organized as follows. Section 2 presents various challenges in big data Analytics and their mitigation techniques by applying various tools and technologies along with various applications in the healthcare domain which uses analytics for providing an effective and efficient solution. A case study on Healthcare Analytics is also included in this section. Detailed description of different Parallel/distributed algorithms and their role in big data analytics are described in Sect. 3. Section 4 focuses on various machine learning algorithms and their application in analytics domain. Section 5 concludes the chapter.

2 Big Data Analytics: Challenges and Mitigation Techniques

Big data is large amount of data, may be structured, semi-structured or unstructured in nature, generated from various sources across the globe. One major source is definitely Internet of Things (IoT) data which the IoT connected devices will produce.

There are three 'V's—Volume, Variety and Velocity which describes the characteristics of Big Data. It's produced in large volume from various sources across the world. Variety describes its heterogeneous sources and multiple data formats. Velocity is all about data streams in at an unprecedented speed from various sources. Another important concern about Big Data is, it's difficult to capture, process and manage by traditional software tools is a cost effective manner. In today's era of big data, it has become a real challenge to extract meaningful insights by applying traditional algorithms/methods from unstructured, imperfect and complex dataset in almost all the domains like Environmental study, biomedical science, Engineering etc. The challenges include understanding and prioritizing relevant data from the huge set, extracting data from master set where 90 % data reflects noise, security threat, costly tools and framework etc. So various innovative tools, technologies and frameworks have been developed to handle these challenges which includes Hadoop a distributed file system and framework for storing and processing huge amount of dataset using the MapReduce programming paradigm, different NoSQL data stores with flexible schema pattern, several big data analytics tool like Pentaho Business Analytics etc. This chapter describes these various tools and technologies in detailed fashion. It also gives the architectural advantage of these advanced technologies over the traditional ones.

2.1 Defining Big Data Analytics

Big data Analytics is the method of processing big data which is huge in volume and containing heterogeneous data types to discover hidden patterns, unknown correlations, market trends, customer preferences and other useful business information with the help of set of innovative tools and technologies.

2.2 Challenges

There are lots of challenges which need to be taken care in a proper way for successful implementation in big data and Analytics. Figure 1 shows the percentage of various challenges in big data and analytics world which came as a survey result. Few major challenges are described below.

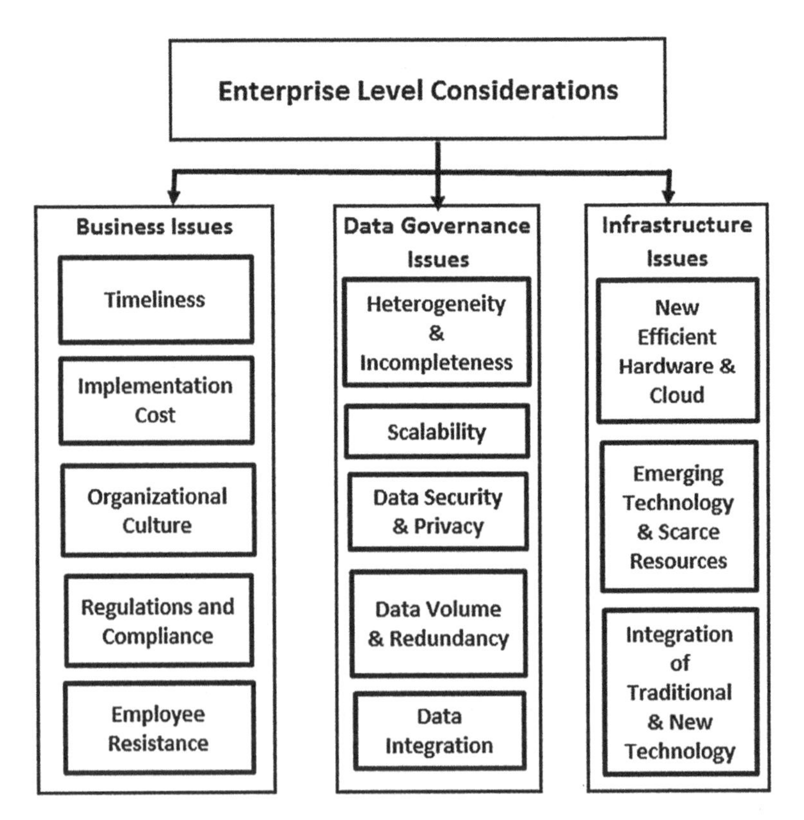

Fig. 1 Biggest challenges for success in big data and analytics

2.2.1 Heterogeneity and Incompleteness

One of the major features of big data is its heterogeneity because of its heterogeneous sources which is basically mixed data, collected based on various patterns or rules. Here the pattern and the rules and the properties of the pattern varies greatly depending on the variation of sources. And data can be both structured and unstructured in nature though 80% of the data is unstructured. So transforming these unstructured dataset into structured readable format for further processing is a major challenge for big data mining. To overcome this challenge, new technologies should be in place to deal with this kind of data. Sometimes data is also incomplete in nature. So integrating these heterogeneous and incomplete data within a specified time line and reasonable cost, is a great challenge. So data quality is a related challenge which comes with data variety automatically. Synchronization of data also another big concern as data is getting migrated from various sources, on different schedules and different rates.

2.2.2 Scalability

Large volume of data is another big concern for handling big data. Adequate processes and tools should be in place to process these huge volumes of data set at an acceptable speed so that important decisions can be made on time.

2.2.3 Timeliness

Time for analysing and deriving meaningful sights from big data is also an issue as it's comes in huge volume. Sometimes the analysis result is required immediately, like a suspected transaction in the credit card. Ideally it should be identified before the transaction completion by preventing the transaction from taking place at all. Full analysis of a user's purchase history may not be possible in real time but a partial analysis can be completed beforehand on base data so that computation on incremental data can be performed quickly to reach a decision on time.

2.2.4 Security and Privacy

The trustworthiness of big data needs to be verified as it's coming from heterogeneous sources. Appropriate techniques should be in place to find maliciously inserted data and to protect them from various security threats like accessing files and sniffing data packets by unauthorized user which are sent to the client, gaining access privilege by the unauthorized user which leads to unscheduled job submission, modification of job priority etc. Information security is a big concern where massive amount of data will be correlated, analyzed and mined for meaningful patterns. Various security measures are available in the market to ensure this information security which should meet the following requirements.

- Basic functionality of the cluster should not be compromised
- Scaling should be done in the same manner as the cluster
- Mandatory big data characteristics should not be negotiated
- Security threats should be addressed in an appropriate manner to big data environments

Various authentication, authorization, encryption and audit trails can enhance the security of big data though the possibility of attack can be there. But that can be reduced by implementing the following techniques.

(a) ***Authentication Techniques***: Authentication is the process of identifying valid user or system before system access, like Kerberos. Access control privileges for user or system is provided by authorization process.
(b) ***Encryption and Key Management***: This process ensures confidentiality and security of user information which is also sensitive in nature. It protects data from malicious user access. Consistent protection is provided by file layer encryption across different platforms regardless of OS/platform type. But file layer encryption is not useful if unauthorized user can access the encryption keys. For these cases, key management service is used as a solution which is responsible for key distribution and certificates and manage different keys for each group, application, and user.
(c) ***Logging***: Managing log files is a solution to detect malicious users, failures etc. It provides a place to look if something fails or if something hacked. And periodical audit needs to be conducted in regular basis to find whether any unusual problem occurred.
(d) ***Watermarking Techniques***: Information hiding is another way of protecting sensitive information from unauthorized users which can be achieved by applying the techniques like Steganography, Cryptography and Watermarking. Among these few techniques, Watermarking plays a vital role in the healthcare domain which is used for protecting medical information as well as secured sharing and handling of medical images [3]. In the current electronic age, telemedicine, telediagnosis, teleconsultation are the new buzzwords where digital medical images need to be shared across the globe among various specialist doctors to obtain its benefit. So the primary concern here is to secure patient's information from the attack of any unauthorised user.

Digital watermarking is the solution to preserve the authenticity and integrity of the content of these medical images. A watermark which is basically a distinguishable mark created on paper at the time of production where as in case of digital watermarking, patterns of bits are inserted into a digital image, audio or video file which uniquely defines the file's copyright information without affecting its look

[4]. Another aspect of digital watermarking is its bit arrangement—here the bits are scattered in the whole file in such a way that it can't be found or manipulated [5].

Various important characteristics of this technique include invisibility, robustness, readability and security. Invisibility is the first visible thing because the watermark is not visible at all. It should be robust enough as embedded watermark should not be affected by any kind of attack or image manipulation. Readability is another major concern as it should convey good amount of information. Security is the primary concern which indicates that a watermark should be secret and must not be detectable by unauthorised user [6]. This requirement is normally achieved by cryptographic keys.

There are several applications of digital watermarking techniques which includes security verification (certification, authentication and conditional access), copyright protection, fingerprinting etc. [7]. For copyright protection, the owner's copyright information is inserted into the digital image which is invisible in nature. Here the authenticity can be proved by extracting that information in case of any dispute. In case of healcare related applications, it opens a new era as most of the stages are performed online. Here the electronic patient report and different medical images are sent to various hospitals for consultation. So by using various watermarking techniques, the confidentiality, security as well as the integrity of these online reports and images can be guaranteed. There are various watermarking techniques are available in the market, out of which two correlation-based (binary logo hiding) and two singular value decomposition (SVD)-based (gray logo hiding) watermarking algorithms are widely used for embedding ownership logo [8]. Reversible watermarking method, also known as Odd-Even method, works for watermark insertion and extraction in a biomedical image. This method has a huge data hiding capability, security and watermarked with great quality. Another remarkable feature is its correlation value which is 1 for both original and extracted watermark. The method is also quite robust as Peak Signal-to-Noise Ratio (PSNR) is high irrespective of the amount of embedded secret data [9].

2.2.5 Skills Availability

Processing and finding decisions from big data requires set of new tools and processes for which enough skilled resource is not available in the market. These new tools include various big data analytics tools along with various NoSQL databases. So project cost automatically increases to hire the available resources in a higher rate. If we consider the statistics regarding the talent gap, we can clearly understand the scenario. According to analyst firm McKinsey & Company, there may be an acute shortage of 140,000–190,000 people in the analytics domain by 2018 in the US itself. And in a report from Gartner analysts in 2012, 4.4 million IT jobs will be created globally in the big data domain by 2015 [10].

2.3 *Mitigation Techniques*

Various innovative tools, technologies and frameworks have been developed to handle big data efficiently which includes Hadoop a distributed file system and framework for storing and processing huge amount of dataset using the MapReduce programming paradigm, different NoSQL data stores with flexible schema pattern, several big data analytics tool like Pentaho Business Analytics etc. Following section gives brief description of these tools and technologies.

2.3.1 Introduction of Parallel Programming Approach: MapReduce

Parallel programming is a methodology where the processing of a particular job is divided into several modules and concurrent execution is performed on the modules. Here modules can run simultaneously on different CPUs where CPUs can be a part of a single machine or they are the part of a network. Improved performance and efficiency are two major motivators of parallel programming. Resource challenge also can be mitigated by using this methodology.

MapReduce, the parallel programming methodology was first developed within Google for huge amount of data processing. Due to its large volume, it was distributed into a set of CPUs for processing within reasonable amount of time. This distribution of data implies the implementation of parallel programming approach as same computation is performed on different dataset on different machine. MapReduce is an abstraction which enables us to perform computation where parallelization details, data distribution, load balancing and fault tolerance are hidden from the users. This programming model is currently adopted for processing large sets of data [11]. The fundamental tenets of this model are Map and Reduce functions. The function of Map is used for generation of set of intermediate key and value pairs, while Reduce function combines all intermediate values with same key. The model provides an abstract view of flow of data and control and the implementation of all data flow steps such as data partitioning, mapping, synchronization, communication and scheduling is made transparent to the users. User applications can use these two functions to manipulate the data flow. Data intensive programs that are based on this model can be executed PaaS. Hadoop which follows MapReduce model, has been used by many companies such as AOL, Amazon, Facebook, Yahoo and New York Times for running their business application. The basic functionality of MapReduce programming is described in the following Fig. 2.

Advantages of MapReduce Programming:

Advantages of MapReduce programming explained and discussed on the basis of scalability, cost effectiveness, flexibility, data processing speed, security management, parallelism, fault tolerance and simplicity in the following.

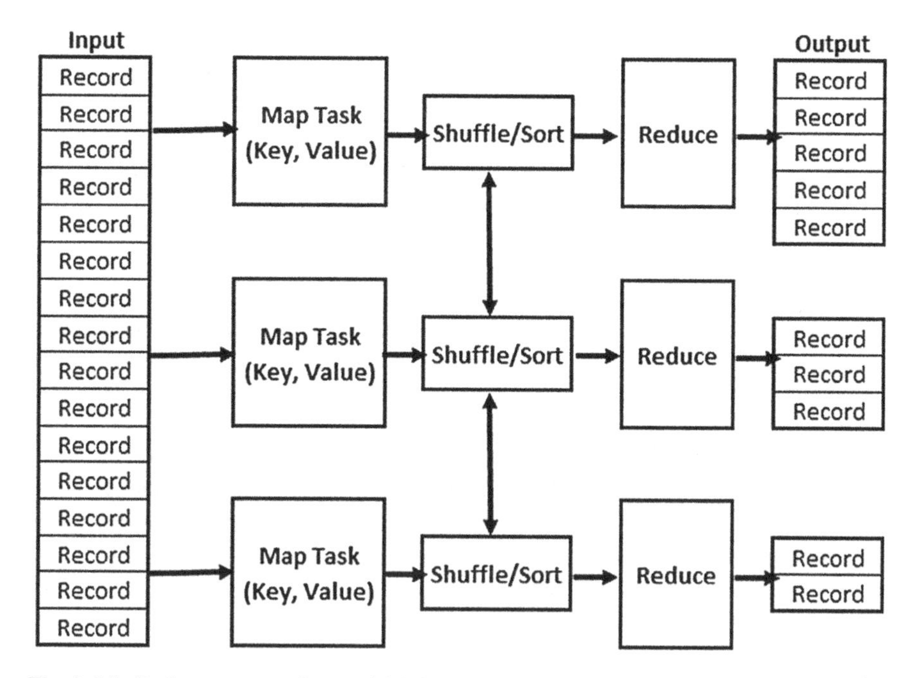

Fig. 2 MapReduce programming model [12]

(a) **Scalability**: MapReduce runs on Hadoop platform which is highly scalable in nature. These Hadoop servers can store and distribute huge dataset across various servers present globally. These servers are inexpensive in nature and parallel operation is acceptable. Depending on the business requirement, new server can be added easily to add more processing power. This advantage is not present in the traditional relational database system which cannot be scaled based on requirement. This MapReduce style enables business to run applications using a large number of nodes which involve huge amount of dataset.

(b) **Cost Effectiveness**: Cost reduction is another big advantage of MapReduce technique over the traditional solutions. Massive cost is associated in traditional system to process the huge dataset whereas implementing Hadoop architecture with MapReduce style reduces the cost to a great extent. It allows storage and huge data processing in an affordable manner.

(c) **Flexibility**: Flexibility is another keyword which made Hadoop MapReduce style so popular. It can be used to access any kind of new sources—structured or unstructured and process them to find the insight from these dataset. It is capable in processing the sources like social media related data, various emails, different log files, marketing related data to find strategic decisions.

(d) **Data Processing Speed**: Faster data processing which is the key requirement in today's e-era can be achievable by implementing Hadoop-MapReduce style. This technique takes minutes to process terabytes of data.

(e) **Security Management**: Managing security is a major aspect of any kind of business data. It is also assured in MapReduce as it works with Hadoop Distributed File System and HBase security which provide permission to the valid user only to access the data stored in the system.
(f) **Parallelism**: Parallel data processing is the primary characteristics of this MapReduce technique which segregates task in such a way that those can be executed in parallel mode. Multiple processors can work on a single task to complete it within shorter time period.
(g) **Fault Tolerance**: Fault tolerance which plays a vital role for business critical data as any kind of data loss leads to major security issues. Hadoop MapReduce methodology is capable of handling this data loss issues as the same data set is copied to various nodes in the network. So if a particular node fails, the data can be retrieved from other nodes which ensure data availability.
(h) **Simplicity**: Simple programming style is another characteristic of this discussed technique which allows programmers to handle task in a more efficient way. This MapReduce is written in java which is easy to learn and already widespread in the market. So mastering this programming style is not a big challenge for the developer community.

2.3.2 Distributed Approach in Cloud Environment—Hadoop Distributed File System for Data Storage and Processing

In reality, cloud computing is used extensively in large data processing applications where data is stored in distributed manner across the globe in various servers and also growing rapidly. Government institutions and large enterprises are leveraging cloud infrastructure to process data in efficiently and at faster rate. Major emphasis is on using parallel programming models to derive extreme capabilities of computing and storage hardware.

Hadoop facilitates a distributed file system and framework which is able to store and process large volume of dataset using the MapReduce programming paradigm. A significant feature of Hadoop is data partitioning and computation across various hosts and the execution of application computations in parallel close to their data. A Hadoop cluster which is a collection of thousands of server can be scaled horizontally by adding more commodity servers based on computation need, storage need and I/O bandwidth. In Hadoop Distributed File System, file system metadata and application data are stored separately. Here metadata is stored in a dedicated server called NameNode and application data is stored in the server called DataNode. All the servers are completely connected and interact with one another by TCP based protocols. In summary, Hadoop framework is the perfect ground to develop applications capable of running on groups of machines, which can perform complete analysis for a large volume of data. So in the world of big data, it appears

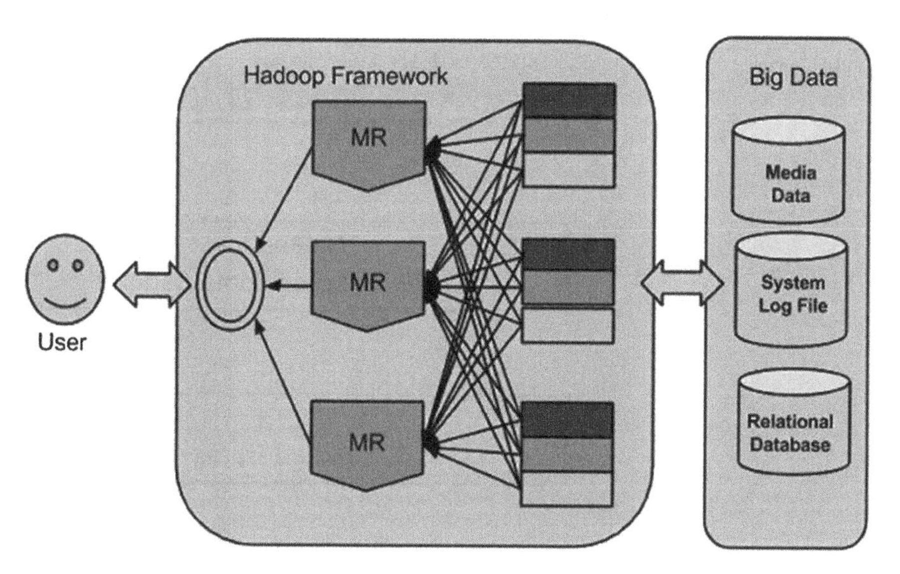

Fig. 3 Basic collaboration among MapReduce, Hadoop and Big data

as an effective solution and accepted across the globe. Figure 3 shows the basic collaboration between Hadoop Framework and Big Data technologies.

A. Hadoop Architecture:

Hadoop framework has mainly four modules which are depicted in the following Fig. 4.

i. **Common Utilities**: These contains the java libraries along with the utilities which is used by other modules of Hadoop.
ii. **YARN Framework**: YARN framework is used for job scheduling and cluster resource management.
iii. **Hadoop Distributed File System (HDFS™)**: It's distributed file system called as distributed storage also, supports master-slave architecture where master contains a single NameNode—responsible for managing file system metadata and one/more slave DataNodes for storing actual data. A HDFS file is the combination of several blocks and those blocks are stored in various DataNodes. The NameNode is responsible for mapping between blocks and DataNodes. On the other hand, DataNode looks after read and write operations with the file system.
iv. **MapReduce**: MapReduce is a software framework, capable of processing huge amount of dataset in parallel on large cluster of commodity servers reliably. It consists of two tasks: Map and Reduce. The functionality of these two tasks are described in the above section. Here the framework takes the responsibility of task scheduling, monitoring and re-execution in case of task failure.

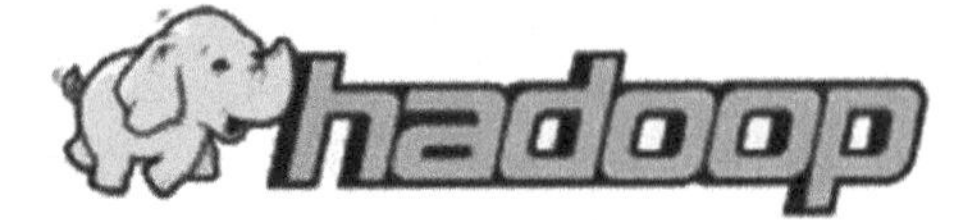

Fig. 4 Basic architecture of Hadoop [13]

B. Advantages of Hadoop Usage:

i. Support of horizontal scalability is one of the beneficial factors of using Hadoop in the big data environment as commodity servers can be added or deleted dynamically from the cluster depending on the business need without interrupting Hadoop's normal operation.
ii. Hadoop library is another unique feature which is enabled for identifying and handling failures at application layer instead of relying on hardware to be fault tolerant and on time availability.
iii. Hadoop framework gives the advantage of writing and testing on distributed environment. Automatic distribution of data and working across various machines are enabled here which utilizes the underlying parallelism of the CPU cores.

2.3.3 Schema Agnostic Data Model: NoSQL

NoSQL database provides a very relaxed approach in the world of data modelling because of its support for the elastic schema pattern and heterogeneous dataset. So management of this large volume of dataset becomes much easier compared to the relational database as data can be distributed automatically with the support of its unique feature—flexible data model. NoSQL database also has the feature of integrated data caching by which data access latency can be reduced.

The main intention is to get rid from strict relational structure and to allow various models to be adapted to specific types of analyses. There are various models, out of which fours models are widely used which are discussed below.

- Key-value stores
- Document stores
- Column stores
- Graph database

A. Key Value Stores

The key value database which basically uses a hash table where a unique key and pointer to a particular item of data exists. The value is stored in the database in the form of a two valued tuple—one is the key which identifies the record and the other is actual data which is basically the value column. So by the key value, we can easily get all information about the object without traversing the whole database. The main features of key value store database are described below.

- The schema less format is ideal for storage of heterogeneous kind of data.
- Key can be any of the type: synthetic or auto-generated.
- A bucket consists logical group of keys—but it may happen that identical keys are present in different buckets. So here the real key is a hash—bucket + key
- Reading and writing operations are very fast as the key is indexed.
- In the light of CAP theorem, key value store structure supports Availability and Partition not Consistency.
- Read and write functionalities are supported by few functions like: Get (key)—returns the and, Put (key, value)—associated which is with the key, Multi-get (key1, key2, keyN), final Delete (key)—is used to remove the value for the key from the data store.
- It does not support the traditional relational database functionalities like atomicity or consistency simultaneously. It should be created as in built functionalities within the application itself.
- Maintaining unique keys may be difficult if data volume increases.
- However, it's not suitable in the scenario where queries are based on the value rather than on the key.
- It's not a good option for transactions or storing relational data.

Figure 5 presents how data is stored in key-value store database where all information about BIT Kolkata (by the key BIT_KOL) or BIT Mesra (by the key BIT_MESRA) can be retrieved in one shot.

B. Document Stores

In this database, data is also collection of key value pairs where value is compressed as a document and it embeds attribute metadata associated with stored contents. Here also data is identified by the key. It's used mainly to store large files such as Videos, music etc. These types of databases allow to fetch the data for an

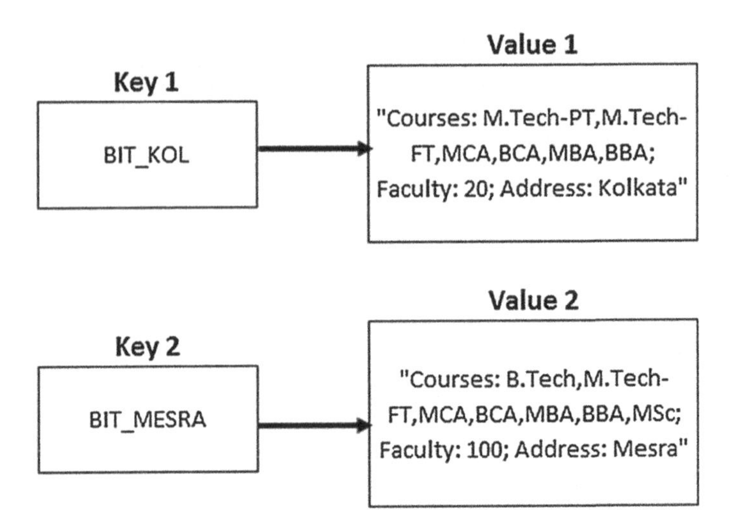

Fig. 5 Example of key—value store

entire page by a single query and most suitable for the applications like Facebook, Amazon.

- Tables do not store data and their relationships.
- Apache CouchDB and MongoDB are examples of document based databases. CouchDB uses JSON and JavaScript along with MapReduce and HTTP.
- It's schema less property makes addition of field in JSON documents a simple task as there is no need to define the changes first.
- Association of metadata with the data fastens the query the data based on the contents.

A single record in MongoDB is a document comprises key and value pairs. The value of these fields may be other documents, arrays and arrays of documents. Figure 6 depicts this kind of scenario.

C. Column Stores

In column store NoSQL database, data is stored in cells grouped together in columns of data instead of rows in relational databases. Here logical grouping of columns is called column families. The main advantage is that there is no restriction on the number of columns which a column family consists and again the columns can be created runtime.

- Here reading and writing operation are executed based on columns instead of rows.
- It stores all the cells corresponding to a particular column in the continuous disk entry instead of storing a single row in the continuous disk space which happens in relational database. For example, querying the conference paper names from the millions of rows is a time consuming task in relational database as it searches

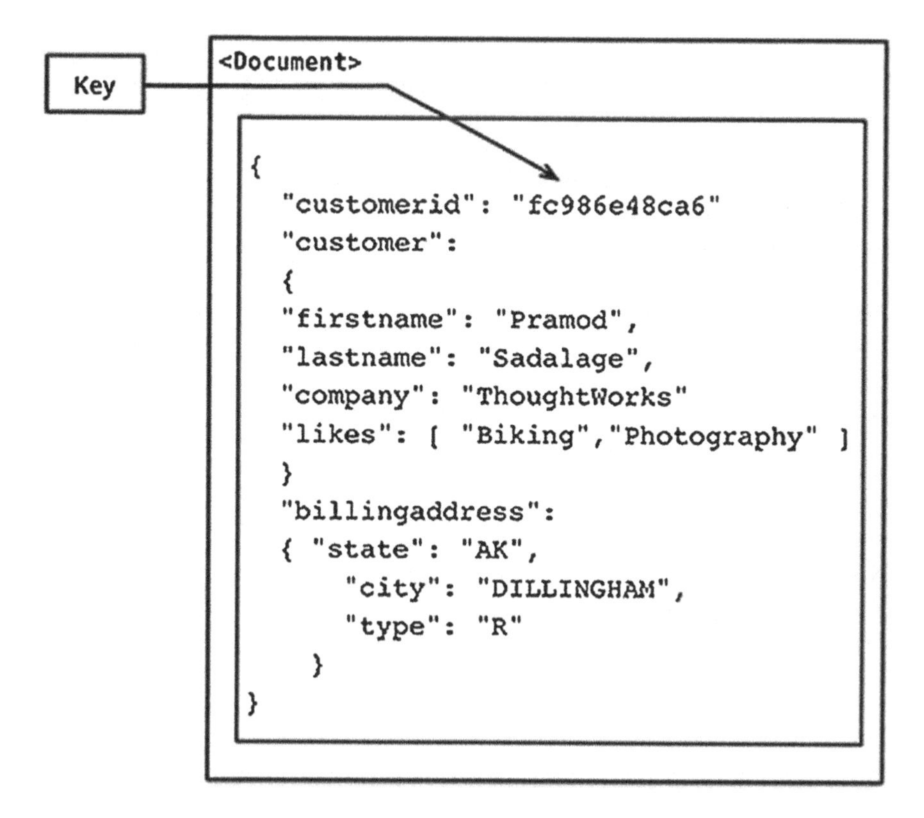

Fig. 6 Example of document store

every location to get the paper name whereas here it can be accessed by reaching one particular disk access as all the values for a particular column are stored in consecutive memory location.

Below is the example of column store database where Course_Information and Address are two column families, represented in Fig. 7. Here if we want to know what the distinct locations of BIT are, we can get it from the column family: "Address", we don't need to traverse the full table but in case of RDBMS, the full table scan is required to get the information.

D. Graph Database

Graph database defines each entry as to how it relates to another item including a pointer to the next item. It stores the relationships directly so that the optimal route between two nodes can be found easily. Here each node consists data about one particular item along with the link of next item.

- Most of the graph databases store value in key-value or document store fashion. In addition to that concept, they store the relationship also which makes the performance faster where data is highly interrelated in nature. This additional

Key	Column Family: Course_Information		Column Family: Address	
	Course Name	Number_Faculty Members	City	PIN
BIT_KOL	M.Tech-FT	8	Kolkata	700107
BIT_KOL	M.Tech-PT	8	Kolkata	700107
BIT_KOL	BBA	5	Kolkata	700107
BIT_KOL	MBA	6	Kolkata	700107
BIT_KOL	BCA	8	Kolkata	700107
BIT_KOL	MCA	7	Kolkata	700107
BIT_MESRA	B.Tech	50	Mesra	835215
BIT_MESRA	M.Tech-FT	40	Mesra	835215
BIT_MESRA	MSc	30	Mesra	835215
BIT_MESRA	BBA	35	Mesra	835215
BIT_MESRA	BCA	35	Mesra	835215
BIT_MESRA	MCA	30	Mesra	835215
BIT_MESRA	MBA	32	Mesra	835215

Fig. 7 Example of column store

feature of storing relationship allows complex hierarchies to be traversed quickly.

- Graph database consists mainly three elements: Nodes, properties and edges. Nodes represent the entities for which we want to keep information like people, business etc., properties holds information related to that node, edges are the lines which creates connection between two nodes, or between nodes and properties and they represent the relationship between the two.
- Graph database is most suitable in the circumstances where data is highly linked to other data in the database and finding relationship among data is a primary requirement including the shortest path between two objects.
- Also very effective for items which vary frequently with time. In those cases change in a particular node will be very easy in this kind of structure.

Figure 8 presents a real life example of graph database where user, page, tag and invitations are the nodes. Login and name are the properties of the node "user", html and create_ts are the properties of node "page" and the arrows indicate the properties. Here the nodes "user", "page", "tag" and "invitation" are interconnected in many ways. So handling these kind of cases by traditional RDBMS is quite complex as every relationship needs to be stored separately which can be easily achieved by the node "property" here. Here every node contains a list of relationship records which indicates the relationship with other connecting nodes. So the database just follows the list and access directly the connected nodes. As a result extensive search or match operation can be avoided compared to traditional RDBMS.

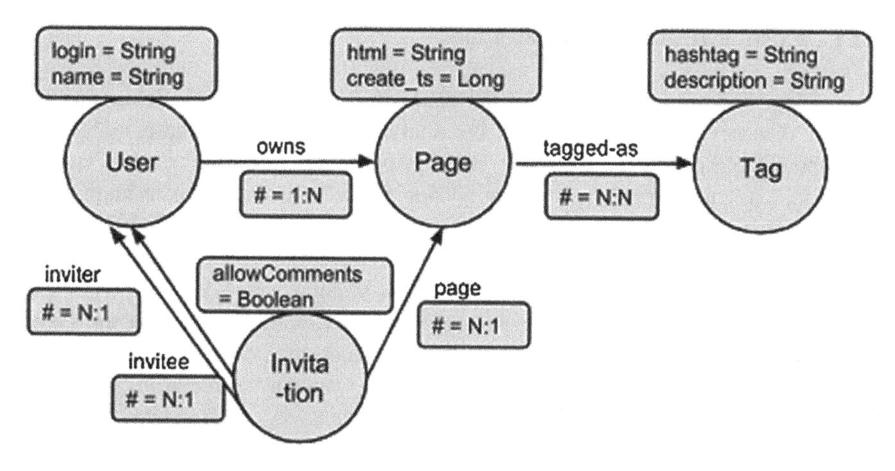

Fig. 8 Example of graph database [14]

2.3.4 Machine Learning Algorithms for Big Data Mining

Machine Learning is a branch which enables computers to learn by their own. No explicit programming is required for this purpose. Here dataset is the source of learning of the algorithms. As a next step, it identifies patterns like trend classification and then automates the output. It may be sorting data into categories or making predictions on future outputs. On the other hand, data mining is the methodology of identifying hidden patterns and features in the data set. The machine learning techniques are used in the data mining domain very often and unsupervised machine learning follows the same principle as data mining. There are various machine learning algorithms which are used for mining large data sets, some of them are Support Vector Machines, Decision Trees, Dimensionality reduction, Neural Networks etc. The brief descriptions of these algorithms are given in the subsequent section.

2.4 Healthcare Analytics—Application for Handling Big Data

In the near future, big data will affect every aspect of our life. There are few areas where already it started to create differences by adding insights from this huge dataset. According to the McKinsey Global Institute, there are four broad areas which deal with big data and can be benefited by analyzing this huge dataset to predict the future. These include applications in public sector, healthcare domain, manufacturing industry and retail domain. Following section briefly describes how big data can be used to add real values in healthcare domain.

2.4.1 Existing Healthcare Applications

Optimizing Treatment and Predict the Risk of Disease: Existing treatments for various diseases can be optimized by analyzing the existing cases which is undoubtedly big data and also risk prediction before appearing of various vulnerable diseases, can be performed by analyzing these huge dataset. The huge computing power of big data analytics help us to decode the complete DNA strings in minute, which also allows us to predict various disease patterns. This will definitely be a great value addition in the field of medical science.

Predicting Early Steps for Premature Newborns: Various big data tools and techniques are already in place to monitor premature and sick babies. These algorithms can predict infections 24 h before they appear by recording and analyzing every heartbeat, breathing patterns etc. In this way, the medical team can intervene early and able to help these fragile babies where time is the most crucial thing.

Prediction of Epidemics and Disease Outbreaks: Big data analytics enable us to predict various epidemics and disease outbreaks on time so that effective measures can be taken to handle the emergency situation if arises. Social media analytics also plays a vital role here for getting various inputs from different people across the country and integrating them to develop the insights.

2.4.2 Healthcare Analytics—Case Study

Big data Analytics is solving various problems and used to meet the business goal across the world in almost every domains like retail, banking, manufacturing, telecommunication, financial sectors. Healthcare Analytics is one such domain where analytics is widely used to obtain any important decision. In the Healthcare domain, huge amount of data has generated from record keeping, compliance and regulatory requirements, patient care in the last few decades which are in paper or hard copy form. Digitization of this large amount of data is the current plan as discovering associations, pattern understanding and trend analysis on this dataset opens a new era in the Healthcare domain which is a crucial part of big data analytics. So applying big data analytics in the healthcare and medical sector is a big step in achieving the facility in lower cost. In this way, it extracts insights from this large dataset which enables to perform various life saving predictions and better decisions on time.

Nowadays, inadequate Medical Facility is one of the primary and vulnerable issues in our society, especially in the developing countries. Our traditional hospital facility is juggling the problems among deficient infrastructure, deficient manpower, unmanageable patient load, equivocal quality of services, high expenditure etc. We are proposing one application, Med-App which intelligently provides the solution for most of the problems occurred due to inadequate medical facilities.

A. Motivation

The primary motivators behind the application includes the following along with some others.

- **Lack of Medical Infrastructure**: Public and private hospitals are incapable to handle the huge population pressure which are increasing exponentially. The main reason of their incapability is inadequate infrastructure and unavailability of medical practitioners.
- **Timeliness**: Another very crucial factor for a sick patient is time, starting the treatment as soon as possible which can save life many times. But too often, access to doctors—and particularly to specialists—can be a difficult challenge. Sometimes, the waiting period in the public hospital is too high that it becomes infeasible for the patients to wait for such a long time as time is the most crucial factor for the vulnerable diseases.
- **Sudden Need of Medical Facility**: Need of Medical facility when user is on the move, it may be suggestion/advice from medical practitioner or availing the medicines or support for immediate hospitalization. So there is an absolute need of an effective and easily accessible health care system which would satisfy the needs of diverse groups within their population.

B. Solution Framework

The proposed medical application—MedApp will address the above issues and can be an effective solution for most of the cases. This is a data analytics based layered framework which has been depicted below by the following Fig. 9. It consists of mainly three layers:

(a) *Source of data*: *Symptoms received from patients*
(b) *Analytics and Knowledge Discovery*
(c) *Visualization and Interpretation*

The layered wise working methodology is described in the following:

(a) *Source of data*: includes various types of symptoms from various patients
(b) *Analytics and Knowledge Discovery*

  i. Preliminary analysis will be carried out from the Medical Solution master database
  ii. More Predictive Analysis or Analytics will be performed to provide the suggestive medicines or necessary measures which should be taken by the patient during the crisis period or before reaching the crisis point. Historical Dataset and Symptom Database both will be treated as two main sources of input generation for better prediction. Registered Practitioner Database, Registered Hospital Database and Registered Emergency Services will provide the list of registered doctors, registered hospitals and registered emergency services like ambulance accordingly who can extend their support during this emergency.

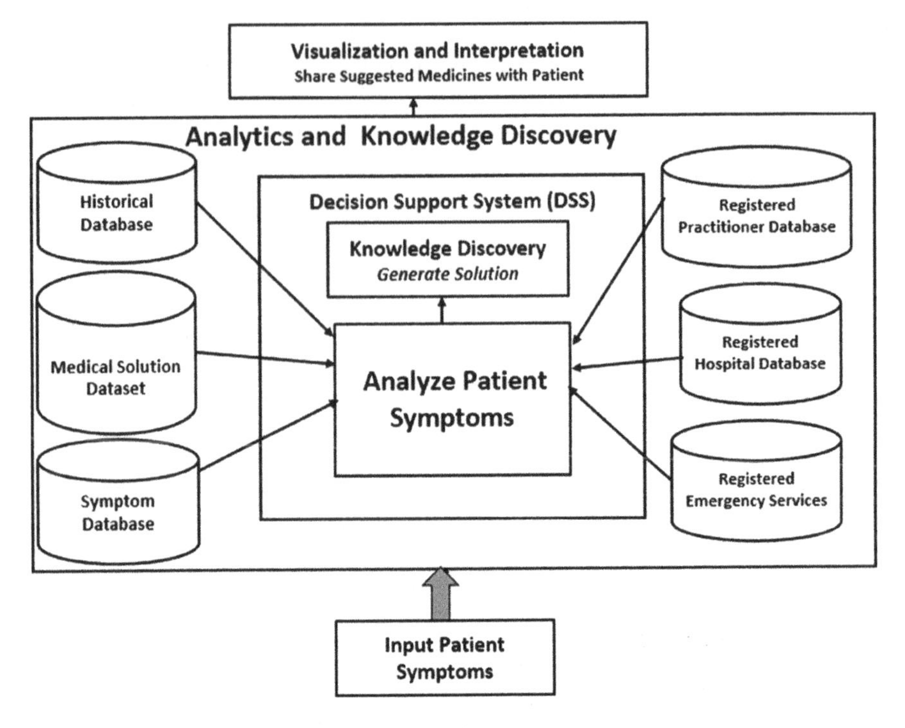

Fig. 9 Solution framework for MedApp application

iii. The next part is Knowledge Discovery which would be performed based on the prediction generated in the previous level.

(c) *Visualization and Interpretation*

The last layer will represent the decision which should be communicated to the user

C. Application Functionality

The brief solution approach of MedApp application is depicted below with the help of flow chart diagram represented by Fig. 10.

The high level details of the above steps are described below.

- **Handling Emergency Situation (Module A)**:

Few databases need to be created which will act as providing necessary inputs to the application. One is Symptom database which will contain various symptoms and corresponding root cause and the other is Medical Solution database which will contain the root cause of the problem and its corresponding solution in terms of medicine and other measures. The next action is populating those databases collecting inputs from patient. The symptom recognizer contains the parameters like Age, Sex, Chief Symptom: (headache/fever/stomach upset/Pain), Onset: (Gradual/Abrupt),

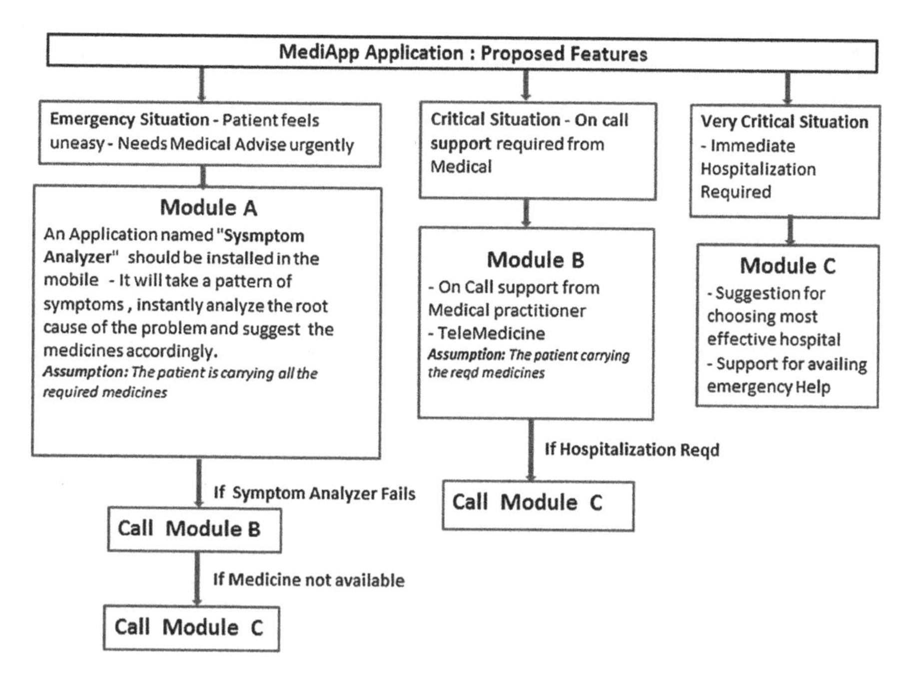

Fig. 10 Basic functionalities of MedApp application

Location of Symptom: (Head/hand/Leg/Abdomen/Neck), Intensity: (Intense/Moderate), Exacerbating Factors (what makes it worse?): (Taking water/taking Food), Ameliorating Factors (what makes it better?), Associated Symptoms etc. Then proper analysis should be done based on the inputs received from the patient and the dataset present in the above mentioned databases. If appropriate solution is not achieved, Module B is called for doctors on call consultation.

- **Handling Critical Situation (Module B)**:

This module describes the functionalities required for on call support of medical practitioner during emergency situation. As a first step of the process, registration needs to be done with set of hospitals, nursing homes and doctors. The application will contain the list of doctors/hospitals along with their contact details who have successfully registered. In the emergency situation, they will be contacted for on call and other support. The patient will receive the list of available doctors/facilitators so that they can be reached for providing help at crisis period. The consultation fees will be paid online to the facilitator.

- **Handling Very Critical Situation (Module C)**:

This module consists the functionalities which are required at the very critical situation like immediate hospitalization. During emergency period, this application finds the closest/closer/close by hospitals/clinics, contact with them for emergency help via messages/E mail and send few important queries which are very crucial at that stage like Ambulance facility, Hospital Bed Availability, Hospital Bed charges, Availability of specialist Doctors, Availability of cashless facility, Advanced Ambulance facility availability etc. The patient will choose the most appropriate hospital based on the query result received through the application. The hospital will arrange a bed and other facilities like ambulance when get the confirmation from the patient. The patient will reach the hospital availing the facility so that time can be saved which is most valuable at that situation.

3 Scalable/Distributed Algorithms and Their Usage in Big Data Analytics

In the era of big data, innovative tools and techniques are required to extract, process and mine enormous volume of data and finding meaningful insight from the dataset. These techniques should be scalable enough to support on demand requirement and also distributed in nature to enable parallel processing. The following section describes few such algorithms briefly.

3.1 *Frequent Item Set Mining—FP-Growth Algorithm*

Frequent pattern searching in large database is a very important as well as expensive task in the data mining world in the last few years. The FP Growth algorithm is an efficient and effective way to mine huge dataset which is also scalable in nature. It was found that this algorithm worked better compared to other similar algorithms like Apriori algorithm and Tree Projection. The main reason of its improved performance lies within its methodology of finding frequent item set without using candidate generation. This is parallel in nature and based on divide and conquer strategy. The main feature of this method is its usage of special kind of data structure which is Frequent Pattern Tree (FP Tree), responsible for keeping item set association information. The brief description of the methodology is described below [15, 16].

- A compressed data structure called FP tree is built using 2 passes by compressing the input database to represent the frequent items.
- As a next step, the compressed database is divided into set of conditional databases where each represents one frequent pattern.
- Finally each conditional database is mined separately. As a result frequent item set can be directly extracted from the FP tree.

(a) ***Frequent Pattern (FP) Tree Construction:***

- Scan the database of Transaction T once to find out the frequent 1-itemset L
- Arrange the support count in descending order to get the L1
- Take the "Null" as the root node when scan the transaction item set for the second time
- construct the FP-tree base on L1

(b) ***Frequent Itemset Generation from the FPtree after constructing the original FP-tree***

- Produce conditional pattern base for every node in the FPtree
- Build the corresponding conditional FP-tree from the conditional pattern base
- Mine the conditional FP-tree recursively and increase the frequent item set belong to it at the same time by producing the involved frequent item set immediately if the conditional FP-tree only contains one path. Otherwise, increase the minimum item of support count if the suffix pattern.
- Then construct the conditional pattern base and conditional FP-tree (The conditional pattern base is the entire branch which takes (E) as their leaf node in the FP-tree. The conditional FP-tree of is a new FP-subtree taking the conditional pattern base as its transaction and constructed in the same way of the original FP-tree).

Fig. 11 Major steps of frequent item set mining algorithm [17]

Following are the major deciding factors to choose this algorithm over the other frequent pattern searching techniques.

- Taking advantages of Divide and Conquer strategy
- No mandate on candidate generation
- Repetitive scan of full database is not required

Major Steps of the Algorithm:

The core methodology of this algorithm is divided into two steps: Frequent Pattern (FP) Tree Construction and Frequent Itemset Generation. The algorithm is depicted below with the help of Fig. 11.

3.2 Deep Learning

Deep learning is a new branch of machine learning whose main objective is moving machine learning nearer to one of its basic goals: artificial intelligence. This learning methodology is responsible for extracting high-level, complex abstractions as data representations with the help of a hierarchical learning process. Complex abstractions are cultured at a specific level depending on comparatively easier abstractions created in the preceding level in the hierarchy. One important feature of deep learning is its capability to analyze huge amount of unsupervised dataset which is extremely required in the big data analytics as the data here is unlabeled and uncategorized. Few well known applications include extraction of complicated patterns from huge dataset, quicker information retrieval, tagging of data etc. The basic advantages are its robustness, generalizability and scalability. In this learning methodology, designing the features in advance is not required, features are automatically learned to be optimal for the specific task. This is also robust to the natural variation of data as learning is automatic. It's also generic in nature as it can be used for several applications and data. Scalability is another very important characteristics of this methodology as here performance improves with the increase of data and it's massively parallelizable. Another big advantage is it can extract representations from unsupervised data without the manual intervention which is extremely effective in the domain of big data as the data volume is huge.

Following are some common applications of deep learning in the big data analytics [18].

Semantic Indexing: Information retrieval is one of the key tasks in big data analytics which is hugely depends on efficient storage and retrieval process. Here the challenge is increased as data volume is huge and also heterogeneous in nature includes text, image, video and audio. In this situation, the semantic indexing is extremely helpful which presents the data in more efficient manner, automatically helps in the process of knowledge discovery and comprehension. Deep learning comes into the picture as it is able to generate high level abstract data representations which can be utilized for semantic indexing. Complex association and factors are revealed by these representations which leads to semantic knowledge and understanding. As data representation plays an important role in data indexing, deep learning is used to provide a semantic and relational understanding of complex data along with a vector representation of data instances which leads to faster searching and information retrieval.

Discriminative tasks and Semantic tagging: Finding nonlinear features from raw data is a challenge in big data analytics to perform discriminative tasks. Deep learning algorithms can be used in this scenario to extract complicated nonlinear features from the huge dataset and then simple linear models are used to perform discriminative tasks by taking the extracted features as input. The main advantages of this approach includes adding nonlinearity to the data analysis and applying comparatively easier linear models on the extracted features which is computationally efficient, automatically a great advantage in the big data analytics. Hence, huge amount of input data is used to develop nonlinear features which is a great advantage for the data analysts as the knowledge present in the data can be utilised effectively. In this way, data analytics can be benefited to a great extent by implementing deep learning techniques.

4 Machine Learning Algorithms and Their Applications in Big Data Analytics

Machine Learning is a methodology in data analytics domain which automates analytical model building. It allows finding hidden insights from large dataset by using appropriate methods which iteratively learns from data without being explicitly programmed.

In the world of big data, large and heterogeneous datasets are two major challenges for the traditional approaches like trial and error to extract meaningful information from this dataset. Also very few tools allow to process this huge complex dataset within reasonable amount of time. Machine Learning, a novel and rapidly expanding research domain provides effective and efficient solution of the above issues by implementing appropriate machine learning techniques which differs from the traditional approaches [19].

4.1 *Classification of Machine Learning Algorithms*

An algorithm can model a problem in various ways depending on its interaction with input data. So choosing the appropriate Learning Style is the first thing which needs to be considered by these machine learning algorithms. There are few learning styles or learning models which a machine leaning algorithm can adopt to get the desired output. The common learning style includes Supervised Learning, Unsupervised Learning, Reinforcement Learning, Transduction, Learning to learn. Brief description of these learning styles are depicted below [20, 21].

4.1.1 Supervised Learning

Supervised learning is a type of learning which is appropriate when correct results are assigned to the training instances that can predict the progress of learning. This is a very common method in classification problems where the goal is mostly to get the computer to learn a classification system that is already created. A very common example in classification learning is Digit recognition. In general, it's most appropriate where classification generation is the main objective and also can be done easily. The most common areas of implementing this methodology is training neural networks and decision trees. For neural networks, it's used to find the error of the network and also for doing necessary adjustments in the network to minimize it. In case of decision trees, classifications are providing information about the attributes which can be utilized to provide the solution of classification puzzle. Figure 12 depicts the basic methodology in supervised learning. The main objective in supervised learning is to build a model which is able to do prediction based on

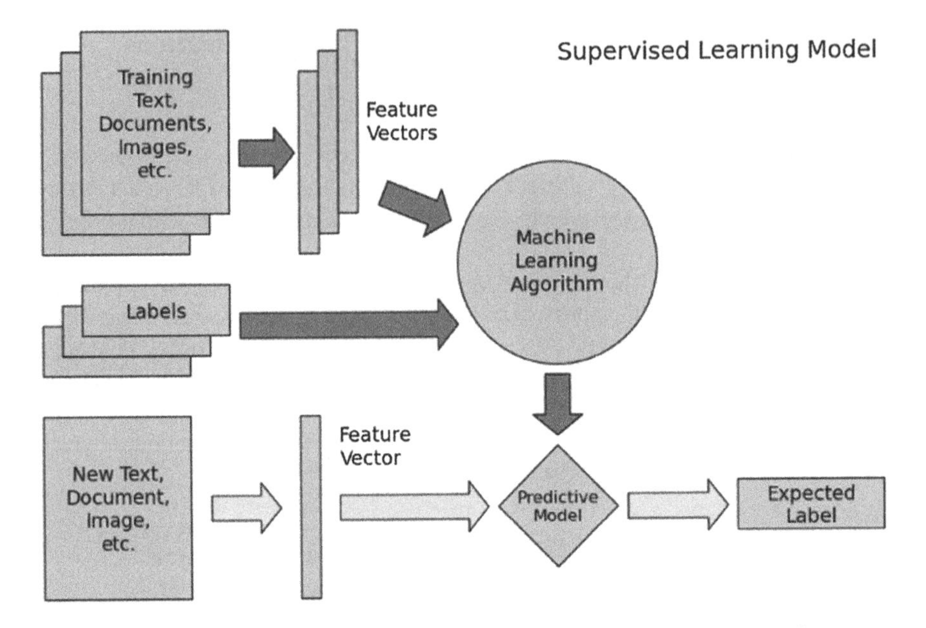

Fig. 12 Supervised learning model [22]

evidence in the presence of uncertainty. For doing this, first it takes known input data along with known responses and based on that it trains a model so that it is able to generate meaning prediction with new set of inputs [23, 24].

Steps in Supervised Learning: The basic steps in supervised learning includes the following [25].

- **Data Preparation**: This is the beginning step of it which starts with input data preparation in some specified format.
- **Choosing appropriate Algorithm**: There are several characteristics of the algorithms which includes training speed, memory usage, prediction accuracy, transparency etc. So appropriate algorithm needs to be chosen based on the requirement.
- **Fit appropriate Model**: Various algorithms have various fitting functions, so fitting function plays very important role in the selection process of appropriate algorithm.
- **Selection of appropriate validation methodology**: There are various validation methods are available which are used to check the accuracy of the resulting fitted model like examine the resubstitution error, cross validation error, out of bag error for bagged decision trees.
- **Test and Update**: After model validation, further tuning can be required to achieve better accuracy, better speed, less memory usage etc.
- **Using final model for prediction**: Final model can be used for prediction of new dataset.

Importance of Supervised Learning Algorithms in Big data Analytics: Machine learning is a very ideal solution for exploiting new opportunities from this huge volume of data as it requires minimum human interaction. Also this methodology is data driven and runs at machine scale. It is also capable of handling huge variety of variables coming from heterogeneous sources. Another big advantage of this method is its improved performance in the presence of large dataset. The machine learning system will provide better prediction if it learns more which is possible if it feeds more data.

Common Algorithms in Supervised learning: The following section describes the commonly used algorithms in supervised learning.

A. Support Vector Machine (SVM)

Support Vector Machine (SVM) is a supervised machine learning algorithm which can be used both for classification and regression problems though mostly used in classification challenges. Here we plot every data item as a point in n-dimensional space where n denotes the feature number. The value of the particular co-ordinate is basically value of the feature. The following example explains it in a better way.

Suppose there is a sample set of population containing 50 % male and 50 % female. We need to create few rules by observing the features of this sample set so that the gender of a new person can be identified correctly based on this ruleset. This is basically a problem of classification domain which can be solved efficiently by Support Vector Machine (SVM). Here the sample features for observation are height and hair length. First we plot the data based on these two features which clearly classify the set into two segments in the following Fig. 13.

Here the circles represent the female population and squares represent the male population. The two rules can be created based on the observation of the above set.

- Male population has the higher average height
- Female population has the longer hair.

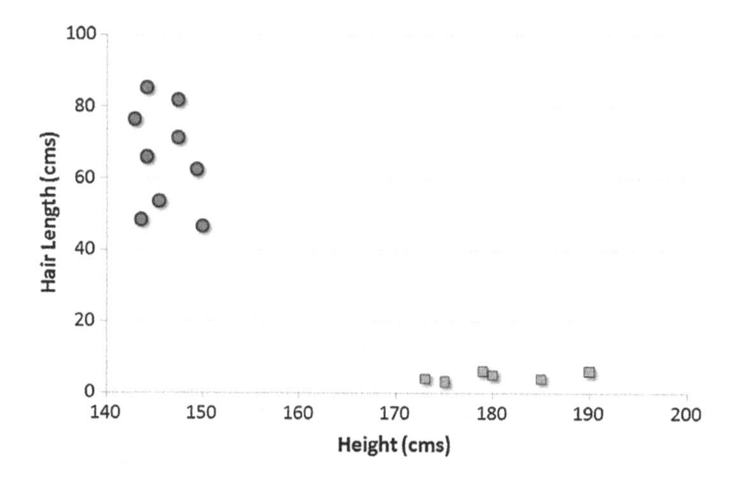

Fig. 13 Mapping of features: hair length and height [26]

Support Vector is the coordinate of individual observation. Here (45, 150) is a support vector which represents a female. Support Vector Machine is a frontier which can segregate the two groups in an optimum way. Various strategies exist in the market which are quiet effective to find the optimum frontier as multiple frontiers can exist in a problem. The simplest way to understand the objective function in a SVM is to discover the smallest minimum distance of the frontier from closest support vector which can belong to any class. After finding all the distances for all the frontiers, we just select the frontier with maximum distance from closest support vector.

B. Naive Bayes Algorithm

Naive Bayes algorithm is one of the fastest classification algorithm which works based on Bayes theorem of probability for prediction of the class of unknown dataset. The basic assumption of Naïve Bayes classifier is that there should not be any relation between the presences of specific feature in a class with the presence of any other feature. This model is very suitable and useful for large data sets.

Posterior probability P(c|x) can be calculated with the help of Bayes theorem based on P(c), P(x) and P(x|c). The following Fig. 14 depicts the formula and meaning of the variables.

There are various advantages of this methodology over the other ones like this is the simplest and extremely fast in prediction of test data set and also capable of multi class prediction. The most common usages include real time prediction, multi class prediction, sentiment analysis etc.

C. Decision Tree Classifiers

Decision tree is a well-known supervised learning method used for classification and regression. A decision tree of a pair (x; y) denotes a function which takes the input attribute x (Boolean, discrete, continuous) and outputs a simple Boolean y. This is basically a predictive model which is used to map the observations regarding an item to conclusion about the item's target value. This can be used to visually and explicitly represent decisions. The ultimate goal of this method is predicting the value of a target variable based on simple decision rules concluded from the data features.

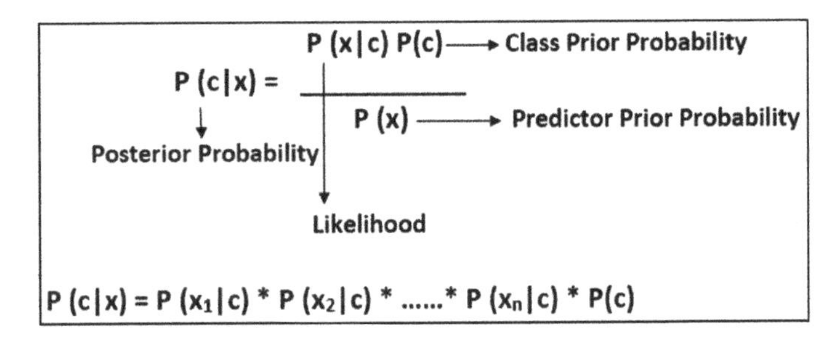

Fig. 14 Bayes theorem

```
buildtree (examples, questions, default)
/* examples: a list of training examples
questions: a set of candidate questions, e.g., "what's the value of feature xi?"
default: default label prediction, e.g., over-all majority vote */
IF empty(examples) THEN return (default)
IF (examples have same label y) THEN return(y)
IF empty(questions) THEN return(majority vote in examples)
q = best_question(examples, questions)
Let there be n answers to q
        – Create and return an internal node with n children
        – The ith child is built by calling
                Buildtree ({example|q=ith answer}, questions\{q}, default)
```

Fig. 15 Outline of decision tree algorithm [27]

A decision tree is also called as classification tree where each non leaf node is denoted with an input feature and the arcs which are joined with the nodes (labelled with feature) are labelled with each of the possible values of the feature. And each leaf of the tree represents a class or a probability distribution over the classes. The outline of the decision tree algorithm is depicted in the following Fig. 15.

4.1.2 Unsupervised Learning

Unsupervised learning is more complicated approach than supervised learning. Here the objective is to learn something by the computer by its own. There are primarily two approaches available in this type of learning. The first approach is teaching the agent with the help of reward system which is an indicator of success. This approach is most suitable into the decision problem framework where the goal is making decisions for maximizing rewards instead of producing a classification. The second type of approach is clustering where the goal is finding similar patterns in the training dataset instead of maximizing a utility function. There are various techniques used in unsupervised learning includes K-means clustering algorithm, dimensionality reduction techniques etc. Few common areas where this type of learning methodology is most suitable are determine the most important feature for distinguishing between galaxies where detailed observation of detailed galaxies are present, for the blind source separation problems etc. [24, 28].

Steps in Unsupervised Learning: The following Fig. 16 depicts the different steps involved in unsupervised learning.

Importance of Unsupervised Learning Algorithms in Big data Analytics: Unsupervised learning is one of the most effective way for analyzing big data as no

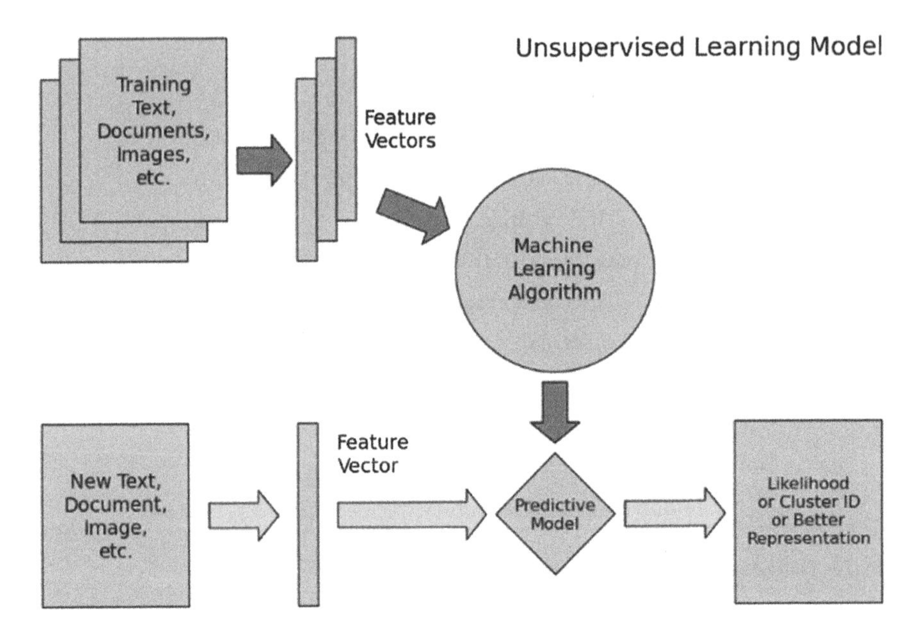

Fig. 16 Unsupervised learning model [22]

training set data is required here. In the big data domain, analysis is normally required on the dataset under exploration where predefined rule set is not available. So in this situation, unsupervised learning is quite effective to find useful patterns above and beyond noise.

Common Algorithms in Unsupervised learning: The following section describes the commonly used algorithms in unsupervised learning.

A. Clustering Algorithms:

Clustering is a popular concept which groups organization of unlabeled data based on similarity. So as a result, similar kind of data belongs to one group and other reside in another group. There are mainly three types of clustering algorithms are available, out of which K-means is the most widely used technique [29].

- **Bayesian Algorithms**: The major goal of this kind of algorithm is to generate a posteriori distribution over the collection of all partitions of the data.
- **Hierarchical Algorithms**: These type of algorithms find successive clusters using the clusters used previously. These algorithms can have two approaches again. First one is Agglomerative algorithms which starts with each element as a separate cluster and combine them into successively huge clusters. Second one is Divisive algorithms which starts with the complete set and continue to split it into successively reduced clusters.
- **Partition Algorithms**: These type of algorithms find all clusters at the same time but can also be used as divisive algorithms in the hierarchical clustering. K-means clustering algorithm resides in this group.

K-Means Clustering: K-means is the easiest unsupervised learning algorithm which is used as a well-known solution of clustering problems. The following figure describes the algorithm briefly. The main idea is to classify a defined data set through a specific number of clusters (let k clusters) fixed apriori. The first thing is defining k centers, one for each cluster. These centers needs to be placed in a cunning way as it various locations lead to various results. So the better choice is to place them in such a way that maximum gap is maintained among them. As a next step, we need to consider each point belongs to a given data set and associate it to the closest center. The first step will be completed when no point is left and an early group age is completed. Now we need to recalculate k new centroids as barycenter of the clusters resulting from the past step. After finding the k new centroids, a new binding needs to be done between the same data set points and the nearest new center. A loop has to be formed. As a result of this loop, it may be observed that k centers change their locations step by step until no more changes are required. Finally, the objective is minimizing an objective function commonly referred as squared error function given by the following Fig. 17.

The brief description of the algorithm is as follows in following Fig. 18.

B. Dimensionality Reduction Techniques:

In the world of big data, the volume of dataset increased tremendously and it leads to lots of redundancy. So it needs a treatment of dimensionality reduction to remove unwanted dimension. These techniques refer to the process of converting data set with higher set of dimensions into lower set of dimensions but ensuring to convey same information. These techniques are very common for achieving better features in classification or regression task in machine learning domain. One very common area of implementing this technique is image processing. There are various methods available in dimensionality reduction, some of them are depicted below in the following.

- **Missing Values**: In big data analytics, we face the problem of missing values very often. It's better to drop the variables if the rate of missing values for those variables are high with the help of appropriate methods.

$$J(V) = \sum_{i=1}^{c} \sum_{j=1}^{c_i} (\|x_i - v_j\|)^2$$

where,

'$\|x_i - v_j\|$' is the Euclidean distance between x_i and v_j.

'c_i' is the number of data points in i^{th} cluster.

'c' is the number of cluster centers.

Fig. 17 Squared error function

Input: Data points D, Number of Clusters k
Step 1: Initialize k centroids randomly.
Step 2: Associate each data point in D with the nearest centroid. This will divide the data points into k clusters.
Step 3: Recalculate the position of centroids.
Repeat Steps 2 and 3 until there are no more changes in the membership of the data points.
Output: Data points with cluster memberships

Fig. 18 Pseudo code of K-means clustering algorithm [17]

- **Low Variance**: We can encounter the constant variable in our data set which has little power to improve the model. In such cases, it's better to drop such variables from the data as it will not explain the variation in target variables.
- **Random Forest**: This is almost similar to the previous technique, decision trees. It's always recommended using the inbuilt feature importance given by random forests to select a smaller subset of input features.
- **Principal Component Analysis**: This technique is used very often in real world. Here variables are converted into a new set of variables which are linear combination of original variables. This new set of variables are referred as principal components.

4.1.3 Reinforcement Learning

Reinforcement learning is a kind of machine learning which is a branch of artificial intelligence. It enables machines and software agents to determine the ideal behaviour in a specific scenario automatically to maximize the performance. Basically this is the learning from interaction with environment. The agent learns here from the consequences of its actions instead of explicitly programmed and determine the new course of actions based on exploitation and exploration. So it can be called as "trial and error" learning also. Based on this learning, the algorithm modifies its strategy to achieve the optimum performance. Various algorithms are available in reinforcement learning to handle the issues. The main advantages include lesser time requirement in designing a solution with slight manual intervention [30].

The following Fig. 19 describes the abstract view of reinforcement learning agent in its environment. At a specific time instant, a state, an event and a reward are observed by an agent from its operating environment, the agent performs learning, takes necessary decision and actions accordingly.

At any time variant t, the agent performs a suitable action so that maximum reward is achievable in the next time instant t + 1. Learning engine which is the most important component, offers knowledge of the operating environment based

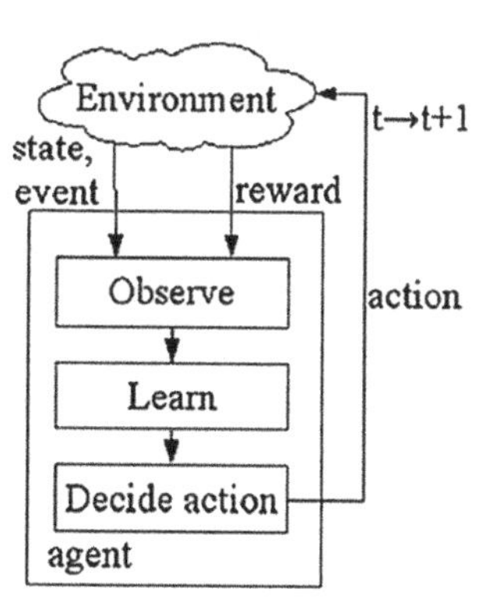

Fig. 19 Abstract view of reinforcement learning agent

on the observation of the consequences of its past actions which includes the state, event and reward.

The following Fig. 20 describes the flowchart of reinforcement learning approach. At time t, an agent chooses a subset of actions to adhere a set of rules. As a next step, it chooses either exploration which is a random action selected to increase the knowledge of the environment or exploitation action which is the best known action derived from Q table. At the next time instant t + 1, it watches the consequences of the past actions including state, event and reward and updates Q tables and rules accordingly.

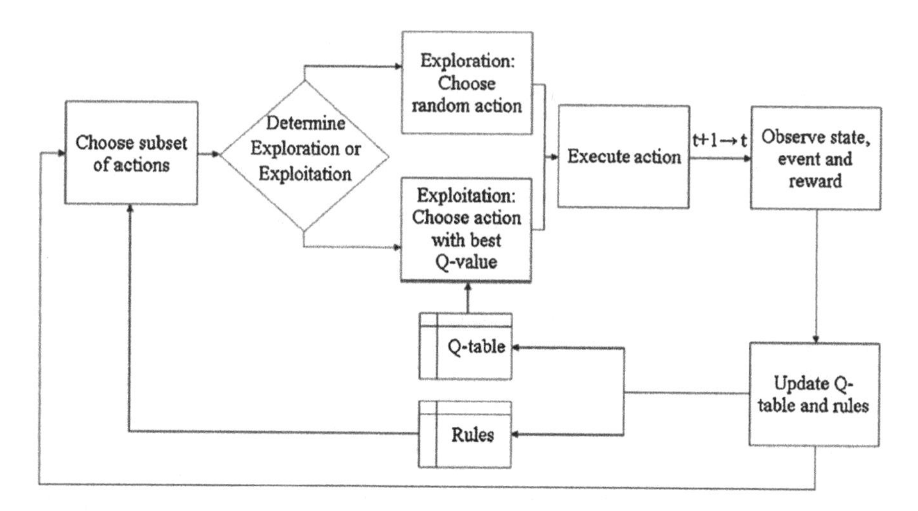

Fig. 20 Flowchart of reinforcement learning approach

Reinforcement learning techniques are extremely useful in big data analytics as it's capable of handling huge amount of data compared to other methods. These techniques automatically learn from past experiences (which is huge in nature) without much manual intervention. It ensures more accuracy in prediction as more examples can be integrated within the predictive model. The following are various real life applications of reinforcement learning.

A. Predictive Voice Analytics in Call Center:

Predictive voice analytics program in call center observes human speech pattern to obtain emotional tone and behaviour and predict future behaviours based on that. Here the reward can be defined as a positive call outcome when the customer agrees to pay for some product. The prediction algorithm explores how the customer speaks based on the voice analysis. It ultimately do the predictive analysis of the customer's future behaviour based on the current one. The reinforcement learning technique will collect data from thousands of calls which includes both positive and negative results and connect individual feature vectors from each call to the end result. After getting the aggregated results data, the efficiency and accuracy of the algorithm is increased. So in summary, reinforcement learning tunes the analytics program in a better way so that it can predict the customer behaviour more accurately which saves human effort to a great extent.

The following Table 1 describes various features and characteristics of the problems based on which we can select the appropriate machine learning algorithm.

4.2 *Applications of Machine Learning Algorithms*

The primary goal of machine learning research is to use the learning algorithms as a solution of real life challenges which includes fraud detection, result of web searching, sentiment analysis, credit scoring, various prediction in the automobile industry, new pricing models, image and its pattern recognition, filtering spam email.

Support vector machines is widely used in mainly in the pattern classification problems and nonlinear regressions. Two such pattern classification problems are cancer diagnosis based on microarray gene expression data and other is protein secondary structure prediction. Here prediction means supervised classification which has two steps. In the first step, a support vector machine is trained as a classifier with a part of the data in a particular protein sequence data set. After that the classifier is used to classify the residual data in the set as a second step.

Nowadays, few innovative techniques are used to determine cancer type instead of the traditional approaches. Traditional approaches are based on the morphological appearances of cancers. Sometimes it becomes really difficult to find clear distinction among the cancer types as it's only based on their appearance. Gene expression based cancer classifiers have achieved satisfactory results for specific type of cancers like lymphoma, leukemia, breast cancer, liver cancer etc. [31].

Table 1 Various parameters for choosing appropriate algorithm

Machine learning types	Algorithm specific comparison parameters
Supervised learning	1. Naïve Bayes, a supervised learning method has the advantage of its *quicker convergence*. If the conditional independence assumption is true, it will converge quicker than the discriminative models like logistic regression and if the assumption is not true, it's still also effective in practical scenario
	2. Support Vector Machine, another supervised technique has the high level of *accuracy*. It's very suitable in the text classification problems where high dimensional spaces are the common practise
	3. Decision Tree is another technique which can handle *feature interaction* quite easily and *non-parametric* in nature. So no need to worry about whether data is linearly separable
Unsupervised learning	1. Cluster Analysis which is used as the most common type of unsupervised learning, works for *explanatory data analysis* to find hidden patterns or data grouping. There are various types of clustering algorithms out of which K-means clustering is the most popular one. The main advantages of K-means clustering is its usage of simple principles which can be explained in non-statistical terms. It's also *highly flexible* in nature and also *adaptable* with simple adjustments. The main advantage lies in its performance for real world applications
	2. Dimensionality Reduction is another popular technique which is used to reduce time and required storage space. The machine learning model is automatically improved with the *removal of multi-collinearity*. Data visualization becomes much easier when dimensions are reduced to 2D or 3D
Reinforcement learning	1. Reinforcement learning can choose an action is response to a data point. This technique is capable of balancing *exploration and exploitation* whereas the supervised techniques are purely explorative in nature
	2. *Minimal manual intervention* is another major aspect of this technique
	3. Capable of implementing *artificial intelligence* as required

Naive Bayes classifier is a type of supervised learning which is used to classify spam and non-spam emails, classify among articles among technology, politics and sports, capable to check a piece of text whether expressing positive and negative emotions etc.

Decision tree classifier is widely used in the domain of astronomy. Noise is filtered from Hubble space telescope images with the help of decision trees. It also helps in star galaxy classification, determining galaxy counts etc. In the domain of biomedical engineering, it's used to identify features to be used in implantable devices. Automatic induction of decision trees is used for controlling of nonlinear dynamic systems in the control system domain. This technique is also widely used in the domain of medicine and molecular biology for diagnosing various disorders. Human Genome project, a great initiate from molecular biology has deployed this technique for analysing amino acid sequences.

K-means clustering is useful for undirected knowledge discovery. It is widely used in the areas ranging from unsupervised learning of neural network, pattern recognition, classification analysis, image processing etc.

It's applied extensively in various problems of data mining domain. In the field of image processing, it's used for choosing colour palettes on old fashioned graphical display devices and image quantization.

Dimensionality Reduction is an important technique in unsupervised learning to achieve better visualization, data in compressed format for efficient storage and retrieval and noise reduction used to gain positive effect on query accuracy. Document classification in a real life problem where this methodology is used widely. Here the objective is to classify unlabelled documents into categories which has thousands of terms. Another area is gene expression microarray analysis where the goal is to classify unlabelled samples into known disease types. Here the main challenge is the presence of thousands of genes along with few samples.

Reinforcement Learning which a very popular technique in today's machine learning world where the agent learns to perform a task based on the past learning experiences from the environment. The basic idea is the reinforcement outcome becomes positive if the goal is achieved and it's treated as negative if obstruction is faced. Video games and Robotics are such fields where there is a wide application of this learning methodology. In general an agent which is a game character or robot is present here which moves within the environment. The agent is allowed to perform task while moving. If it faces obstacles while moving, the outcome is negative and if goal is achieved, the outcome is positive.

This learning technique is also used in optimization of anaemia management among the patients who are undergoing hemodialysis. This is a very well-known problem in Nephrology where optimal Erythropoietin (EPO) dosages can be obtained by proper administration for an adequate long tern anemia management. The suitability of this methodology here its way of tacking the problem for obtaining long term stability in patients' haemoglobin level. If the patient is in a certain state, this technique suggests the sequence of actions which guides the patient to the best possible state [32].

Another real life application of this learning is the optimization of a marketing campaign. The basic approach is using data from marketing campaign to provide suggestion to the company policy for achieving long time organization goals which is achieved by implementing this type of learning [32].

Discussion and Future Scope:

The fundamental aspect of machine learning is to provide analytical solutions which can be created based on studying past data models. Data analysis is supported to a great extent where past data models, various trends and patterns work as the learning inputs whereas automated algorithmic systems is the final outcome. In today's world, data analytics and prediction are the keywords, without which it will be difficult for us to sustain in the future. As per the future prediction across the globe, machine learning will remove human intervention from the world of analytics which is completely dependent on prebuilt algorithms for doing various predictions and analysis. There are various learning procedures which has the capability to study and learn from past experiences and based on that it simulates the human decision making process. It acts as an effective solution making tool in the domain of demand forecasting also. It removes the human intervention as well as biasness in demand planning activities. As it has the inherent capability of learning from past and current data, it's capable of handling challenges arise due to demand variation.

The Internet of Things has given a new leash to the traditional machine learning techniques. Some common machine learning applications include customer feedback in Twitter, self-driven Google car, various fraud detection systems which are capable of handling huge amount of heterogeneous data. According to future prediction across the globe, the global community will be witness a remarkable growth in the near future in smart applications, digital assistants and various usage of artificial intelligence. Machine learning will take the lead in these emerging technologies. Vendors will be pushed to provide new machine learning tools to cope up with the increased demand. Though these ready products will be available in the market, there will be a huge requirement to customize them and create more advance model according to the specific need. Machine. According to McKinsey, the implementation of this emerging technology will enable the business to work with reduced manpower which will definitely help them in reducing operational cost. Global investment banks are welcoming automated trading which increases the probability of making profits by at least 30 %. As a result, more data scientists and big data experts will be required for making the business successful. In Germany, an algorithm for reading street sign has achieved 99.4 % success rate where for human it's 5 % only. Google and Amazon are some big names whose reliability increases on machine learning instead of domain experts to make more profit in the business. In summary, machine learning will work a major differentiator in the all kind of industry.

5 Conclusion

In today's era of big data, it has become a real challenge to extract meaningful insights by applying traditional algorithms/methods from unstructured, imperfect and complex dataset in almost all the domains like Environmental study, biomedical science, Engineering etc. The challenges include understanding and prioritizing relevant data from the huge set, extracting data from master set where 90 % data reflects noise, security threat, costly tools and framework etc. So various innovative tools, technologies and frameworks have been developed to handle these challenges which includes Hadoop a distributed file system and framework for storing and processing huge amount of dataset using the MapReduce programming paradigm, different NoSQL data stores with flexible schema pattern, several machine learning algorithms includes supervised, unsupervised and reinforcement learning etc. This chapter describes these various tools, technologies, machine learning algorithms along with their application in the analytics domain in detailed fashion. These applications help to gain clearer picture on the usages of these machine learning algorithms in the world of big data.

References

1. Clifton, D.A., Niehaus, K.E., Charlton, P., Colopy, G.W.: Health informatics via machine learning for the clinical management of patients. Yearbook Med. Inform. **10**(1), 38 (2015)
2. Moazeni, M.: Parallel Algorithms for Medical Informatics on Data-Parallel Many-Core Processors (2013)
3. Acharjee, S., Ray, R., Chakraborty, S., Nath, S., Dey, N.: Watermarking in motion vector for security enhancement of medical videos. In: 2014 International Conference on Control, Instrumentation, Communication and Computational Technologies (ICCICCT), pp. 532–537. IEEE (2014, July)
4. Bose, S., Acharjee, S., Chowdhury, S. R., Chakraborty, S., Dey, N.: Effect of watermarking in vector quantization based image compression. In: 2014 International Conference on Control, Instrumentation, Communication and Computational Technologies (ICCICCT), pp. 503–508. IEEE (2014, July)
5. Rathi, S.C., Inamdar, V.S.: Analysis of watermarking techniques for medical images preserving ROI. In: Computer Science & Information Technology (CS & IT 05)-open access-Computer Science Conference Proceedings (CSCP), pp. 297–308 (2012)
6. Coatrieux, G., Lecornu, L., Sankur, B., Roux, C.: A review of image watermarking applications in healthcare. In: Engineering in Medicine and Biology Society, 2006. EMBS'06. 28th Annual International Conference of the IEEE, pp. 4691–4694. IEEE (2006, August)
7. Abd-Eldayem, M.M.: A proposed security technique based on watermarking and encryption for digital imaging and communications in medicine. Egypt. Inform. J. **14**(1), 1–13 (2013)
8. Suri, J., Dey, N., Bose, S., Das, A., Chaudhuri, S.S., Saba, L., Nicolaides, A.: 2084743 diagnostic preservation of atherosclerotic ultrasound video for stroke telemedicine in watermarking framework. Ultrasound Med. Biol. **41**(4), S133 (2015)
9. Pal, A.K., Dey, N., Samanta, S., Das, A., Chaudhuri, S.S.: A hybrid reversible watermarking technique for color biomedical images. In: 2013 IEEE International Conference on Computational Intelligence and Computing Research (ICCIC), pp. 1–6. IEEE (2013, December)
10. Manyika, J., Chui, M., Brown, B., Bughin, J., Dobbs, R., Roxburgh, C., Byers, A. H.:. Big Data: The Next Frontier for Innovation, Competition, and Productivity (2011)
11. Kamal, S., Ripon, S.H., Dey, N., Ashour, A.S., Santhi, V.: A MapReduce approach to diminish imbalance parameters for big deoxyribonucleic acid dataset. Comput. Methods Programs Biomed. **131**, 191–206 (2016)
12. A presentation on MapReduce. http://www.slideshare.net/nishantgandhi99/map-reduce-programming-model-to-solve-graph-problems
13. A tutorial on "Introduction to Hadoop". http://www.tutorialspoint.com/hadoop/hadoop_introduction.htm
14. A whitepaper on "Graph Database". http://lambdazen.blogspot.com/2014/01/from-entity-relationship-to-property.html
15. Sidhu, S., Meena, U.K., Nawani, A., Gupta, H., Thakur, N.: FP Growth algorithm implementation. Int. J. Comput. Appl. **93**(8) (2014)
16. A whitepaper on "Data Mining Algorithms In R/Frequent Pattern Mining/The FP-Growth Algorithm". https://en.wikibooks.org/wiki/Data_Mining_Algorithms_In_R/Frequent_Pattern_Mining/The_FP-Growth_Algorithm

17. Verhein, F.: Frequent Pattern Growth (FP-Growth) Algorithm. School of Information Studies, The University of Sydney, Australia (2008)
18. Najafabadi, M.M., Villanustre, F., Khoshgoftaar, T.M., Seliya, N., Wald, R., Muharemagic, E.: Deep learning applications and challenges in big data analytics. J. Big Data **2**(1), 1 (2015)
19. Brownlee, J.: A Tour of Machine Learning Algorithms. A post available at http://machinelearningmastery.com/a-tour-of-machine-learning-algorithms/
20. Qiu, J., Wu, Q., Ding, G., Xu, Y., Feng, S.: A survey of machine learning for big data processing. EURASIP J. Adv. Signal Process. **2016**(1), 1–16 (2016)
21. Oberlin, S.: Machine learning, cognition, and big data. CA Technology Exchange, 44 (2012)
22. A learning material on "Machine Learning 101: General Concepts". http://www.astroml.org/sklearn_tutorial/general_concepts.html
23. Machine Learning—What it is & Why it Matters. http://www.sas.com/en_id/insights/analytics/machine-learning.html
24. Machine Learning, Part I: Supervised and Unsupervised Learning. http://www.aihorizon.com/essays/generalai/supervised_unsupervised_machine_learning.htm
25. Supervised Learning Workflow and Algorithms. http://in.mathworks.com/help/stats/supervised-learning-machine-learning-workflow-and-algorithms.html?requestedDomain=www.mathworks.com
26. A blog on "Understanding Support Vector Machine Algorithm from Examples". http://www.analyticsvidhya.com/blog/2014/10/support-vector-machine-simplified/
27. A lecture note on "Machine Learning: Decision Trees". http://pages.cs.wisc.edu/~jerryzhu/cs540/handouts/dt.pdf
28. Ray, S.: Essentials of Machine Learning Algorithms (with Python and R Codes). A post at AnalyticsVidhya available at http://www.analyticsvidhya.com/blog/2015/08/common-machine-learning-algorithms/
29. Cios, K.J., Swiniarski, R.W., Pedrycz, W., Kurgan, L.A.: Unsupervised learning: clustering. In: Data Mining, pp. 257–288. Springer US (2007)
30. Yau, K.L.A., Komisarczuk, P., Teal, P.D.: Reinforcement learning for context awareness and intelligence in wireless networks: review, new features and open issues. J. Netw. Comput. Appl. **35**(1), 253–267 (2012)
31. Wang, L. (ed.): Support Vector Machines: Theory and Applications, vol. 177. Springer Science & Business Media (2005)
32. Martín-Guerrero, J.D., Soria-Olivas, E., Martínez-Sober, M., Serrano-López, A.J., Magdalena-Benedito, R., Gómez-Sanchis, J.: Use of reinforcement learning in two real applications. In: European Workshop on Reinforcement Learning, pp. 191–204. Springer Berlin Heidelberg (2008)

Co-creation and Participatory Design of Big Data Infrastructures on the Field of Human Health Related Climate Services

P. Fdez-Arroyabe and D. Roye

Abstract Co-creation of scientific knowledge based on new technologies and big data sources is one of the main challenges for the digital society in the XXI century. Data management and the analysis of patterns among datasets based on machine learning and artificial intelligence has become essential for many sectors nowadays. The development of real time health-related climate services represents an example where abundant structured and unstructured information and transdisciplinary research are needed. The study of the interactions between atmospheric processes and human health through a big data approach can reveal the hidden value of data. The Oxyalert technological platform is presented as an example of a digital biometeorological infrastructure able to forecast, at an individual level, oxygen changes impacts on human health.

Keywords Co-creation · Sustainability · Interdisciplinarity · Transdisciplinarity · Morbidity · Climate services · Digital divide · Big data · Apps · Oxyalert

1 Introduction

Global change and sustainable development and its related issues such as loss of biodiversity, the human dimension of global change or environmental changes such as climate change are nowadays of global concern. Weather and climate are extremely connected to many human being's activities and people's wellbeing in many different ways. Understanding the relationships between climate, weather and human health is an ancient topic. Hippocrates was able to establish multiple connections between meteorological variables and diseases [1, 2] using observational

P. Fdez-Arroyabe (✉) · D. Roye
Department of Geography, Urbanism and Planning, University of Cantabria, GEOBIOMET Research Group, Avda. de los Castros S/N Santander, PC 39005, Spain
e-mail: fernandhp@unican.es

D. Roye
e-mail: dominic.roye@unican.es

C. Bhatt et al. (eds.), *Internet of Things and Big Data Technologies for Next Generation Healthcare*, Studies in Big Data 23,
DOI 10.1007/978-3-319-49736-5_9

methods. Medical topographies became a systematic approach to survey, map and describe the links between the physical elements of a specific location (lithology, minerals, air, water, plants, animals, materials used for housing) and the existing diseases in this geographical site. They were more abundant between the seventeenth and nineteenth century. Medical topographies [2] are a clear example of how human health has been related to the ecosystem's health for ages. Biometeorology is a scientific discipline that has studied the relationships between the atmosphere and living organisms (plants, animal and human beings) for decades, and now climate change is putting this concern on the table in a very strong way.

Climate change appears linked to an increase in extreme events and to new and emerging diseases in different places of the world, according to the last IPCC reports [3]. Each new version of these reports has added new models and datasets to the previous ones (atmospheric models, oceanic models, biophysical models, economic scenarios…). Predictions and risks are based on models which use huge amounts of digital data in order to facilitate projections and predictions of potential impacts of changes and their statistical uncertainties. Global warming has become an example of a real threat of global concern with the COP21 agreement [4] signed in Paris.

The interaction between living organism and the atmosphere has been continuous for ages, even before climate change became "*vox populi*" on the global community. Anomalous weather variability is probably the main expression of climate change which affects human being's health daily.

Many scientific disciplines have started to develop weather/climate related health warning systems to prevent citizens from extreme and anomalous meteorological impacts which are presumably becoming more diverse, frequent and intense in the near future. Moreover, at a different temporal scale, climate induced changes in ecosystems can promote modifications on the spatial distribution of diseases and the arrival of emerging diseases at different geographic locations. Massive volumes of information are required to study the complexity of the interactions among physical and social phenomena.

Simultaneously, the technological revolution is transforming rapidly many things while people are now living in a new digital society which construction is taking place daily, based on concepts such as virtual reality, big data, social networks, users, geolocation or digital divide [5, 6] among many others. The use of massive data sets and multiple electronic devices by citizens is a reality that cannot be stopped. The consumption of services based on these new technological infrastructures represents each day a higher percentage of the economic sectors in the developed countries. A new digital culture [7] is being created. Technological transformations are affecting multiple dimensions on the natural, social and economic systems in which the world is organized and research is produced.

During last decades, we have progressively moved towards the knowledge society where lifelong learning becomes a must in terms of competitiveness and wellbeing. Knowledge has been recognized as the driver of economic growth and productivity by the Organization for Economic Cooperation and Development (OECD) [8]. The knowledge-based economy has been related to education and innovation and to the use of Information and Communication Technologies (ICTs). Creation and production of new knowledge is a constant need of human beings in order to reach a higher understanding of things and processes at the social, bio-physical, psychological, natural or technological spheres to better explain complexity of reality. The acceptances of global interactions where natural and human ecosystems are fuzzily connected at different spatial scales are breaking the limits of the traditional system theory. A new comprehension of reality appears when known and new factors, processes and technologies that were not included before in our interpretations become now considered rationally under innovative approaches. The generalization of this practice into a collaborative environment can take us to co-creation and co-production processes as new methods of thinking and researching able to generate new understandings.

This chapter initially presents a brief approach to the concepts of co-creation and co-production of knowledge in the field of global change and sustainable development linked to transdisciplinary and citizen's science.

Co-creation at the European research agenda is briefly presented in relation to global change and sustainability issues under the Future Earth European movement. Some applied methods and techniques of knowledge co-creation are also mentioned.

The second section of the chapter is focused on the need to study the interaction between weather, climate, diseases and human health. The Environmental Protection Agency (EPA) has produced a detailed list [9] of the main climate change impacts on human health in the United States of America: temperature-related impacts; air quality impacts; extreme events impacts; vector-borne diseases impacts; water related illnesses; food safety and nutrition; mental health impacts and other health impacts. These big groups of impacts are applicable to the regions of the world with different considerations for each place. Extreme heat has been linked to cardiovascular, respiratory and cerebrovascular diseases and also to mental diseases. Water can act as a hazard in many different ways. An increase in the number of flooding can provoke direct impacts on mortality and morbidity. Indirectly, outbreaks of communicable diseases take place after inundating events when the risk of infections is increased. Waterborne diseases (cholera, typhoid fever, leptospirosis, hepatitis A…) and some vector borne diseases (malaria, dengue, yellow fever, West Nile Virus…) can spread widely after a flooding event. On contrast, the lack of water in some regions of the world is linked to the scarcity of food and big famine episodes. Water and air pollution are also issues of global concern in terms of impacts on mortality and morbility and morbidity for citizen. Air pollution is perhaps one on the most visible examples of the global dimension of the environmental problems where local emissions of pollutants have health impacts on remote regions from the original source.

The development of the new umbrella of the Global Framework for Climate Services [10] tries to confront most of these impacts. This joint initiative of the WHO and WMO is presented and specific emphasis is given to the relevance of having free access to massive digital data and complex technological infrastructures in order to co-produce useful health related climate services. The necessity of transitioning from traditional databases to climate datasets and health care big data expansion is presented in the chapter with abundant references to the existing limitations of this process in the field of climate-related health services development. Some of them come from the traditional disconnection between disciplines with a lack of mutual understanding. Another important limitation is related to the temporal and spatial scales in which datasets has been traditionally registered. Some examples of traditional earth systems and medical systems data are given to shown how relevant the development of unstructured systems can be in this scientific area. The existence of ecological fallacies is also a big concern in the traditional approaches of collecting datasets and the use of big data can be useful to solve this limitation. Nevertheless, some legal issues of accessing to confidential information will also arise in this field, especially in the health sector. Further than these legal, methodological and technical issues, the section is finished attending to the concept of digital divide in relation to the development of big data systems for climate services developers and users what can appear as a big wall for a real implementation of these new health-related climate services.

Finally, a case study of a preliminary early warning system based on a biometeorological model and a technological platform is presented as an example of an open knowledge co-creation process based on transdisciplinary research where academia, investigators, public administration, companies, technology and citizens are getting together in order to co-produce and facilitate a free global human health related climate service. The biometeorological data infrastructure is presented as a combination of different elements such as: a biometeorological conceptual model or initial hypothesis; a technological infrastructure formed by a server and a mobile application; a relational database management systems and a group of datasets; a sequence of procedures developed by the main server and by the mobile application; products and services provided by the infrastructure such as global and regional risk maps; users feedback as an important component of the infrastructure that facilitates the final elaboration of customized early warning systems to each citizen.

1.1 Co-creation and Scientific Knowledge

Co-creation on global change and sustainability scientific research starts with identifying societal concerns in this field in order to define topics which should be studied to solve specific problems. Co-creation is a learning process and must be active, creative and based on collaboration between scientists, citizens, users, stakeholders and decision makers considering the aims and the added value of the process itself. Mauser et al. [11] speak on the integration of different dimensions of global problems through transdisciplinarity in relation to environmental sustainability where stakeholder and academic involvement get together, with different degrees of participation, in a circular process of co-design and co-production and dissemination of results. Figure 1 presents a summary of this process based on Mauser theory which has been adapted by the Future Earth Initial Design Report [12].

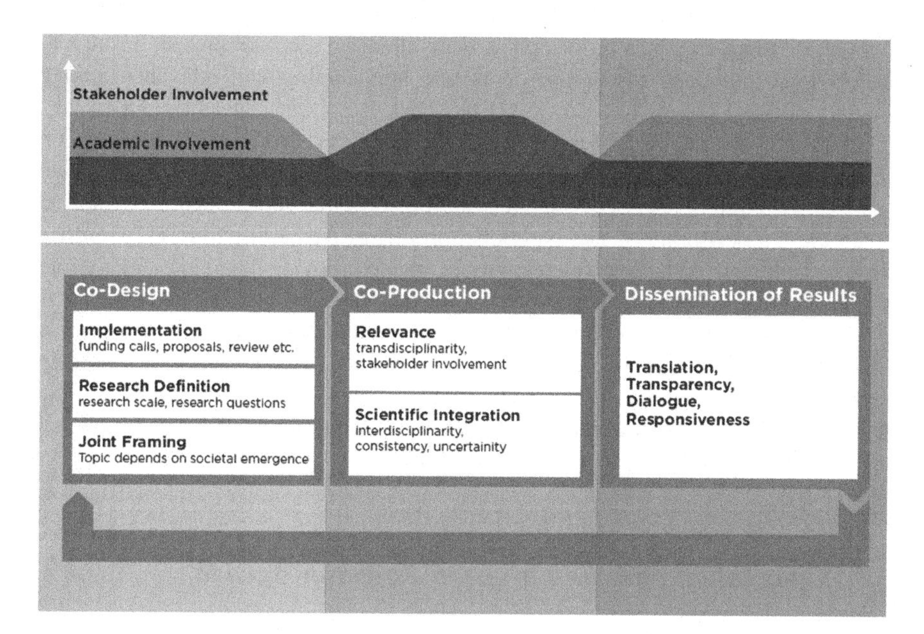

Fig. 1 Steps in co-design and co-production of scientific knowledge. *Source* Future Earth Initial Design Report inspired on Mauser et al. (2013)

In general terms, the first step refers to the research agenda definition through sectorial integration where is specified the topics definition, the research scale, the funding call proposal and the reviewing processes. A second stage, co-production of knowledge, is based on stakeholder integration through transdisciplinary and scientific integration based on interdisciplinary actions. Tress et al. [13, 14] define these two concepts in relation to the co-creation process in environmental sustainability under an integrative approach in the following way:

- interdisciplinary studies: *projects that involve several unrelated academic disciplines in a way that forces them to cross subject boundaries to create new knowledge and theory and solve a common research goal.*
- transdisciplinary studies: *projects that both integrate academic researchers from different unrelated disciplines and non-academic participants, such as land managers and the public, to research a common goal and create new knowledge and theory. Transdisciplinary combines interdisciplinary with a participatory approach.*

Nonaka and Toyama [15] defined knowledge creation [16, 17] as a process based on contradictions and interactions among individuals, the organization, and the environment. They also argue that knowledge is created in "*a spiral that integrates opposing concepts such as:* "*order and chaos, micro and macro, part and whole, mind and body, tacit and explicit, self and other, deduction and induction, and creativity and efficiency*".

Finally, there is a dissemination process that is used to present results to stakeholders and open discussion on results applicability and relevance among different societal groups in order to get feedback from them and maintain an iterative open cycle on the process. This integrative circular learning process can generate innovative concepts such as Global Health, Healthy Cities, Climate Services, Ecosystems Services that are widespread on the society and used later on to represent a new point of view of global problems. According to LSE Enterprise [18] co-creation is collaborative creativity to enable innovation and integrates a mix of management, marketing, psychology and group decision making processes. It is a facilitated process where the quality of the interactions among people is as important as technology in order to facilitate learning. From a business company point of view, the customer must be always considered a co-creator of value. In the field of researching the customer is the full society what means that each individual has a co-creator role.

1.2 Co-creation and the European Research Agenda

The European Alliance of Future Earth National Committees is trying to spread over the old continent this new philosophy of developing and producing science. Concepts such as co-creation, participatory design, interdisciplinary and transdisciplinary or citizens science are defining a new conceptual frame to develop scientific research in Europe in relation to global change studies and environmental sustainability. This a clearly presented in the Future Earth Design Report documents [12] where the global sustainability within earth system boundaries is presented as a priority for scientific research attending to cross-scale interactions from local to regional and global scales. In this sense, this has become an important scope at the European Commission where a funding initiative oriented to create a "*European map of knowledge production and co-creation in support of research and innovation for societal challenges*" has been recently opened through the *Research and Innovation* program. The participation of many actors in the process of knowledge creation and innovation is considered a key point at this level. The research agenda in Europe is being redesign attending to the principals of co-creation mentioned before (Fig. 2).

The Science and Technology Alliance for Global Sustainability is acting as sponsor of Future Earth on a Global Scale. Its members consist of the International Council for Science (ICSU), the International Social Science Council (ISSC), the Belmont Forum of funding agencies, the United Nations Educational, Scientific and Cultural Organization (UNESCO), the United Nations Environment Programme (UNEP), the United Nations University (UNU), and the World Meteorological Organization (WMO) as an observer. According to Melissa Lech [19], Vice-Chair of the Future Earth Science Committee:

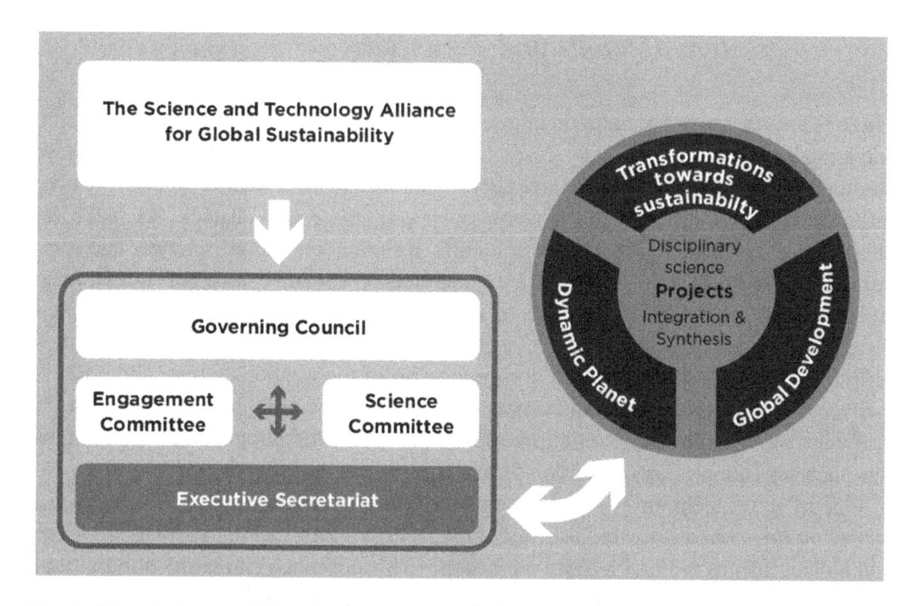

Fig. 2 The initial governance structure of Future Earth. *Source* Future Earth Initial Design Report

- "*getting involved in co-design and co-production is also a way of getting involved in the politics of knowledge, and the politics of delivering versions of sustainability that speak to particular groups' agendas. Science needs to be designed and produced in ways that speak to and are relevant to the perspectives, priorities and interests of particular groups, and being involved in shaping questions and delivering science is one way of ensuring that happens*"

The main challenges of Future Earth are defined in its corresponding booklet [20] and can be synthesized in the idea of delivering water, energy and food for all in a context of a decarbonized socio-economic world with healthy, resilient and productive cities and rural areas compromised with sustainable consumption and production patterns. Inside this widespread goal, there are two specific challenges that fit very well the content of this chapter which are:

- "*to improve human health by elucidating, and finding responses to, the complex interactions amongst environmental change, pollution, pathogens, disease vectors, ecosystems services and people's livelihoods, nutrition and well-being*"
- "*to increase social reliance to future threats by building adapatative governance systems, developing early warnings of global and connected thresholds and risks, and testing effective, accountable and transparent instutions that promote transformations to sustainability*"

It is at these points where co-creation of new knowledge on the interactions between the atmosphere and the human health and digital data structures development become essential to design and produce customized early warning systems at an individual scale [21].

1.3 Co-creation Methods and Techniques

There is a wide range of methods and techniques to co-create knowledge in science and research arena but in many cases the main difficulty to use them is that these methodologies and techniques are deeply unknown in scientific spheres where research proposal are written. This is obviously the main obstacle to make an effective co-creation approach on scientific research on global change and sustainability. Many of these methods are generated on social science and humanities, and there are important difficulties to introduce them further than the associated disciplines. Abdul Samad et al. have grouped a list of thirty methods/techniques [22] to co-create knowledge considering the aim of the methods (share and collect; measure and analyze; plan and improve), the type of techniques that are used (software tools; networking; communities of practice; workshops) and the period of time needed (hours; days; months; years) to develop the experience.

One of these techniques is proposed by Cüneyt Budak and refers to *building a global on line community* and is based on websites or any specific software to share and collect information with daily periodicity. This approach can correspond in part to the case study presented later in this chapter, where a mobile application is used to promote participation of the citizens from the world on sharing information about their health state in those specific moments where anomalous weather changes happen in the place where they are. In this sense, Suter et al. expressed clearly that "*we can even predict that a global online community, collaborating at a portal with an adequate design for a specific content, being easily accessible for a much wider public anytime can be much more effective than many international conferences*".

Another co-creation method that could also be related to the design and implementation of a health related climatic/meteorological service is described by Swaran Shandu under the name of "*Social software tools for personal knowledge management*". The main characteristic of this method is that it is based on the power of social software tools that usually consist of Weblogs, Wikis and a Tagging service. The service proposed here has a final aim of using citizens feedbacks based on the software of the application to facilitate biometeorological information to each individual about how much meteo-sensitive they are for specific atmospheric variables. In other words, to increase their own knowledge in relation to how the weather affects their own wellbeing.

There is a third example of a knowledge co-creation technique to "*Collect and Share existing knowledge on collaborative multidisciplinary scientific research processes*" proposed by Ayalew Kassahun et al. This method can also fit very well to the development of biometeorological early warning systems due to the fact that the implementation of any warning systems requires collaborative and multidisciplinary research based on stakeholders and user feedback to avoid previous mistakes and improve the efficiency of the warnings.

2 Climate Services and Data Infrastructures

Society is confronted with an increasingly complex environment which is especially visible under the challenge of global change and the increase vulnerabilities of ecosystems and people. This manifest dependence of our activities with respect to environmental and especially atmospheric conditions is continually brought into our daily life. Its influence in economic or leisure activities is largely determining our lifestyles. In order to improve and optimize the response and management of the risks and opportunities arising from climate variability and change it is important to design and produce new climate services in the field of human health.

2.1 Climate Services and Human Health

Climate services are based on the need to give added value to the climatic and meteorological information available in a growing digital world. Furthermore, the services should be built in a most appropriate way for decision makers to be able to use them properly. After the World Climate Conference-3 held in Geneva in 2009 and organized by the World Meteorological Organization, the Global Framework for Climate Services (GFCS) [10] was founded to coordinate, strengthen and develop initiatives and infrastructure for climate services [23, 24].

The GFCS established five main objectives: (1) reduce the vulnerability of society to climate-related hazards through better provision of climate information; (2) advance the key overall development goals through better provision of climate information; (3) the use of mainstream climate information in decision-making; (4) strengthen the engagement of providers and users of climate services; and (5) maximize the utility of existing climate-service infrastructure [10]; also it defined five priority areas: agriculture and food security, disaster risk reduction, energy, health and water.

It is undeniable that the environment influences directly and indirectly the state of human health. The human body and the atmosphere are in a physical and chemical equilibrium of constant exchange. All human beings are forced to react to the atmospheric elements to ensure correct and optimal organ function. Environmental effects on human health have different responses in the sense of an Illness-Wellness Continuum [25]. Mortality is, on the one hand, a premature consequence, and on the other affects a smaller part of the population than the possible effects in morbidity [26]. The circumstances associated to morbidity can be very diverse (Fig. 3). Depending on the seriousness of the response, there is more or less population affected. Obviously, many of the impacts of atmospheric changes on human health do not end with death or with a hospital admission. A large part can be manifested through a visit to the doctor or self-medication. However, in the lower levels of morbidity a lack of administrative records appears in the health system due to the loss of relevance. These kinds of low level weather-related effects

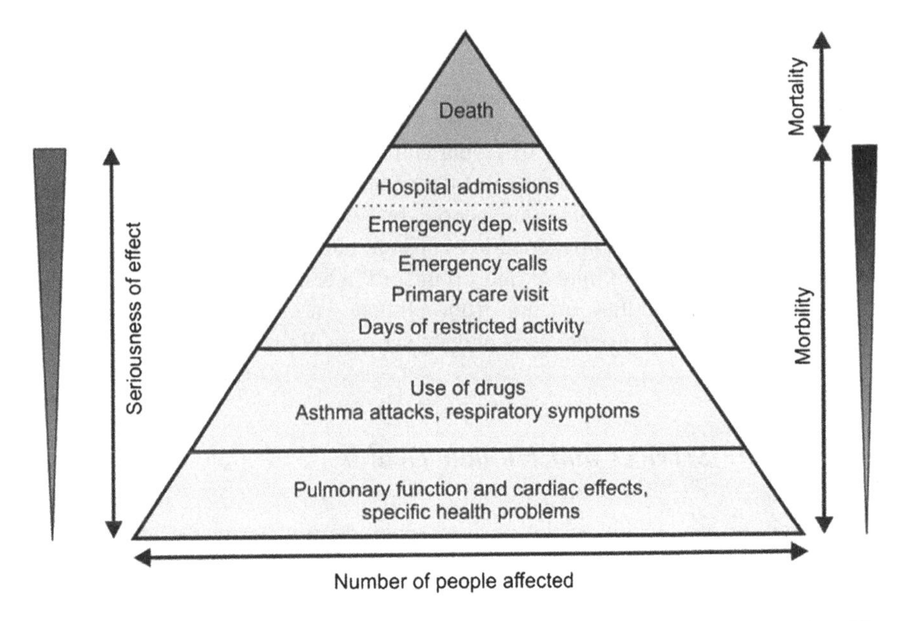

Fig. 3 Environmental effects on cardio-respiratory diseases. *Source* Modified according EEA (2013)

in morbility, restricted activity or experience some discomfort, are managed by citizens themselves. In consequence only the direct participation of population can provide useful information into a system. It is at this point, where moving from structured data systems to unstructured ones such as big data becomes a need to improve the health related climate services in the future.

One aspect that should be emphasized is that neither the weather nor climate makes people sick "per se" in most cases. The improvement and the worsening in relation to the health status is a reaction due to a specific atmospheric change or situation [27]. Consequently, the confusing use of the terms "climate" and "weather" in the context of impacts on human health should be clarified even if they are used indifferently in many cases. The weather describes the conditions and atmospheric changes in a short period of hours or days at a given location. Instead, the climate is a theoretical concept that contains the set of conditions and atmospheric processes in terms of a wide spatial temporal distribution of climatic elements. Variations and extreme events that characterized a region or a place are also included. Moreover, climate is defined through statistical parameters of atmospheric elements in a long time period (by convention 30 years). Furthermore, it is possible to describe climatic features through the irregular succession of circulation weather types, which individually would not constitute the climate of a region.

Due to this statistical characterization of climate, it would not be possible to say that climate influences human health [28], even if, in reality, it has effects and clearly impacts. Nevertheless, the sum and frequency of these atmospheric situations and circulation weather types allow us to characterize precisely climate at a place over an extended period because climate is the long term of weather. In conclusion, the concept climate can be understood in two ways. The first is the one that corresponds to the term "weather", in relation to the direct effects of particular atmospheric situations; however, the second relates to the effects of frequent exposure to such situations.

Another aspect that must be taken into account is that climate and weather-related impacts can be direct or indirect [23]. The first refers to weather elements or atmospheric phenomena, such as temperature, humidity, solar radiation, atmospheric pressure, cold and heat waves or other extreme events such as droughts, floods, etc., which exert environmental pressure on human beings with certain frequency and intensity. Indirect effects, on the other hand, are the result of anomalous changes of natural processes or of human activities. For example, the unusual alteration of natural systems processes can prolong periods of pollination, change the spectrum of allergens, spread infectious vector-borne diseases and reduce food production or oscillations on drinkable water availability.

Furthermore, the complexity of the atmospheric environment increases when it is considered how atmospheric elements interact simultaneously among themselves (air temperature, atmospheric pressure, solar radiation, etc.) and produce synergic impacts on human health. Consequently, a problem arises in trying to reduce the impact to one or more relevant or dominant parameters [29, 30]. It should also be mentioned that aside from the mentioned negative effects, there are also climate and weather-related positive ones. A good example is climate-therapy as a part of preventive medicine and rehabilitation for the improvement of many, especially of atopic, diseases. The purpose is to cure and improve the health status through the exposure of appropriate climatic conditions which can generate calming and toning effects. This requires looking for places that meet favorable climatic conditions for the therapy of these kind of pathologies that we want to improve [31]. For example, climate therapy is common in regions of medium-high mountains. These areas are characterized by clean air, pollution-free, reduced air humidity and a minimum concentration of aero-allergens, which is favorable for atopic asthma or dermatitis [32–35].

Given these complex relationships between human health and the environment, there is an important gap between climate services developers and health communities [36]. A kind of disconnection has been observed between these two spheres of knowledge which is expressed in many cases by a lack of mutual understanding, coordination and different approaches or terminology. It is especially important that actors of both sectors start sharing knowledge and information to produce effective climate services in terms of being useful in public health management. A good example of a development of a health-related climate service can be seen in the context of the heatwaves effects on morbi-mortality that led to the development of heat warning systems in many countries around the world [37]. However, there are important limitations in order to close this gap between climate services and health communities in the future.

An important limitation is the different spatial-temporal scales in the data registered and used by the respective actors. These approaches are derived on the one hand of scientific knowledge and skills, and on the other of needs. For the study and understanding of environmental health the geographical scale is essential. Health and climate are characterized by unique spatial and temporal patterns, which combine the different factors at multiple scales. For example, there is a temporary discrepancy in the flu cases data available which are reported in epidemiological weeks, but the weather-related effects on health occur with the daily atmospheric conditions. In addition, medical information is usually summarized in administrative units which do not coincide spatially with climatic regions, or more generally, with environmental spaces.

Hence, the challenge is to combine very heterogeneous databases of high quality (environmental, meteorological, socioeconomic and medical) at international, national, regional and local levels. The information should be combined to express risks and human vulnerabilities in short, medium and long temporal terms. Historical and real time data should also facilitate the development of climate and weather related health services. However, in relation to health data, we find a legal problem of sensitivity due to confidentiality of the information, a barrier that complicates particularly the implantation of climate services in administrative terms.

Future services are tightly linked to the availability and the access to health information. This fact brings us another problem which is that climate and weather-related impacts on human health are particularly concentrated in the Least developed Countries (LDCs) where the vulnerable population is very high and do not have proper infrastructures to provide or even use climate services [38]. According to the WHO [39], it is essential to understand the health effects of climate change within the overall context of global health and health equity. Ultimately, the lack of population's health competence is very linked to equity differences [40] in these countries, but also in highly developed countries it can be observed. In addition and complementary, there is an increasing gap also in relation to digital competence [41].

2.2 From Traditional to Big Data Infrastructures

Information systems have traditionally been designed and constructed on structured databases systems which are mainly based on relational database design. The Entity Relation (ER) model defines the conceptual view of a database based on entities or real world objects and the existing associations or relationships among entities. Each entity can be described with attributes which are used to define the degree of the relationship among entities. At the present time, Big Data is becoming widely used in a society of increasing data volume, as a result of an exponential evolution of information of different types. The term Big Data refers, foremost, to volumes of large, complex, linkable information. In many ways, size is the only dimension that is conspicuous when we mention Big Data but according to Gandomi and Haider [42] there are six basic characterizing features:

- Volume, the magnitude of data.
- Variety, as structural heterogeneity.
- Velocity, generation and analyzing rate.
- Veracity, the lack of reliability.
- Variability, variation in the data flow rates.
- Value, low value density.

2.2.1 Earth System Data

Given the main features, the Earth System Data represent a clear example of Big Data. It is mainly heterogeneous information with a diverse spatial-temporal range, based on observations, modeling, forecasting, and simulation from multidisciplinary perspectives (Climatology, Oceanography, Geology, Geography, etc.) of the Earth as a system [43]. Just one of these elements, such as the atmospheric forecasting, requires an extraordinary amount of empirical data and continuous modelling of the information.

Different systems are capturing and storing remote data in order to understand physical and chemical processes related to the climate change problem. The World Climate Research Program (WCRP) is acting in this direction with the Core Projects initiatives (CliC, CLIVAR, GEWEX, SPARC and CORDEX) and with other co-sponsored activities. An important feature is that many Earth Science datasets are freely available for all users, an essential requirement when referring to climate services [24, 38]. Furthermore, the increase of spatial-temporal resolution of data is becoming a key element in Earth Science disciplines such as Climatology and Meteorology, but also in many others. Earth Science datasets formats have spatial-temporal large capacities (netCDF, HDF5 or GRIB) and an interface for scientific data access which allow a multidimensional structure and the exchange of data independently of the operating system used.

The indoor environmental information is also essential to understand environmental related health patterns. This is less considered even though in many cases, people are exposed very few hours per day to the outdoor conditions. It should be noted that the methods, computation and visualization require other approaches; various tools, techniques and frameworks given the mentioned features of Big Data. The complexity of Big Data, which are mostly unstructured data, has consequences in databases that change to a no-relational model. One of the databases used for Big Data is Hadoop, an Open-Source-Framework that allows applications to work with multiple nodes in parallel [44]. Besides the data management, the procedures are much linked to find patterns among datasets, analytics which include new forms of visualization, machine learning and artificial intelligence [44, 45]. In medical diagnostic procedures, where pattern are crucial, machine intelligence, probabilistic neural network, support vector machine or classic methods such as principal component analysis become increasingly important for better diagnosis [46–49].

2.2.2 Medical System Data

Any study based on transdisciplinary interactions demands access to a wide variety of datasets. One of the most difficult sectors to access information is the sanitary community. This access is even much more complicated when access in real time is required. For example, the disease codification is based on the International Classification of Diseases (ICD), but in many cases, two versions of the classification must be considered simultaneously. This classification is formed by big groups and many subgroups that correspond to specific diagnostics of multiple diseases. Certain types of diseases are especially relevant in terms of the global impact they can have. They belong to the infectious diseases such as influenza or meningitis and real time data are essential to prevent major impacts. An important characteristic to emphasize in health information, and similar to the Earth Science, is the scale or the different levels of health informatics (for example, molecular, tissue, patient or population) [50].

In the area of health, a well-known example Big Data is "Google flu" that makes use of search queries to estimate the trend of influenza activity in 25 countries, although there are large errors in the prediction compared to official records [51]. However, it is important to note that the quantity of data does not imply to waive, especially in science, traditional methods nor the disappearance of issues of measurement, validity construct, reliability or dependencies among data [51, 52], since in many cases, these data do not have controlled the output of instruments that involve precisely the validity and reliability, which is considered the basis of scientific analysis.

Moreover, even if robust patterns are found through Big Data, it is necessary to obtain evidence of causality and health-related utility. For example, possible medical treatments based on Big Data need to be tested in controlled scientific studies [53]. However, in the context of health-related climate services, sanitary databases present several problems:

- First, the health information is unstructured or not digitized for use by external users. Some of the diagnostics are literal descriptions which imply that there is a subjective component in the codification.
- Second, closely related is the high sensitivity of the data due to the protection of personal data. In addition, security issues are also linked, which can be significant in the Big Data domain and require new approaches such as biometric authentication, encryption or watermarking [54–61]. Precisely, this aspect changes when it comes to data derived from public applications in which citizens actively participate such as social networks.

- Third, the state of the information in the health system is not necessarily optimal or sufficient for the development of climate service since its creation has a different purpose, mainly administrative and management. This fact leads us to the need to create new specific records.
- Fourth, in some cases, health data are not standardized for exchanging and, access to standard formats through administrative channels can be very complex. Moreover, the information is not always centralized and can be split into multiple different administrations levels or institution in a particular country. The problem is even greater when it comes to health information beyond the borders of a country.
- Fifth, there are problems of definition and/or criteria for much health data. For example, in the case of hospital admission, you can find patients with clinical symptoms of influenza who enter in a hospital with the primary diagnosis of influenza but in another hospital they are admitted with a primary code correspondent to other cardiovascular or respiratory disease.
- Sixth, it is related to the number of people affected by climate-weather impacts and the degree of severity of the effect. There are no records when severity is low even if many people are affected. These circumstances are more frequent than extreme events but they do not leave any trace in the health system. The relevance of these particular cases for the administration is practically poor. Eventually, the cost to the health system of less severe effects with most affected population may exceed those that are more serious but with less affected population [62].

Apart from earth and health data, it is also necessary to incorporate other data sources for the development of climate services including socio-economic, financial, geographical data and even population data since the health status of the population is determined by social and individual factors such as attitudes, engagements, social resistance, emotional and psychological states. In this context, collecting observational data becomes a major concern because they have many *biases* due to selection, confounding variables and even the lack of generalization. In epidemiological research, this problem is known as the unsolvable dilemma of generalization-individualization [31]. This dilemma illustrates a well-known fact: the results represent an average of one specific group and are little reliable for extrapolations at individual levels.

Regardless of the use of big data or more traditional sources, it is imperative for the creation of any climate service that the objective be specifically formulated to know where to look at in order to validate the work hypothesis. Some concluding aspects to think about in relation to the creation of climate services would be: changing policies in order to make data and services more easily available, deepening in risk management, constructing a framework for active participation of the population, intensifying research on climate-weather-related effects and the implementation of corresponding services, supporting inter- and transdisciplinary work groups with all actors, creating new climate-weather and health data, and homogenizing and building spatial-temporal datasets.

2.3 The Big Wall of Digital Divide

Despite the development of the information society or precisely of this new form of society, we are faced a big wall of increasing digital divide in all socioeconomic, cultural, geographical scales. The term 'digital divide' describes the discrepancy between individuals, households, business and geographic areas regarding their access and usage of Information Communications Technology and the variety of Internet [63]. The concept also describes the gap between those with the skills, knowledge and abilities, or the digital competence [41, 64] to use the new technologies and those without them. There are two competences that have been considered essential by the European Center for the Development of Vocational Training [66] (CEDEFOP):

- ICT skills as the ability to use a computer or the Internet
- Scientific technological skills as the ability to use scientific and technical tools.

The technological revolution, digital culture and competence are essential to implement co-design theory and co-production at any level. The technological revolution and digital society require circular knowledge where thinkers, workers and user speak the same language to avoid breaks in the synergies that are generated by the use of digital tools (Fig. 4).

Despite the fact that most of the developed countries have and are preparing their national e-government and e-health platforms [53] in the health community a good example is the use of electronic medical records that patients must be able to interact, but at the same time many older people, or other vulnerable groups, may be unprepared for this kind of new digital interactions. Furthermore, low health competence is associated with significantly less use of the Internet for health information among older people [67]. The increasing digital services, in this context the climate health-related, could exacerbate the digital divide.

Eventually, the local context and the geography is the key element to understand and reduce the disparities between multiple communities and groups.

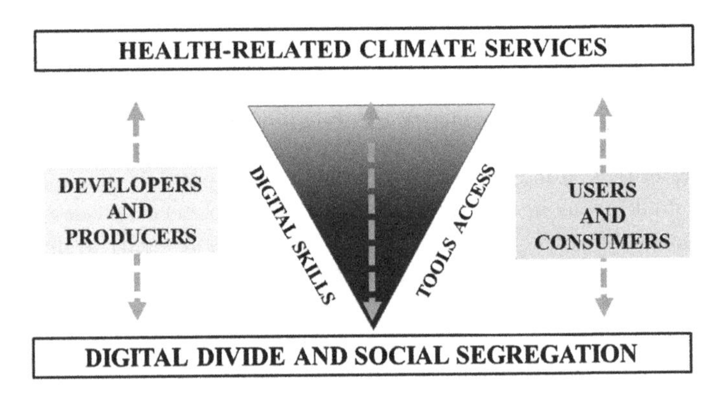

Fig. 4 Digital divide and health related climate services

3 A Case Study: A Climate Relate Health Service

The example presented here is just an example of a climate/weather relate health service in the field of Biometeorology that has been created under the co-creation approach and concepts mentioned in the previous sections.

The main components of the biometeorological data structures are a scientific conceptual model; a technological infrastructure and platform; a relational database management system with a structured datasets and procedures; different groups of users (Fig. 5).

This work has been designed under the circular learning philosophy and the systems must be updated permanently in its conceptual and technological dimensions. Users and stakeholder feedback is useful to:

- re-think the original scientific concepts
- update the technological infrastructure and new procedures
- incorporate new unstructured sources of datasets
- improve the existing services to stakeholders and users
- increase the efficiency of the early warning system

The main limitation of the proposed system radicates on the lack of monitorization of biophysical parameters of citizens nowadays on real time but this an ongoing process. A second limitation is related to accuracy and precision of the temporal and spatial resolution of meteorological data collection. In many cases, empirical values of the closet atmospheric environment of a person are based on false geostatistical assumptions. On the other hand, complexity of studying how changes of meteorological variables at a very high temporal resolution (miliseconds, hectoseconds, deciseconds or minutes) can affect our health through their impacts on basic microorganisms such as enzimes, bacterias or viruses becomes an unexplored world yet.

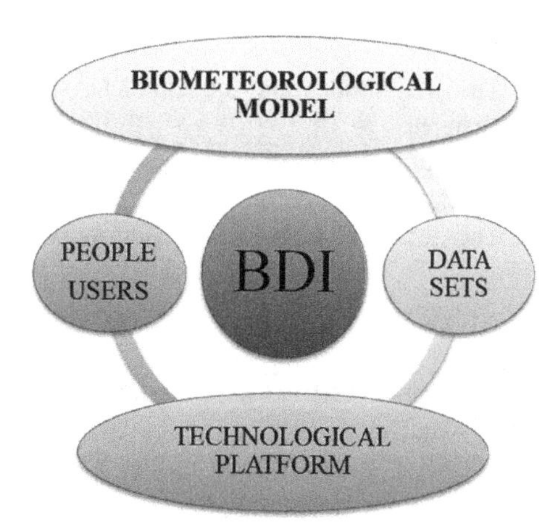

Fig. 5 Biometeorological data infrastructure

The future scope of the Oxyalert system is to be able to define the biometeorological vulnerability of each user of the system in relation to each meteorological factors change (sun radiation, air temperature, air humidity, oxygen changes, heat persistance…). In this sense, a individualized biometeorological profile will be elaborated for each human being in the same way a genetic map can be produced nowadays in biological science. Artificial intelligence and machine learning will be essential in reaching this future scope.

3.1 The Scientific and Conceptual Model

The scientific hypothesis represents an example of a weather-related health service. The conceptual model has been developed attending to the partial density of atmospheric oxygen inter-daily changes and it is the result of a much more complex process of knowledge integration from different scientific disciplines, such as Geography, Medicine, Ecology, Climatology, Cartography, Biometeorology and Biophysics.

Some previous studies [21, 68, 69] indicate that changes in the amount of oxygen at the horizontal surface layer in the atmosphere can have the same impact on human health as those which occur when a person moves to a very high altitude in a short period of time without considering any previous acclimatization process. In this sense, changes in the amount of oxygen in the atmosphere are constantly impacting quietly on citizen's health all around the world based on the same principle.

A quick increase in the oxygen availability produces hyperoxia conditions and a sudden decrease of oxygen availability implies hypoxia conditions. Depending on the type of variation, impacts can affect different social targets in terms of public health.

The harmfulness of the impacts of these changes will also be determined by three parameters that are usually considered for the assessment of any geophysical risk:

- The magnitude and the characteristics of the impact generated by oxygen changes
- The vulnerability of each person to each meteorological factor and to each type of change
- The degree of exposure of each individual to oxygen changes (Fig. 6).

3.2 The Technological Infrastructure

The technological infrastructure is formed by a group of electronic devices, different software and procedures. It represents the seed for the future development of

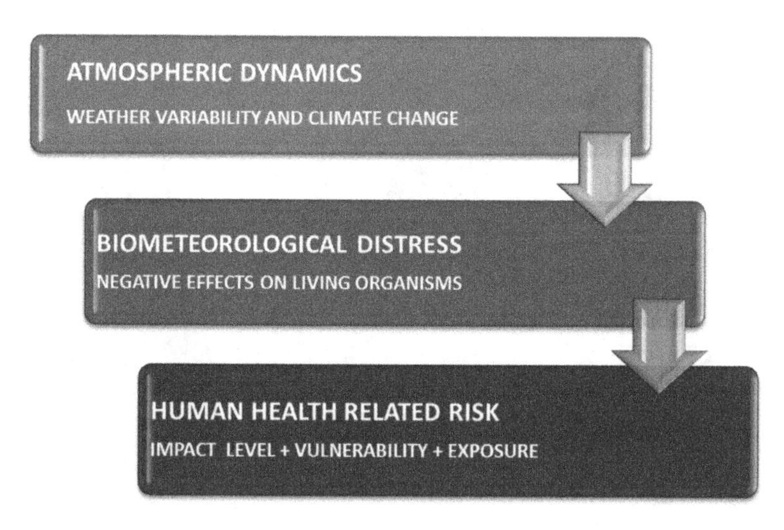

Fig. 6 From atmospheric dynamics to human health risk

a big data infrastructure for the development of climate services related to human health. The main component of the system is a mainframe which is in charge of searching for global meteorological information in the North American Ocean Administration (NOA) center to download the Global Forecast System meteorological datasets which are facilitated every six hours for several days in advance. A de-codification process of the GRIB format in which the obtained meteorological information is stored is carried out, and the biometeorological model is applied to compute the partial density of the atmospheric oxygen for the whole world at a spatial resolution of 0.25°. Resulting grids with the oxygen forecasting values are split and saved automatically into multiple files (Fig. 7).

The second element of the infrastructure is a mobile application called Oxyalert Beta [70] which can be freely downloaded from Google Play. The App Oxyalert offers an early warning system based on the results of the biometeorological model computed in the server. When the App is started, a list of complex processes of checking services, identifying users, registering geopositioning, accessing to oxygen data for the registered X, Y coordinates and transferring the forecasting information from the server to the mobile device take place in a short period of time (Fig. 8).

Next, the computed parameters are transferred to the citizen's mobile devices where the forecasting for the following three days is presented graphically in two different figures where relative changes every 6 h and the oxygen evolution curve can be seen.

There is a widget in the application that constantly shows the oxygen difference in grams per cubic meters (gr/m^3) at the user location:moreover, the warning system presets alerts to the user by changing the color of the widget depending on the risk level generated by the change at each geographical location. It is important to

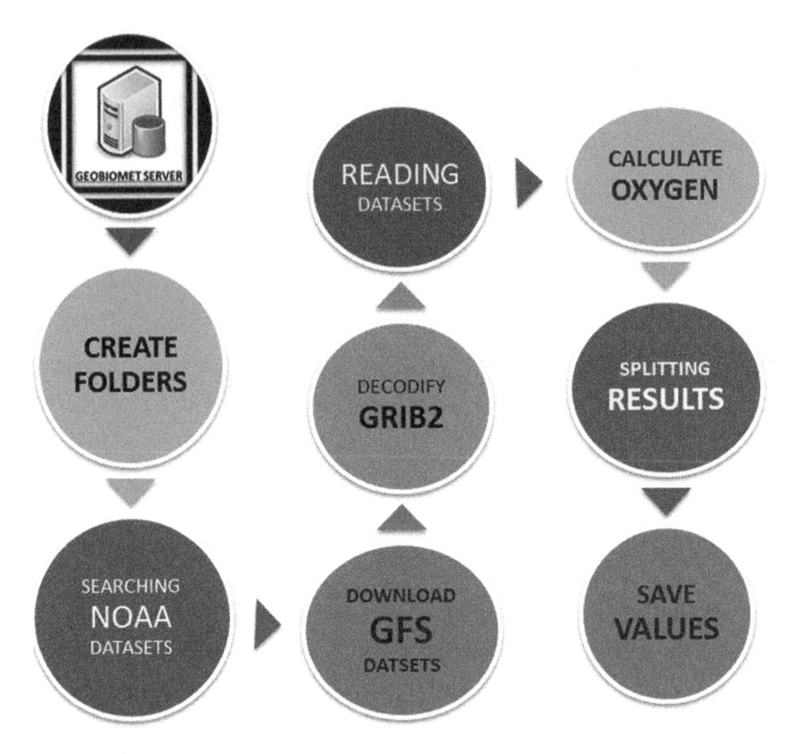

Fig. 7 Sequence of procedures develop by the central server to compute partial density of atmospheric oxygen values

indicate that risk levels are relative. This means that the same warning level responds to different values of change depending on the geographic location of the user (Fig. 9).

The platform registers user feedback to biometeorological oxygen warnings through a questionnaire that is opened automatically in the smartphone when certain thresholds of impact are reached in the closest physical environment of the users. This is an essential part of the co-production model in order to re-think and re-design the scientific theories and the technological tools that are used. The questionnaire can be started and filled in by users also at any time if they want to inform the system about their health state even if there is no biometeorological warning.

Users facilitate important information in relation to headaches, muscular pain, and emotional state or sleep quality among other issues. This information is stored in the relational database management system in the technological platform. Citizens also facilitate personal information such as date of birth or gender or the existence of previous diseases when they register to download the application which is very useful in later analysis. Registration and questionnaire forms are shown in Fig. 10.

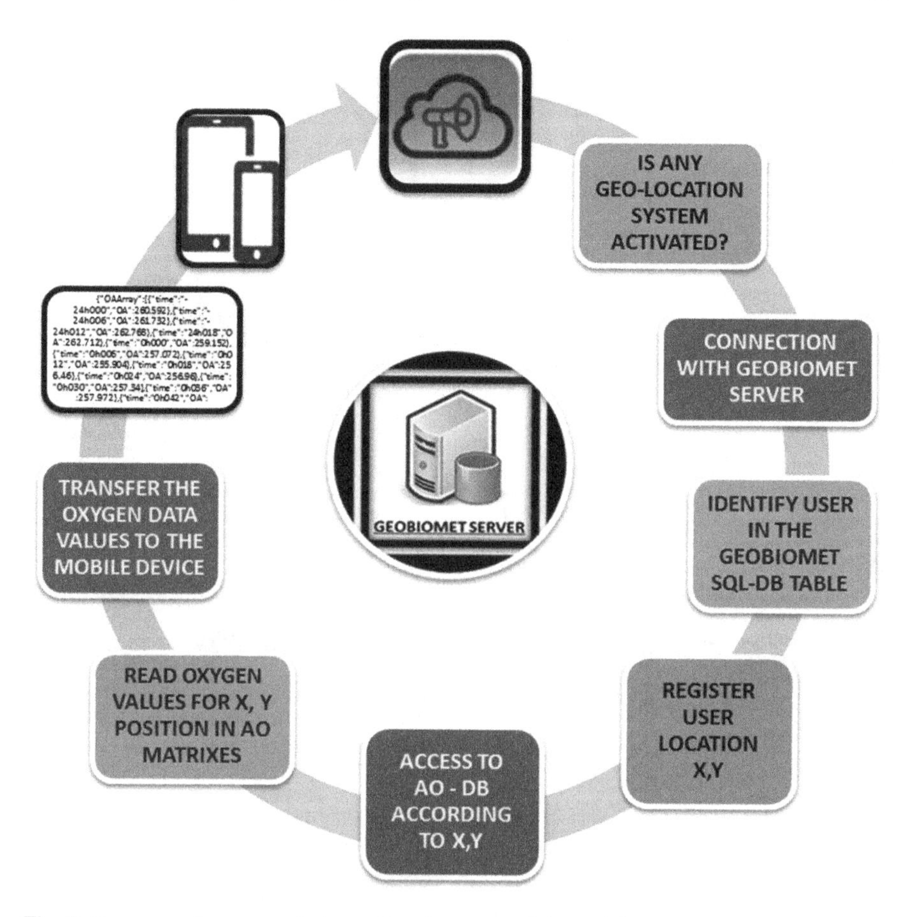

Fig. 8 Sequence of processes between Oxyalert app and the mainframe

3.3 Products and Services Provided

The main services facilitated by the systems respond to a wide range of scientific social and personal needs. On one hand, four global oxygen maps (GOM) are produced automatically daily. This information can be an extraordinary input for other biophysical studies related to global change and sustainability such as biodiversity and deforestation, fires spreading or deoxygenation of oceans and phytoplankton production, among other topics. Moreover, global risks maps are also defined based on the oxygen differences over 24 h.

Secondly, personal alerts are given to each user when oxygen changes are over the limits for the place where they are and information on the forecasting of changes for the following three days is also facilitated. This can be extremely useful for meteo-sensitive people who have some respiratory or cardiovascular chronic

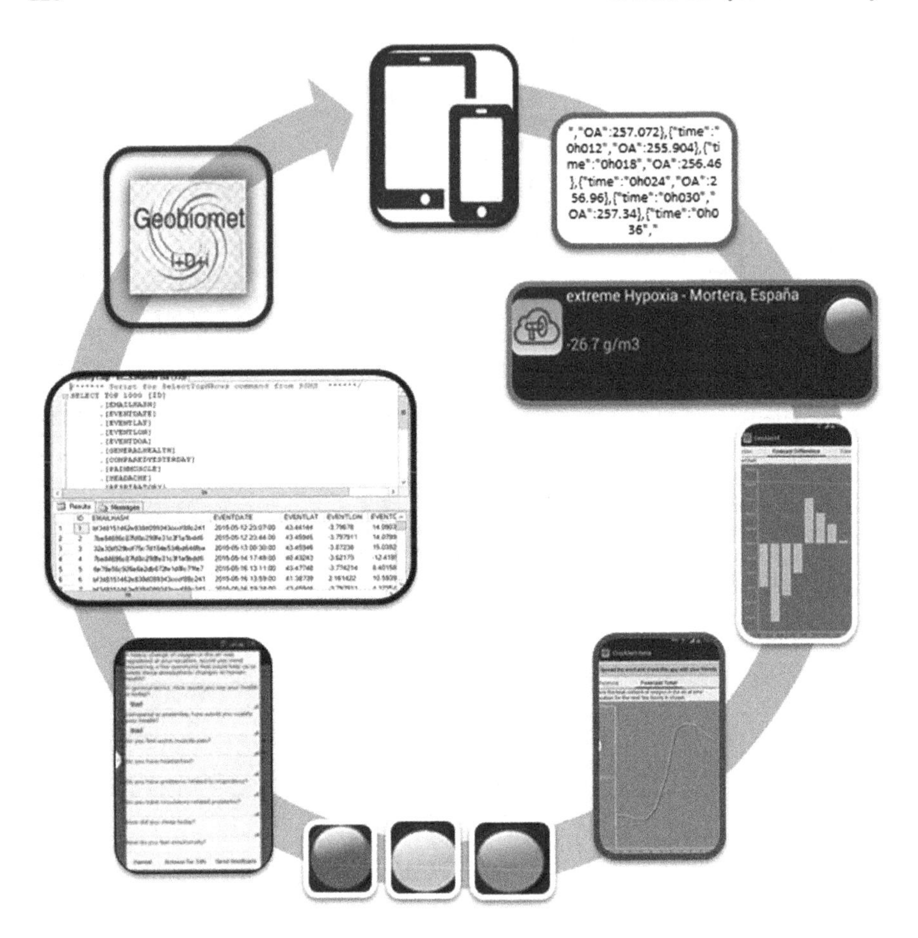

Fig. 9 Computation of oxygen differences and alerts in the App

disease or the elderly for whom hyperoxia or hypoxia changes can represent a serious health hazard.

Finally, people who commit to the project by sending daily reports can receive his/her own biometeorological profile in relation to oxygen changes after 1 year through the mobile application. This is a clear example of citizen science where user participation through a social software tool can provide personal knowledge management.

It is important that preliminary results have confirmed an initial theory that says that in temperate areas of the world, autumn is a season when stronger changes on the partial density of the atmospheric oxygen take place compared to summer time. Apart from the ability to anticipate impact colectivily, the system offers us the possibility to give personal advice to users who have reported how they feel with

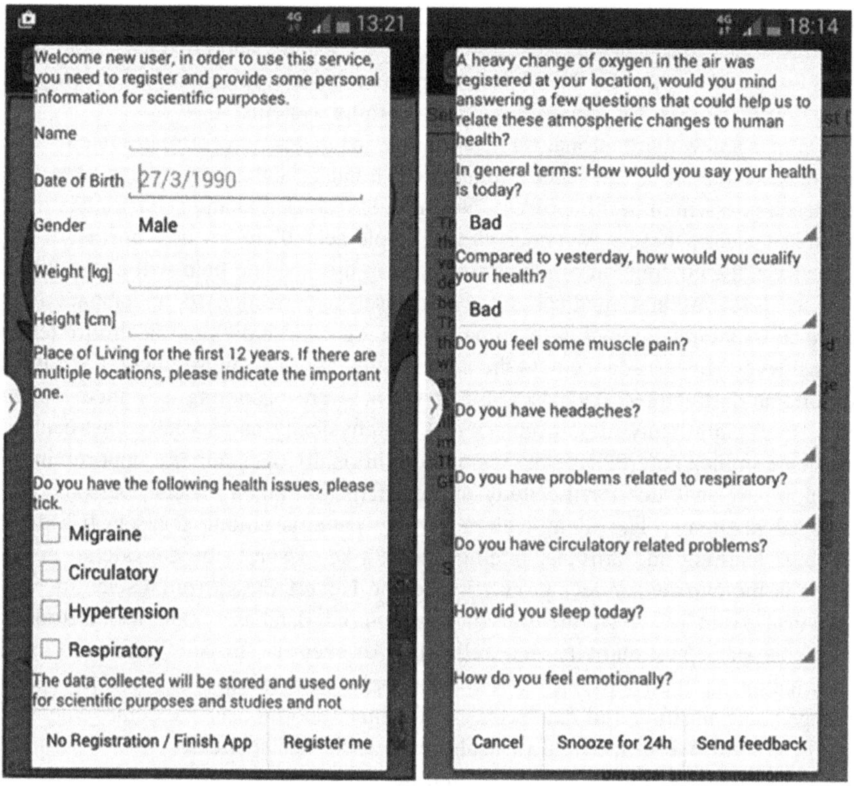

Fig. 10 Users registration and health reports forms

each change. This is what has been called previously Customized Early Warning Systems which consist of adapting the general risk warning to the specific vulnerability of each user.

4 Conclusions

Co-creation and co-production of knowledge are essential in the definition and implantation of global and personalized health-related climate services based on earth and health information. Interdisciplinary and transdisciplinary are two characteristics of these studies, and scientific design should be part of this circular process. The European Union has included the issue of co-creation in science on the research agenda at the highest level, and bottom-up initiatives, such as Future Earth national committees, have already been created in several European countries.

Many subtle effects of weather changes or situations on human health go unnoticed for society and citizens, especially for the administration. Climate change has brought this topic onto the daily agenda of politicians. Decision-makers, health systems, meteorological services, researchers, companies and citizens should confront this problem through the development of a transdisciplinary biometeorological approach that leads, for example, to early warning systems.

There is a new international framework (GFCS) to develop warning systems able to forecast the climate/weather impact on human health, and the co-creation approach is essential in this process. Nevertheless, academia and stakeholders must be able to learn these new concepts and implement them in their normal work. Otherwise, the co-creation of new knowledge in this specific field will not succeed.

Earth systems and medical massive datasets are needed to understand how physical structures interact with human physiology and individual health to define impact levels. In accordance with the increasingly complex environment, the related systems and structured databases used until now are becoming a limited tool in order to explain many circumstances that are physically and socially unstructured by their complex nature. Big data seems to additionally open a major opportunity to develop new analytics for the study of the interaction among social, personal and physical phenoma. The identification of new patterns among datasets based on machine learning and artificial intelligence is a key issue to be considered in the future in the climate services production sector. Nevertheless, from a scientific and statistical point of view, the use of unstructured databases can also introduce problems of representativity and reliability of records. In any case, real time information is indispensable to define people vulnerability to meteorological changes, and unstructured databases can facilitate enormously the achievement of this new challenge in the field of health-related climate services.

Undoubtedly, the technological revolution plays an important role in this process but it can also be a very serious limitation if people, at all levels, are not able to overcome the digital divide that this kind of revolution implies.

The Oxyalert infrastructure is an ongoing project that offers a climate/weather related health service under the co-creation philosophy where citizen participation is essential to re-think and re-design the technological platform, the early warning systems and the conceptual biometeorological model. It is an example of constructing new knowledge based on a participatory process of users and stakeholders where individual experiences become the raw material to define, on the one hand global alerts and, on the other, a customized service based on information on how each person's health and well-being is affected by a specific physical factor, such as the atmospheric oxygen. It is therefore necessary to generalize the recording of health reports from people as an essential way to describe the well-being of citizens and the population in general.

Acknowledgments Funding support has been received from the Spanish Minister of Economy and Competiveness through the National Funding Budget applied to the national project CSO2013-46153-R. The Geobiomet Research Group would like to thank this institutional support in the field of Biometeorology.

References

1. Teich, M., Porter, R., Gustafsson, B.: Nature and Society in Historical Context. Cambridge University Press. ISBN 0521498813 (1997)
2. Barona, J.L., Cherry, S. (eds.): Health and Medicine in Rural Europe (1850–1945) Seminari d'Estudis sobre la Ciencia. Universitat de Valencia ISBN 84-370-6334-5
3. IPCC Fourth and Fifth Assessment Report: Climate Change 2007 Working Group II contribution to AR4 "Impacts, Adaptation and Vulnerability" and to AR5 "Impacts Adaptation and Vulnerability"
4. COP21 Climate Action, United Nation Framework Convention on Climate Change. http://www.cop21paris.org/ (2015). Accessed June 2016
5. Drucker, P.: The Age of the Social Transformation. Atlantic Mon, p. 274 (1966)
6. Servon, L.J.: Bridging the Digital Divide, Technology, Community and Public Policy. Blackwell Publishing (2002)
7. Warschauer, M.: Technology and Social Inclusion. Rethinking the digital divide. The MIT Press, Massachusetts (2004)
8. OECD (1996) The Knowledge-Based Society. Paris
9. EPA https://www3.epa.gov/climatechange/impacts/health.html. Accessed 12 Jan 2016
10. Gobal Framework for Climate Services http://www.wmo.int/gfcs/. Accessed 5 May 2016
11. Mauser, W., Klepper, G., Rice, M., Schmalzbauer, B.S., Hackmann, H., Leemans, R., Moore, H.: Transdisciplinary global change research: the co-creation of knowledge for sustainability. Curr. Opin. Environ. Sustain. **5**(3–4), 420–431 (2013). ISSN 1877-3435
12. Future Earth Initial Design Report http://www.icsu.org/future-earth/media-centre/relevant_publications/future-earth-initial-design-report. Accessed 20 June 2016
13. Tress, B., Tress, G., Fry, G.: Potential and limitations of interdisciplinary and transdisciplinary landscape studies. In: Tress, B., Tress, G., Van der Valk, A., et al. (eds.): Interdisciplinarity and Transdisciplinarity in Landscape Studies: Potential and Limitations. Delta Program, Wageningen, pp. 182–192. Delta Series no. 2 (2003)
14. Tress, B., Tress, G., Fry, G.: Integrative studies on rural landscapes: policy expectations and research practice. Landscape Urban Plan. **70**(1/2), 177–191 (2005)
15. Nonaka, I., Toyama, R.: The theory of the knowledge-creating firm: subjectivity, objectivity and synthesis. Ind. Corp. Change **14**(3), 419–436 (2005). doi:10.1093/icc/dth058
16. Nonaka, I.: A dynamic theory of knowledge creation. Organ. Sci. **5**(1), 1437 (1994)
17. Nonaka, I., Takeuchi, H.: The Knowledge Creating Company: How Japanese Companies Create the Dynamics of Innovation. Oxford University Press, New York (1997). (1995)
18. Humphreys, P., Samson, A., Roser, T., Cruz-Valdivieso, E.: Co-creation: New Pathways to Value. An Overview, LSE Enterprise, Promise Corporation (2009)
19. Leach, M.: Co-design for relevance and usefulness. Future Earth Blog by Sayer L. http://www.futureearth.org/blog/2014-jul-23/co-design-relevance-and-usefulness-qa-melissa-leach (2014). Accessed 14 May 2016
20. Future Earth Booklet http://www.futureearth.org/media/future-earth-booklet-what-future-earth. Accessed 15 May 2016
21. Fdez-Arroyabe, P.: Climate change, local weather and customized early warning systems based on biometeorological indexes. J. Earth Sci. Eng. **5**(2015), 173–181 (2015). doi:10.17265/2159-581X/2015.03.002
22. Samand, A., Wohlfart, L., Wolf, P.: Hands-on Knowledge Co-creation and Sharing: Practical Methods and Techniques. ISBN 978-951-6350-0 (2007)
23. McMichael, A.J.: Globalization, climate change, and human health. (Review article). The New Engl. J. Med. **2013**(368), 1335–1343 (2013). doi:10.1056/NEJMra1109341
24. Hewitt, C., Mason, S., Walland, D.: The global framework for climate services. Nat. Clim. Change **2**, 831–832 (2012)
25. Gavidia, V., Talavera, M.: La construcción del concepto de salud. Didáctica de las Ciencias Experimentales y Sociales **26**, 161–175 (2012)

26. Laschewski, G., Jendritzky, G.: Effects of the thermal environment on human health: an investigation of 30 years of daily mortality data from SW Germany. Clim. Res. **21**, 91–103 (2002)
27. Schuh, A.: Angewandte medizinische Klimatologie. Grundlagen und Praxis. Sonntag Verlag, Stuttgart (1996)
28. Eis, D., Helm, D., Laußmann, D., Stark, K. (eds.): Klimawandel und Gesundheit—Ein Sachstandsbericht. Robert Koch-Institut, Berlin (2010)
29. Kalkstein, L.S.: A new approach to evaluate the impact of climate upon human mortality. Environ. Health Perspect. **96**, 145–150 (1991)
30. Jendritzky, G.: The atmospheric environment—an introduction. Experientia **49**, 733–740 (1993)
31. Jendritzky, G., Bucher, K., Laschewski, G., Schultz, E., Staiger, H.: Medizinische Klimatologie, en: Handbuch der Balneologie und Medizinischen Klimatologie, ed. Por Gutenbrunnere Hildebrandt. Springer, Heidelberg (1998)
32. Rijssenbeek-Nouwens, L.H., Bel, E.H.: High-altitude treatment: a therapeutic option for patients with severe, refractory asthma? Clin. Exp. Allergy **41**, 775–782 (2011)
33. Schuh, A., Nowak, D.: Klimatherapie im Hochgebirge und im Meeresklima. Evidente Akut- und Langzeiteffekte—ein qualitativer Review. Dtsch. Med. Wochenschr. **136**, 135–139 (2011)
34. Rjissenbeek-Nouwens, L.H., Fieten, K.B., Bron, A.O., Hashimoto, S., Bel, E.H., Weersink, E.J.: High-altitude treatment in atopic and nonatpic patients with severe asthma. Eur. Respir. J. **40**, 1320–1321 (2012)
35. Massimo, T., Blank, C., Strasser, B., Schobersberger, W.: Does climate therapy at moderate altitudes improve pulmonary function in asthma patients? A systematic review. Sleep Breath. **18**, 195–206 (2014)
36. Jancloes, M., Thomson, M., Máñez Costa, M., Corvalan, C., Dinku, T., Lowe, R., Hayden, M., Hewitt, C.: Climate services to improve public health. Int. J. Environ. Res. Public Health **11**, 4555–4559 (2014)
37. Toloo, G., FitzGerald, G., Aitken, P., Verrall, K., Tong, S.: Evaluating the effectiveness of heat warning systems: systematic review of epidemiological evidence. Int. J. Public Health **58**, 667–681 (2013)
38. Connora, S.J., Omumbo, J., Green, C., DaSilva, J., Mantilla, G., Delacollette, C., Hales, S., Rogers, D., Thomson, M.: Health and climate—needs. Proc. Environ. Sci. **1**, 27–36 (2010)
39. WHO: Protecting Health from Climate Change: Global Research Priorities. World Health Organization, Geneva (2009)
40. WHO (2012) Health education: theoretical concepts, effective strategies and core competencies. A foundation document to guide capacity development of health educators. World Health Organization. Regional Office for the Eastern Mediterranean
41. Janssen, J., Stoyanov, S., Ferrari, A., Punie, Y., Pannekeet, K., Sloep, P.: Experts' views on digital competence: Commonalities and differences. Comput. Educ. **68**, 473–481 (2013)
42. Gandomi, A., Haider, M.: Beyond the hype: big data concepts, methods, and analytics. Int. J. Inf. Manage. **35**, 137–144 (2015)
43. Baumann, P., Mazzetti, P., Ungar, J., Barbera, R., Barboni, D., Beccati, A., Bigagli, L., Boldrini, E., Bruno, R., Calanducci, A., Campalani, P., Clements, O., Dumitru, A., Grant, M., Herzig, P., Kakaletris, G., Laxton, J., Koltsida, P., Lipskoch, K., Mahdiraji, A.R., Mantovani, S., Merticariu, V., Messina, A., Misev, D., Natali, S., Nativi, S., Oosthoek, J., Pappalardo, M., Passmore, J., Rossi, A.P., Rundo, F., Sen, M., Sorbera, V., Sullivan, D., Torrisi, M., Trovato, L., Veratelli, M.G., Wagner, S.: Big data analytics for earth sciences: the earth server approach. Int. J. Digit. Earth **9**, 1 (2016)
44. Sagiroglu, S., Sinanc, D.: Big data: a review. In: 2013 International Conference on Collaboration Technologies and Systems (CTS), San Diego, CA, 2013, pp. 42–47 (2013)
45. Krumholz, H.M.: For A learning health system big data and new knowledge in medicine: the thinking, training, and tools needed. Health Affairs 33(7):1163–1170 (2014)

46. Chatterjee, S., Ghosh, S., Dawn, S., Hore, S., Dey, N.: Optimized forest type classification: a machine intelligence approach. In: Third International Conference on Information System Design and Intelligent Applications, Vishakhapatnam. Springer AISC (In press)
47. Kriti, V.J., Dey, N., Kumar, V.: PCA-PNN and PCA-SVM based CAD systems for breast density classification. In: Hassanien, A.-E., Grosan, C., Fahmy Tolba, M. (ed.) Applications of Intelligent Optimization in Biology and Medicine: Current Trends and Open Problems, pp. 159–180. Springer International Publishing (2016)
48. Thein, H.T.T., Tun, K.M.M.: An approach for breast cancer diagnosis classification using neural network. Adv. Comput. Int. J. (ACIJ) **6**, 1 (2015). doi:10.5121/acij.2015.6101
49. Samanta, S., Choudhury, A., Dey, N., Ashour, A.S., Balas, V.E.: Quantum inspired evolutionary algorithm for scaling factors optimization during manifold medical information embedding. In: Bhattacharyya, S., Maulik, U., Dutta, P. (eds.) Quantum Inspired Computational intelligence: Research and Applications. Elsevier (2016)
50. Herland, M., Khoshgoftaar, T.M., Wald, R.: A review of data mining using big data in health informatics. J. Big Data **1**, 2 (2015)
51. Lazer, D., Kennedy, R., King, G., Vespignani, A.: The parable of google flu: traps in big data analysis. Science **343**, 1203–1205 (2014)
52. King, G.: Ensuring the data-rich future of the social sciences. Science **331**, 719–721 (2011)
53. Khoury, M.J., Ioannidis, J.P.A.: Big data meets public health. Science **346**, 1054 (2014)
54. Nandi, S., Roy, S., Dansana, J., Ben, W., Karaa, A., Ray, R., Chowdhury, S.R., Chakraborty, S., Dey, N.: Cellular automata based encrypted ECG-hash code generation: an application in inter-human biometric authentication system. Int. J. Comput. Netw. Inf. Secur. **6**(11), 1–12 (2014)
55. Biswas, S., Roy, A.B., Ghosh, K., Dey, N.: A biometric authentication based secured ATM banking system. Int. J. Adv. Res. Comput. Sci. Softw. Eng. **2**, 4 (2012)
56. Bose, S., Madhulika, Acharjee, S., Chowdhury, S.R., Chakraborty, S., Dey, N.: Effect of watermarking in vector quantization based image compression. In: Control, Instrumentation, Communication and Computational Technologies (ICCICCT), International Conference Proceedings, pp. 503–508 (2014)
57. Dey, N., Bose, S., Das, A., Chaudhuri, S.S., Saba, L., Shafique, S., Nicolaides, A., Suri, J.S.: Effect of watermarking on diagnostic preservation of atherosclerotic ultrasound video in stroke telemedicine. J. Med. Syst. **40**(4), 1–14 (2016)
58. Dey, N., Ashour, A.S., Chakraborty, S., Banerjee, S., Gospodinova, E., Gospodinov, M., Hassanien, A.E.: Watermarking in bio-medical signal processing. In: Dey, N., Santhi, V. (eds.) Intelligent Techniques in Signal Processing for Multimedia Security. Springer SCI series, (2016)
59. Pal, K., Dey, N., Samanta, S., Das, A., Chaudhuri, S.S.: A hybrid reversible watermarking technique for color biomedical images. In: Computational Intelligence and Computing Research (ICCIC), 2013 IEEE, International Conference Proceedings, pp. 1–6 (2013)
60. Dey, N., Mukhopadhyay, S., Das, A., Chaudhuri, S.S.: Analysis of P-QRS-T components modified by blind watermarking technique within the electrocardiogram signal for authentication in wireless telecardiology using DWT. IJIGSP **4**(7), 33–46 (2012)
61. Acharjee, S., Ray, R., Chakraborty, S., Nath, S., Dey, N.: Watermarking in motion vector for security enhancement of medical videos. In: Control, Instrumentation, Communication and Computational Technologies (ICCICCT), International Conference Proceedings, pp. 532–537 (2014)
62. EEA: Environment and human health, Joint EEA-JRC report Nr 5 (Report EUR 25933 EN), inf. téc., European Environment Agency (2013)
63. Pick, J.B., Sarkar, A.: The Global Digital Divides Explaining Change. Springer, Progress in IS (2015)
64. Fernández de Arroyabe Hernáez, P.: Virtual divide, Bologna education model and geographic information technologies, GeoFocus **6**, 39–51, ISSN: 1578-5157 (2006)
65. Mardikyan, S., Yıldız, E.A., Ordu, M.D., Şimşek, B.: Examining the global digital divide: a cross-country analysis. Commun. IBIMA 2015(592253) (2015). doi:10.5171/2015.592253

66. CEDEFOP: Lifelong Learning: Citizens' Views in Close Up. Center for the Development of Vocational Training (2004)
67. Levy, H., Janke, A.T., Langa, K.M.: Health literacy and the digital divide among older Americans. J. Gen. Intern. Med. **30**, 284–289 (2015)
68. Fernández de Arróyabe, P.: Climate services and human health: a niche of opportunities for economic growth. Scientific Annals of Alexandru Ioan Cuza Geography Series, University of Iasi, Vol. LIX nº 2, Rumania, ISSN: 1223–5334 (printed version), (online version) eISSN 2284-6379 (2013)
69. Fernández de Arróyabe, P.: Meteorological conditions and human health. In: Carlos Garcia-Legaz Martínez y Francisco Valero Rodriguez (eds.) Adverse Weather in Spain. WCRP Spanish Committee & CCS. ISBN: 978-84-96709-88-1 (2013)
70. App OxyAlert Beta (2014) Geobiomet Research Group UC. https://play.google.com/store/apps/details?id=es.geobiomet.oxyalert&hl=es

Part III
Health Informatics

Information and Communication Emerging Technology: Making Sense of Healthcare Innovation

Heru Susanto and Chin Kang Chen

Abstract Information and communication technology (ICT) has contributed a lot of things to support the health system in many aspects and has an impact positively. Information technology even changed on how hospital order stocks activities. E-health system is a stage that uses the ICT to interface different clients; it was intended to convey social insurance. Mobile health information system and internet support public health and clinical care-offers and also it is widely available and can enhancing electronic health for healthcare organization at different level; such as regional, community, and individual levels. Telematics has ease people from afar to do medical check via media usually. One part of e-Health is electronic medical record that contains patients information and accessible by healthcare staff. Clinical decision support system is a system that helps to make a decision regarding their patients matter. Management and maintenance of server should also be watch after as it affects many things in the information technology. Administrative staff also record their patients clinical record and organizing their financial management by using IT. Even robots have replaced some of the position such as doing surgery in health organizations. This study is an attempt to provide a picture of preferences over the information and communication emerging technology to enabling healthcare innovation through big data perspective. The results are interesting. Healthcare innovation through ICT and big data are indispensable elements of a multifaceted approach to forestall medication errors and enhance the patient safety. Clinical staff play a major role in the health organizations as information system in health organization. Improvisation of uniformity and recognition of the design aside from implementation of such systems should also be advantageous to the ICT though big data. Likewise, generating an economic and policy environment

H. Susanto (✉)
Department of Information Management, Tunghai University, Taichung City, Taiwan
e-mail: susanto.net@gmail.com

H. Susanto
Computational Science, The Indonesian Institute of Sciences, Serpong City, Indonesia

C.K. Chen
School of Business and Economics, University of Brunei, Bandar Seri Begawan City, Brunei Darussalam

C. Bhatt et al. (eds.), *Internet of Things and Big Data Technologies for Next Generation Healthcare*, Studies in Big Data 23,
DOI 10.1007/978-3-319-49736-5_10

conducive to the financial intention of hospitals and physicians will facilitate wider adoption of such technology in the health information system sector.

Keywords Mobile health · Health information technology · Clinical decision support system

1 Introduction

As we approach the twentyfirst century, noteworthy changes in data innovation that occur will influence lives. Information system is an arrangement of interrelated parts that gather, control, store and scatter information, data and give a criticism system to meet a goal [1]. Information system nowadays has become the most crucial part in any organization including daily lives, for example health organizations such as hospitals and private clinic use information systems to operate their work such as record their patients' personal information, billing, financial management and many more. In health organizations it turns out to be more vital to arrange social insurance in a patient-driven consideration. PC and data innovation of ICT have been utilized to enhance customary general well-being honed for a long time. The existing literature on information technology in health system suggested that the information technology have a huge impact on the health systems in terms of the efficiency, quality and safety. Murray-weir et al. [2] stated that implementation of ICT in health care industry has been regarded as essential to the reduction of medical errors and increased patient safety. Also, health information technology promises to deliver the right information at the right time and the right place (Benson 2012) not to mention that a variety of mechanisms through which health ICT can improve quality, including more accurate documentation, rapid retrieval of information, management of complex information, and enhanced communication.

The most significant barriers to the implementation of the technology is the lack of appropriate incentives. Healthcare in developing countries faces a number of challenges due to economic constraints, poor infrastructure, a shortage of trained clinical staff, extreme climate and geographical barriers among others. Furthermore, individuals who are older and with less education and lack of technology experience are less likely to use a electronic health as patient portal that may lead to them low accessible electronic health management tasks ([3]).

Health Information Technology (HIT) improves the quality, patient safety and reduces the cost of healthcare. HIT can be introduced such as Electronic Health Record (EHR), Electronic Medical Record (EMR) and Clinical Decision Support System (CDSS). Health information management (HIM) is the main focus on managing medical records and since it became electronic, the overlaps between informatics grew. Moreover, the most frequently used HIT is the electronic medical record (EMR) but, it has been replaced by electronic health record (EHR) that shows more extra information about the patient. Changes in health information technology play a major role in enhancing the quality of health system especially in terms of health care.

2 ICT Emerging Technology

ICT on health system has long been established. Since 1991, the improvement of data innovation has denoted the new era of organized innovation, which influenced all ranges including social insurance administration and innovation. The compelling utilization of wellbeing data innovation by essential consideration practices to encourage quality change can offer practices some assistance with improving their capacity to convey fantastic care and enhance persistent results. In the twentyfirst century technology is becoming more advanced, it has made the system more efficient and effective. Before the existence of information technology, a lot of paperwork was involved.

Before information technology was implemented, patients' appointments were only written on paper or card. Therefore, appointments are usually missed by patients as people are rather forgetful or had other commitments. The newly implemented system helps patients to be reminded of their appointments. For example, the framework additionally offers patients the decision of having short message service (SMS) reminders for their consultation.

The inconvenience where patients were advised to go the nearest hospitals or clinics with their homes due to records not able to be in other hospitals or clinics. As records were mostly recorded on paper and it would usually take days to be transported. Therefore, information technology makes it easier for doctors and nurses to access patient's health records from the system. As in the twentyfirst century where technology is considered as the most innovative, technology is always up to date hence making every process quick. Therefore, the waiting time for patients is reduced as system keeps all patients' records. Technology is indeed efficient and effective but it comes with a price. The cost of maintaining and installing the system is expensive.

Information Technology is now widely used because population of every country is constantly growing. Therefore, information technology in health system is not recently developed. It has been used since the existence of PC or portable computers that was in the 1990s. Ever since, it has been evolving to be able for people to get the most efficient and effective health care. Due to that, this can help save paper because the amount of paper that would be used will dominate storage of folders. With that the information technology can save space for organizations and to have an efficient healthcare.

3 Big Data for Healthcare: An Critical Issues

The concept of big data for healthcare organization has been widespread within computer science since the earliest days of computing. It is defined as large quantity of data which includes new technologies and architectures so that it becomes likely to abstract value from it by seizing and analysis process. Due to such large size of data it becomes very challenging to achieve effective analysis using the existing traditional systems. Big data due to its several characteristics such as volume, velocity, variety, variability, value and complexity put onward many challenges. Each time a different storage medium was created, the quantity of data accessible exploded because it could be simply retrieved. While Big Data can be certainly perceived as a big consecration, big tests also arise with wide-ranging data sets. The original definition focused on structured data, but most researchers and practitioners have come to understand that most of the world's information resides in massive, unstructured information, mostly in the form of text and imagery. These innovative technologies have presented significant changes to the way communication takes place between companies, people, and the community at large.

The explosion of data has not been accompanied by a consistent different storage medium. Big Data for healthcare organization also stated that as the amount of data just beyond technology's capability to store, manage and process efficiently. These imitations are only discovered by a robust analysis of the data itself, explicit processing needs, and the capabilities of the tools (hardware, software, and methods) used to analyze it. As with any new problem, the conclusion of how to proceed may lead to a recommendation that different tools need to be forged to perform the new tasks. As little as 5 years ago, we were only thinking of tens to hundreds of gigabytes of storage for our personal computers. Today, we are thinking in tens to hundreds of terabytes. Thus, big data is a moving target. In another way, it is that quantity of data that is just beyond our immediate grasp. The recent growth rate in the quantity of data collected is staggering.

One of the issues in big data is the diversity and incompleteness of data where machine analysis algorithms expect homogeneous data. Moreover, the larger set of data, the longer it takes to analyse. It is difficult to design a structure when data is growing in a very high speed. Some organizations are willing to share some information for public to use, so technical mechanism need to verify the source of external data used so that the data do not give wrong information to society. However, provenance of data may be doubtful, the ownership of the data may be subject to dispute, the classification of information discovered may not be realistic until after analysis. In order to solve thousands of unorganized data on the internet, Apache Hadoop software has been introduced. This software is an open source software that is available for any organizations to organize a large data across any servers. Apache Hadoop can handle all types of data from disparate system whether if the data is unstructured, structured, log files, pictures, video or email regardless of its built-in format. Apache Hadoop software is flexible as it helps to links together the file system on many local network and compile them into one area. The software also has high tolerance for hardware failure where the system can track down missing files and redirect work to another location. Moreover, Apache Hadoop system is cost effective as it charge the cost per terabyte of storage. It is highly known for highly scalable storage and automatic data replication. Apache Hadoop software ensure the quality of data available is reliable.

Second issue is storage. In order to keep data, we need an excessive and large space to store them as internet and websites have explosive amount of information. Data and transaction logs are stored in multi-tiered storage media. Cloud computing would be the most common used application by public or an organization. Cloud computing can be accessed anywhere, it employs visualization of computing resources to run numerous standardized virtual servers on the same physical machine. However they charge the cost based on small time intervals, hourly. For business who wants to keep their data private, private cloud are one of the option that can be used by an organization where their database are can be accessed internally or externally. Private cloud on the other hand separate an organization's data storage and prevent incidental access through shared resources.

Third issue is regarding privacy and security, modern technology these days require us to use mobile devices technology to make payment anywhere and anytime. Online businesses are practically spreading globally, for example Zalora and Alibaba Express are the commonly visited websites. In order to make payment, we have to transfer our money by using credit or debit card where we usually type our account number and password into the system. The saved information are now kept on the websites database. However, the database can be breached by hackers. Customer need to be very careful about purchasing from online businesses. Another example would be, making payment by swiping debit card to the cash registrar machine, the organization have the access to personal and sensitive customer data and information for instance; social security numbers and purchase history. However, there are some of the people in the organization who breaks the law regarding personal data and commit crime of stealing money. An organization have to pay public relation and financial price when their database are compromised. One case where a business Target was involved in a serious financial and security breached where the retailer's payment system was hacked and lost millions of credit card number, in response Target paid $61 million for the incident. Business need to take care of their databases carefully and place more value on protecting that data.

Fourth issue is about endpoint input validation and filtering. Endpoint is a device that is linked to the local area network (LAN) or wide area network (WAN) and allows communications across the network. An endpoint device is being used only for the internet-connected PC hardware on a transmission control protocol or internet protocol. Other users can go through the information that their network provides when they have their own endpoint devices. Input validation and filtering is an intimidating challenge posed by untrusted input sources. The case about endpoint input validation and filtering data retrieved sent by an iPhone application that shares with the same validation problem from weather sensors and feedback votes. Rivals can create fraud virtual sensors or trick iPhone to provide the results.

Fifth issue is about real time security monitoring. Real time data monitoring (RTDM) is a process in which an administrator can analyze and modify things such as the addition or deletion of a data when using a software, database or system. It ensures that the database administrator to analyze the overall functions and processes accomplished on the data in real time. It consists of monitoring Big Data infrastructure and using the similar processing of data infrastructure. Example for monitoring Big Data infrastructure is when the performance and health of all data intersection is being monitored that make up the big data infrastructure. An example of using the similar processing of data infrastructure would be a health care provider that is being applied as monitoring tools to seek fraudulent claims.

4 Featuring of Health Information Technology

The main advantages of Health Information Technology improves the quality, patient safety and reduces the cost of healthcare. Health Information Technology can be introduced such as Electronic Health Record, Electronic Medical Record and Clinical Decision Support System. Clinical Decision Support System, as tools for decision maker, is a complicated process that relies upon human ability to provide undivided attention and to memorize, recall, and retrieve big data which are susceptible. Pieces of information can be accessed and organized while the links can also be distinguished by the ICT systems.

ICT emerging technology is effective in bridging this 'knowing–doing' gap through relevant information provided. In other side, bar codes have been used widely for arrays of systems, for example in the distributing of drug and automated dispensing cabinets, which tends to diminish dispensing errors by packaging, dispensing, and recognizing medications using bar codes. One of the contemporary evaluation of the effects of bar-coding drugs in pharmacy have been carried out, checking them before they are sent to patient care units. The results have indicated that the dispensing error decreases by 31 % after bar-code implementation whereas the rate of adverse events fell up to 63 %.

Bar-coded medication administration (BCMA) systems require supervision of the medication at the bedside by the nurse whereby there is a scanning of the patient's identification bracelet and the dose of the medication before given out. The system ensures vigilance in the nurse to any discrepancy on patient name to the route of administration of the medication. BCMA reduces could reduce errors by: ensuring the precision of patient, dose, route, and duration. BCMA systems allegedly results in a 54–87 % reductions in administering errors of medication. In a London teaching hospital, implementation of a 'closed-loop' system including CPOE and BCMA reduced prescribing and medication administration errors.

5 The E-Health Innovations and Challenges

The innovation in health was introduced through National Health Information Infrastructure (NHII). Here, NHII improved the quality of data, information, and knowledge to enabling decisions through ICT emerging technology in all domains of the health areas [4]. The NHII technology, empowering and enhanching clinicians and patients on their role *such as; health threats, enable patients to receive laboratory results promptly and reliably, allow healthcare staff to monitor disease and coach patients with chronic conditions, transform individual data elements into pools of anonymous data for research and public health needs, allow researchers from around the country to collaborate without leaving their labs, link a new medical advance to an individual patient, speed new useful knowledge to clinicians, and automate routine tasks so that chances of human error are greatly reduced* [4].

NHII as implementation of health information technology is very important part to introducing electronic health more broaden for patients and healthcare organization. Moreover, There several reasons, why Health Information Technology may poses threat to the health system. Firstly, there are insufficient evidences to support the prospect on impact of such systems on clinical outcomes. Most of the evidences available recently merely depends either on extensive collegiate hospitals that have developed a single site which uses these systems both privately and publicly, or on substantial economic models relying on projections. The former is understated by skeptical generalization of the discovery findings, as there is constant enforcement of commercially developed systems with little or no resources for customization. The latter, on the other hand, seemingly overestimate benefits of ICT by making calculations based on superiority of the cases. Assessment of these problems in more recent reports were conducted whereby the advantageous effects of distinctive ICT and their clinical implementations, across numerous institutions, on a vast area of clinical outcomes such as inpatient mortality, length of stay, complexity, and expenditure have been determined by methods of high precision.

A second concern is raised by the fact that ICT systems can rather have negative impacts on patient safety. ICT has an adverse effect on clinical care by generating extra or new workload for clinicians, causing workflow problems, or even creating new kinds of errors. These reports undermined the fact that ICT systems are necessary to be devised in order to enhance clinical workflow and improved technically. One perspective to addressing this problem is that clinical ICT systems in the markets should have standardized rules whereby they should be tested and authorized by a certification agency, such as the Certification Commission for Healthcare Information Technology (CCHIT—http://www.cchit.org). This recognition process assures a buyer that a system is permitted to carry out activities in the domains of functionality, interoperability, and privacy and security as they conform to the minimum standards of the system.

Thirdly, it is also strongly perceived that albeit the significance in impediment of medication errors in the IT system itself, the focal point should be on implementation, in alternative words, the way that it has been integrated into clinical processes, and workflow and how users literally use it in conventional clinical care, occasionally depicted as the sociotechnical environment of the clinical workplace. For instance, a recent result has indicated a threefold increase in mortality in infants after implementation of CPOE notwithstanding that in another study there was a decreasing rate of 36 % in standardized mortality utilizing the same software, but with implementation that varies in strategy. The current approach to IT standardization and certification is focused on the functionality of the system, but does not address its implementation or usability by clinicians.

A fourth concern is raised by the fact that IT systems can rather have negative impacts on patient safety. IT systems can have an adverse effect on clnical care by generating extra or new workload for clinicians, causing workflow problems, or even creating new kinds of errors. These reports undermined the fact that IT systems is necessary to be devised in order to enhance clinical workflow and improved technically. One perspective to addressing this problem is that clinical IT systems in the markets should have standardized rules whereby they should be tested and authorized by a certification agency, such as the Certification Commission for Healthcare Information Technology (CCHIT—http://www.cchit.org). This recognition process assures a buyer that a system is permitted to carry out activities in the domains of functionality, interoperability, and privacy and security as they conform to the minimum standards of the system.

Furthermore, it is also strongly perceived that albeit the significance in impediment of medication errors in the IT system itself, the focal point should be on implementation, in alternative words, the way that it has been integrated into clinical processes and workflow and how users literally use it in conventional clinical care, occasionally depicted as the sociotechnical environment of the clinical workplace. For instance, a recent result has indicated a threefold increase in mortality in infants after implementation of CPOE notwithstanding that in another study there was a decreasing rate of 36 % in standardized mortality utilizing the same software but with implementation that varies in strategy. The current approach to IT standardization and certification is focused on the functionality of the system, but does not address its implementation or usability by clinicians.

The main obstacles to pervasiveness in adoption are due to the costly systems and an environment of enticements that were disorganized, whereby hospitals and physicians pay for the systems whereas the insurance companies will be beneficial financially. One mechanism that is vital on evacuation of this barrel is financial incentives to healthcare organizations. The Obama Administration has already proposed incentive payments to Medicare and Medicaid providers and hospitals for using CCHIT-certified EHRs in the widely anticipated 2009 economic stimulus bill. For years, US federal law, commonly called the Stark law, made it illegal for hospitals to assist outside physicians financially in acquiring EHRs.

5.1 *Computer Provider Order Entry (CPOE)*

With the quick emergence of information technology in the healthcare industry, there is a high possibility that hospitals or clinics would have less demand on the use of paper-based information while increasing the use of electronics. Various types of information technology that has been implemented and one of the types of information technology that is used is Computerized Provider Order Entry known as the CPOE. Computerized Provider Order Entry (CPOE) is a system that enables the medical professional to enter the medication orders or other specialist doctor instructions into the computer system. The aim of the Computer Provider Order Entry (CPOE) was to achieve the patient satisfaction. This has replaced the traditional way of how the medication order is done in the hospital which includes paper prescriptions and verbal as they can read and analyze all the information through the computer system. CPOE serves as a tool to increase standardization, quality, and efficiency in the delivery of care provided to patients in healthcare organizations [5]. However, the implementation of CPOE can change not just the information technology in the healthcare industry but also in healthcare systems in the organization in terms of the clinical and ancillary department which also include the change in clinical processes. But apart from that, it could bring benefits to the health systems. By which the benefits include the minimized medication error, potential human error, handwritten error, improve communication and avoided the waste of time in gaining the data.

One of the benefits stated is reducing the medication error. Medication errors have been retaining as one of the major problems that is faced by some of the medical professional as this is a very common mistakes made by every hospital. Therefore, it could be essential for the hospital to implement the CPOE system to minimize the error to ensure the patient safety. Medication errors can also be related to potential human error. Human error can be a very common human behavior in the healthcare industry due to the busy schedules of the medical professional and the doctors whereby this could lead to a high risk of making error. Yet, each human being is capable of making an error, even on a good day [6]. So with the availability of the CPOE, it can reduce the human error to as minimal as possible. This could also leads to saving time of accessing the data without the need to search through the pile of paper or documents as the data of the patients or the hospital are extremely vast. The system in this case plays a part in enabling the doctors to receive the data or information they want by just a few clicks in the CPOE.

A reduction of medication error can also help the hospital in cost saving which literally means that it could reduce the cost of the patients care. Therefore, with the right medication order provided to the patients, it could help the patient to recover more quickly. As a result, it could lead to the reduction of the length of stay of a patient as it required a high expenditure of the patient staying at the hospital such as the medicine, food and others.

Handwritten error can also cost quite a big impact to the health organization as it is the main source of errors found in health department, especially the pharmacy where they select the patient medicine through what is written on the paper by the doctor which might not be clear. Poor handwriting to lack of attention to details causes medication errors to happen in anyplace [5].

However, CPOE does not always bring benefits as there are also drawbacks in implementation of CPOE which is the cost to implement it. The cost of implementation and the maintenance of the CPOE is high as it might cost an estimate of total of millions of dollars. A good example is in the United States where they are slow to adopt the CPOE due to the high cost, Estimated costs to implement a system at a 500-bed hospital without network upgrades is $8 million, with ongoing maintenance costs of more than $1 million a year [2]. Therefore, this shows that it could be a barrier for some hospital or clinics who have financial difficulties to implement this CPOE system.

Another drawback is the time taken for the implementation of CPOE in every department in the hospital as it may sometimes take years to complete the installation of CPOE which shows its quality of time-consuming. Other than that, it is also needed to provide CPOE training to operate the Computerized Provider Order Entry as the implementation of CPOE in the newly hospital has affected the workflow of the healthcare department. For example, in the hospital that has been using the handwritten order for years or so, acquiring doctors to operate the computerized order entry would be a major change in the workload. Therefore, this could affect the productivity and the efficiency of the hospital as they are still new to the system and may need to take a longer period of time for them to be efficient in the CPOE system.

5.2 E-Health System

A system is a set of procedures that organized in order for the things to run smoothly. E-health system focuses on how the communications and managements have change in medical practices from a traditional method. Today, the information technology plays a vital role in health system. The doctor will use internet and computer as a tool and medium to interact with their patients. However, this system still cannot be adopted around the world especially in most developing countries because of the cost and Information Technology knowledge which act as a barrier, according to Sharez et al. [7]. World population increases over the years, currently there is about 7 billion people in the earth today. It is estimated about tens of millions patients die every year due to unsafe medical care [8]. With a proper health system implementation, this problem may be reduced in the future. Many health organizations like World Health Organizations and health industry technology try to improve the medical technology system in order to make people much healthier. In the USA, the government spends almost 38 billion dollars over the 10 years just to support health information technology [9–11].

Aside from that, E-health is a platform for medical staff to interact with the patients. E-health is a step forward for delivering a health care to the society. An increase in internet users and rapid technology improvement drives many health organizations to implement e-health system in their organization. Rising in the number of aging people mostly in the Europe region is another issue why e-health is important today. E-health helps the medical staff to manage the hospital better. E-health shows that the internet plays a vital role to support the health care today. Implementing e-health is not easy and cheap. E-health system may have some disadvantages, but it gives more benefits to the society, therefore e-health system need to be improved. This actually requires the management of server and maintenance. This is to ensure there are no unexpected events that will happen such as website traffic as there might be a lot of people updating their information online. Therefore, without proper server management and maintenance, all online related works might halt or perhaps can be hacked by someone [10, 11].

5.3 Mobile Health

Recently, mobile technology is evolving rapidly. Mobile technology is a portable gadget that is relatively easy to carry anywhere and it connects with the internet. Therefore, mobile technology is one of the other initiative to deliver health care. Recently, many people decided to use mobile health system as tools for health care. Mobile health is much cheaper than other health care technology. Mobile health connected through internet as a medium. Internet is a powerful tool that connects people. With internet, people can communicate from different places in just a second. It is assumed that in the future, face-to-face interaction amongst doctor and patient will become less common [12]. Rather than visiting the doctor, patient can do an interaction through video conferencing or communicate through email instead of visiting the doctor. With electronic communication, a doctor can monitor their patients through video conferencing if the patient prefers to stay at the comfort of their own home. Mobile health can reduce the cost of consultations since the patient does not have to visit the medical staff. The management can be fasten through internet communication rather than the manual. Any appointment with medical staff or doctor can be done online to prevent clashes with any patient. Furthermore, online appointment application is quicker rather than the manual ways where it takes a time. This is supported by the fact that online appointment is working 24 h per day.

Although it is assumed that face-to-face interaction will be less common in the future, it still stands as the best method for consultation. Mobile health is not really suitable for delivering health care since it has a limit in connection. Communication through video conferencing will not work if the internet is down. The appointment that was sent through email may not be read by the patient as not all people have a connection to the internet and not all people check their email frequently. Online application appointment is much better than the manual ways, although it is defeated by the fact that the system will not work if the server is down. This is because communicating via internet is less time-consuming.

5.4 Health Telematics System

20 or more decades ago, to meet or to get a treatment from a doctor is not easy. People must travel to the city to get a treatment. But with modern information technologies, it is not a problem anymore. For some countries, people who live in rural area can make a consultation with a medical staff through telemedicine or health telematics system. It is another type of health information system. Telemedicine is an electronic device that transfer complex data from one place to another, basically the data are in video or multimedia form [13]. According to Chandwani and Yogesh [14], telemedicine may reduce the cost of health care delivery since the isolated communities do not have to visit the medical staff at hospital. Telemedicine has been used for treatment, diagnosing and preventing

disease from spreading to other areas [14]. Telemedicine is usually used by rural hospital or clinic to communicate with specialists at other hospitals. Telemedicine can also be a medium for medical staff to interact with patients that were diagnosed with spreadable diseases or parasites and monitoring patients in the Incentive Care Unit.

It seems difficult for medical staff or doctor to monitor their patient through the screen. Probably it may take more times as compared to the traditional method where patient have to faces the doctor. Other problems that may rise are the quality of the data and the transmission or the connection. The image quality or video that are transmitted from the telemedicine is crucial for the medical staff to make decisions. If the image or video quality are bad it seems that the specialist will take more time to make a decision for the patient and it may lead to a risk. Telemedicine is not suitable for any emergency problem where treatment is needed instantly for patient. Telemedicine relies on the connection and source of power to transmit the data information. Without the power the telemedicine will not be working. Giving treatment via telemedicine is not easy since the only thing the medical staff can do is just talking and monitoring. Telemedicine is type of information technology, the cost of equipment telemedicine is not cheap. Most African countries cannot afford to implement a health technology such as telemedicine. Perhaps, only developed countries have the potential to use this health information technology.

5.5 Electronic Medical Record

Every organizations today will keep their data in digital form and prevent it from leak. Today, health organizations are implementing electronic medical record (EMR) system to store all the data information from the patients. Patients in the UK today can have an access to their health record (Fisher et al. 2009). The record not only can be accessed by the staff within the organization but with this system, the patient can look through their record. It records all the health record which includes the laboratory result, medicine prescription and appointment schedule. With this system, data will be stored safely without worrying that it can be lost like paper records. Compared to paper records, staff can get the patient's record quickly. Electronic medical record make specialists easy to analyze and retrieve the data information in order for them to pursue a better treatment for the patients. Furthermore, this system is crucial in order to make the decision making effective. This system will fasten the process of management, for instance, pharmacist can give the medicine to the patient just by accessing through the patient's health record instead of reading the description from the doctor.

Implementing this system may reduce the organization expenses since the use of paper is decreased. With electronic medical record, error can be prevented and detected through the system. Recording any information on the paper will lead to many risks compared to recording data in the digital form since some handwriting is difficult to understand and read.

5.6 Clinical Decision Support System

Computer plays a vital role today for medical staff either for management or decision making. Clinical decision support systems (CDSS) is a computer program that is designed to help the medical staff to make a good decision making for patients according to Bright et al. [15]. CDSS is link to EHR to get a patient health record. This system basically helps the physicians to calculate the drug dose. CDSS helps the medical staff to analyze the data or lab result. Medical staff cannot totally rely on this system because CDDS is programmed to give the doctor advice or alert on something. There is possibility that the data recorded in the EHR may not correct.

As mentioned above, e-health system gives many advantages to the society. The most important thing is e-health system is very effective for a better decision making amongst the specialist. With this system, distance is not a barrier to get a better health treatment anymore. But to implement it is not easy. The medical staff had to understand and have a good knowledge about how the e-health system works. The rapid changes in technology cannot be prevented. The health technology industry keeps improving and innovating new system. But the medical staff are struggling and stressed with the continuous health care system changes according to Yan et al. [16]. Implementing the e-health is not easy since the cost of maintenance is expensive and it requires an expert technician. Furthermore, not all patients have the knowledge on the information technology therefore only certain patients know how to use the technology.

6 The Emerging Technology to Enabling Innovation

As doctor's facility data framework has been secured in the substance of all healing center operations and administration, and the creations contain programming, equipment, system and other subsystems, administration and upkeep workload is critical and troublesome. This includes server upkeep, information reinforcement, client administration and system security and upkeep [17]. Hospital information system framework are numerous and scattered in destinations, the users include doctors, attendants, therapeutic specialists, administration faculty, budgetary, and so on., on the toll framework and money related information with high security and secrecy prerequisites [17]. Framework utilizes the working arrangement database and application level of client consent to run the utmost of the triple control instrument to give a brought together role based client administration devices in the framework so that every client has an exceptional account number, password, and given diverse levels of authorizations, so they can just work on their own strategies and call-related information, and cannot simply access to the information without knowing the document. In the meantime, we have the client control program as an addition. Through these measures, we can successfully keep the illicit intrusion of system clients, to guarantee the sheltered operation of the system.

6.1 Management and Maintenance of Network Security

System security is firmly related with the application of engineering, system security for the most part alludes to the system when clients get to the application server and database server, and this guarantee server security. From all levels of utilization and security investigation, the information needed of exceptional insurance layer, cannot give direct links. Application server layer is additionally the requirement for security and the need to control client access. To build up a strict system security administration framework, from the administration of system gear and lines to the server, workstation utilize, the client's login detail has been stricten. This has been done chiefly in the accompanying measures: utilization of firewall innovation to counteract illegal access to the machine; strict control of the interior location of the management; the utilization of complex secret word framework, thorough character verification.

At present, dependability of PC programming and equipment system has been incredibly enhanced, likewise, disk arrays and other gear can be utilized to enhance framework adaptation to internal failures. These procedures enhance the unwavering quality of the framework, however, this cannot ensure framework security idiot proof, just to a specific degree, to decrease the misfortunes brought on by media disappointment. For unexpected mistakes or deliberate dangerous operation, computer virus attacks, framework disappointments brought on by standard database reinforcement is to guarantee the security of alternate things re-measure [17]. At the point when a misfortune happens, we can depend on the reinforcement to restore information. We have taken the reinforcement programs as it is takes after: at least once every morning and evening to reinforce hard drive that was ready on the server and disk arrays.

Server maintenance
Day to day server maintenance, server support concentrates on programming upkeep, including customary or incidental observing of memory, disk space monitoring, security access control, PC infection checking etc.

Reinforcement of data information is an essential issue that is a must to be considered in the framework safe operation, the framework cannot ensure solidity without any issues, equipment disappointment, programming crash, infection impact and the powerful or unusual catastrophe, this might bring about the disappointment of the framework, undermining the information security [17]. Hardware reinforcement is the best intends to recover from a catastrophe and accident. They did this to fulfill the ongoing administrations and information insurance necessities and to acknowledge high information accessibility, as a consequence, the framework is exchanging and have a least recuperation in time to outline framework reinforcement program.

Privacy and Security Awareness
Protection and security dangers are a worry because of programmers, fraud, unapproved access and defilement (adjustment) of patient information [3, 18–20],

making EMRs accessible to far-flung medicinal services suppliers fundamentally makes them more open to the world on the loose. Nevertheless, issues, for instance, dangers of security introduction, versatility in key administration, adaptable access, and productive client disavowal, have remained as the most essential difficulties towards accomplishing fine-grained, cryptographically implemented information access control [21, 22–24].

6.2 Clinical Information System

These are one of the most vital parts in the health system which is recording and updating patient's health record. Clinical and administrative data are related to each other because it might be impossible to make or develop a clinical system without any various types of administrative data. For instance the most essential part that can be found implemented in the system is issuing a letter to patient to request for their update of address which requires the latest patient's address details and any related information in order to follow-up. Considered rather straightforward, the center of a coordinated healing facility and clinical data framework is just an 'expert record' comprising of the most fundamental part of patient points of interest ('administrative data'), giving links to different clinical frameworks. Each departmental clinical framework then permits people to set up extra research data sets for particular exercises.

The aim for clinical and administrative system is to give a common wellspring of data around a patient's wellbeing history. The system needs to keep information in secure place and controls who can achieve the information in specific circumstances. These systems im-prove the capacity of social insurance experts to organize care by giving a patient's well-being data and visit history at the spot and time that it is required. Patient's research center test data additionally for visual results, for example, X-beam might be reachable from experts. Hospital information system gives interior and outside correspondence among human services suppliers.

The advantages of using information system in recording patient's health record are it allows health-care providers to record tolerant data electronically as opposed to utilize paper records. It likewise has the ability to perform different undertakings that can help with medicinal services conveyance while keeping up models of practice.

6.3 Financial and Clinical HIS

Hospitals around the world today might not use traditional method to record all the transaction made, for instance, doing book keeping and stock checking manually. Nowadays people do all the transactions by using an application such as UBS to record transaction and check the stocks using computers.

Billing patient

Private hospitals or clinics used mobile technology such as computer to bill their patients. For instance in the United States, computers are used widely by US hospitals and physician to bill their patients [3]. In the hospitals, they utilize electronic frameworks to track supplies, calculate profit and losses, controlling stock and process finance. Maybe no industry faces such a mind boggling errand regarding to charging as it does with the human services vertical. Medicinal charging mechanization is not exclusively a matter of expanding efficiencies. It is additionally a basic piece of enhancing income and the general patient experience.

Accounting systems in healthcare

A cost bookkeeping framework is a framework for recording, investigating and dispensing expense to the individual administrations given to patients [25]. Finance department plays a big role in the medical welfare. However, most costing is done on an expected premise based after allotting the aggregate costs reflectively or more regularly, on past years costs. As the foundation of the association, the bookkeeping division permits the association to work at its fullest potential. Without a bookkeeping division, it would be unthinkable for an association to work in a financially savvy way (Hicks, n.d). At the point when working inside a medicinal office, the bookkeeping office is essential to its prosperity.

Material management and stock control

Stock control is a piece of numerous industry-neutral bookkeeping bundles. Human services associations have some particular prerequisites, however, for instance, the capacity to build charge catch (charging for things utilized as a part of treatment) is a neglected hotspot for overhead cost lessening in therapeutic associations. On the other hand, robotics such as bar-coding and RFID can expand the straightforwardness with which stock is overseen and enhance charge catch. Managing perishable solutions is another one of a kind component of medicinal materials administration. Moreover, elements, for example, parcel and termination following are not just monetarily invaluable; they give an imperative well-being related part.

Creditors and purchasing

Successful money administration depends on wise records of payable handling. Creditor liabilities modules handle the dispersal of installments to merchants. Propelled money administration highlights incorporate the capacity to enhance installments. This can be proficient through an assortment of means keeping so as to incorporate trade out procuring positions until installment dates arrive, diminishing mistakes and late installments, and notwithstanding exploiting economies of scale through clumped orders or early installment rebates. Electronic installment strategies, for example, electronic assets exchanges (EFT) are helping associations to deal with their payables with lower handling costs and enhanced unwavering quality. Complete acquiring frameworks give the capacity to oversee extensive scale buying reliably and with the fitting endorsements and control. Reporting components can enhance seller administration and interest computation. Mechanization elements, for example, programmed acquiring taking stock limits into account can promote and enhance effectiveness.

6.4 Medical Robotics

Medical robotics has become increasingly important part of the healthcare system around the world. Robots are already beginning to affect medicine (the application of science and technology to treat and prevent injury and disease) and health care (the availability of treatment and prevention of illness) [27]. The technologies in medical robotics keep on advancing therefore there would a possibility that there is a potential to trigger the development of the new treatments for the wide variety kind of disease and also the rehabilitation systems. Most of the medical robotics are mostly implemented in the surgery section in the health industry. With the implementation of medical robotics, this has help the hospital to perform difficult procedures and more patients can be rehabilitated as most of the task or treatment are limited by the human abilities that were handling them.

One of the medical robotics that has been used are surgical robotics. The surgical robotics functions are to carry out the process of the surgery procedures during the ongoing surgery which was controlled by the computer systems. This benefits the surgeon as the surgeon can program the robot motion precisely about the procedure of the surgery which results in high accuracy in making the surgery and increasing velocities with no overshoot. Surgical robotics also eliminate the tremors of the surgeon whereby this avoid any surgical error or mistakes as this could result in the injury of the patient.

However, surgical robotics can also have disadvantages as well which includes surgical robotics do not have the hesitant to make any move during surgery as it was computerized completely. This can have a great risk of making errors if the surgeon did not input the right procedure to the robot.

Computer-assisted surgery

Computer assisted surgery (CAS) is a technology that have the possibility to empower the healthcare services to improve proficiency of diagnosis, treatments and clinical administration. The introduction of computer-assisted surgery was to enhance the performance of surgical interventions with electronic instruments and software [26]. The computer assisted surgery has been increasingly used worldwide in wide variety of surgical processes. It is also regularly considered an image guidance such as 3D image which is mostly used in computer tomography (CT) or magnetic resonance imaging (MRI) and navigation as this acts as a guidance for surgeon during the surgery. With the availability of this technology surgeon can now be able to plan the surgery carefully and precisely and able to match the goal of the surgery [10].

The benefits of the computer assisted surgery (CAS) are surgeons can acquired a better visualization of the internal infrastructures of the body by using the MRI or CT. Therefore, this allows the surgeon and the medical professional to have a better and accurate diagnostics of the patients. CAS can also provide simulations to the physicians to perform difficult surgery before handling the real surgery. The rising in public demand for patient safety and the complicated operations, the necessity of operative training outside the operating room is not a question any longer [28].

This can help to improve their skills and surgical knowledge needed during the surgical. However, the disadvantage of CAS is the cost as the machines of the CAS can be very costly therefore it can be hard for hospital that has a tight finance to invest on the machines. CAS may also sometimes cause error which can lead to wrong or inaccurate diagnostics of the patients [11].

Computer assisted surgery is greatly demanded by all the health care authorities as it has become machine that is used on a daily basis in the hospital or clinics. With the CAS, there is a reduce in the risk of making wrong diagnostics, it has improved the safety of the patient care significantly and improve the health of the patient. Therefore, the case of the limitations of the high cost of the machines may not have really affected the healthcare industry.

7 Managing Change and Innovation

To proceed further, it is necessary to have a straightforward yet dynamic perception for navigation of investments in Health Information Technology. Nowadays, people can go online and have an instant access for the sake of managing their personal financial information. With a few clicks of a mouse, people can move their money and even have bank accounts transferring from one institution to another. This has been impossible with most of electronic health records, but there has been an innovation recently.

For the determination of accomplishing an exceptionally competitive health-care marketplace, the focal point should be shifting electronic health information to the patient rather than staying in the hands of an individual provider.

Health IT systems should also be relatively easy to use whereby instead of hindering it, the systems facilitate the work of clinicians. User interfaces should be identical enough that a clinician working in one health system can instinctively distinguish how to use another without the need of large-scale training. For instance, car manufacturers offer an assortment of models, however, the control indicates a persistence and enable a customer to drive any vehicle off a rental lot without instruction are more crucial. Comparatively, Health IT should make no distinction.

Health IT systems with low complications will not only be less oppressive on suppliers and patients, but they will also be ensured of the secureness of the system. Lately, there has been an imposition of laws by the Institute of Medicine Department of Health and Human Services whereby providers are obliged to report on health IT vendors and volunteers to identify correlation between Health IT inimical events and uncertain circumstances. Establishment of domestic report and monitoring instruments would instantaneously causes an upsurge of our understanding towards the finest practices for high security adoption and implementation of health IT.

8 Limitation and Future Research

This study incorporates two main issues of electronic health innovation: ICT emerging technology and Health Information Technology. ICT emerging technology refined the authorization of information, trigger the business process reengineering, and the collaboration within the healthcare organization. It is not just simply supporting process reengineering but it also has a strong impact in improving efficiency and effectiveness of healthcare organization. Health Information Technology improved the quality of health data, information, and knowledge used to support decisions at all levels and in all domains of the health sector; i.e., personal health, health care delivery, public health, and research.

The study triggers a future research direction in health information technology strategy which would focus on enhancing patient and healthcare organization, change management associated with the implementation of paperless cultures; support decision making for clinicians and patients, empowering patient and allow clinicians to monitor disease and coach patients with chronic conditions.

The future direction of this study can also accommodate and customise for integration of more complete and robust security support features, particularly the integration of an information security decision for electronic health for support system, an expert system and a security pattern recognition system, complemented with a knowledge inference and learning system to emulate the decision-making ability of a human expert. This software ability could solve compliance barriers, create an early warning system for suspected security breaches and help enhance strategic planning of electronic health.

9 Conclusions

IT systems ICT emerging technology are indispensable elements of a multifaceted approach to forestall medication errors and enhance the patient safety. Nonetheless, we need to be observant of their capability of adverse effects on clinical workflow with consequential complexity. Improvisation of uniformity and recognition of the design aside from implementation of such systems should also be advantageous to the IT system. Likewise, generating an economic and policy environment conducive to the financial intention of hospitals and physicians will facilitate wider adoption of such technology in the health information system sector. Staff that are in-charge of clinical and administrative information system also play a major role in the health organizations as information system in health organization requires a lot of skilled staff in IT so that the technology used in administration are useful wherein it helps the finance sector in the health organizations in their stocks update. However, the factor cost may need to be considered such as the installation, overheads and the training.

References

1. Stair, R., Reynolds, G.: Principles of information systems. Cengage Learning (2013)
2. Murray-Weir, M., Magid, S., Robbins, L., Quinlan, P., Sanchez-Villagomez, P., Shaha, S.: A computerized order entry system was adopted with high user satisfaction at an orthopedic teaching hospital. HSS J. **10**(1), 52–58 (2014)
3. Herrick, D.M., Gorman, L., Goodman, J.C.: Health Information Technology: Benefits and Problems. National Center for Policy Analysis (2010)
4. Detmer, D.E.: Building the national health information infrastructure for personal health, health care services, public health, and research. BMC Med. Inform. Decis. Mak. **3**(1), 1 (2003)
5. Kruse, C., Goetz, K.: Summary and frequency of barriers to adoption of CPOE in the U.S. J. Med. Syst. **39**(2) (2015)
6. Smith, P.: Making Computerized Provider Order Entry Work. Springer Science & Business Media (2012)
7. Sharez. U., Innayatullah. S., Shah. A.: E-health futures in Bangladesh. Foresight **15**(3), 177–189 (2013)
8. World Health Organizations: Summary of the Evidence on Patient Safety: Implications for Research. World Health Alliance for Patient Safety, Genava (2008)
9. Lustria, M.L., Smith, S.A., Hinnant, C.C.: Exploring Digital Divides: An Examination of eHealth Technology Use in Health Information Seeking, Communication and Personal Health Information Management in the USA. Florida State University, Florida (2011)
10. Suri, J., Dey, N., Bose, S., Das, A., Chaudhuri, S.S., Saba, L., Shafique, S., Nicolaides, A.: 2084743 Diagnostic preservation of atherosclerotic ultrasound video for stroke telemedicine in watermarking framework. Ultrasound Med. Biol. **41**(4), S133 (2015)
11. Virmani, J., Dey, N., Kumar, V.: PCA-PNN and PCA-SVM based CAD systems for breast density classification. In: Applications of Intelligent Optimization in Biology and Medicine, pp. 159–180. Springer International Publishing (2016)
12. Weiner, J.P.: Doctor-patient communication in the e-health era. Israel J. Health Policy Res. http://www.ncbi.nlm.nih.gov/pmc/article/PMC3461429/ (2012)
13. Beaumont, R.: Type of Health Information Systems. http://www.floppybunny.org/robin/web/virtualclassroom/chap12/s2/systems1.pdf&sa=U&ved=0ahUKEwjIhIbYvY3LAhWBgw8KHZtyDKcQFggLMAA&sig2=oFYr6frzvfUKH8-6TgUCyQ&usg=AFQjCNEeQ6FO-Y_2NAQJ7sv2t_vXDaqysw (2011)
14. Chandwani, R.K., Yogesh, K.D.: Telemedicine in India: current state, challenges and opportunities. Trans Govern People Process Policy **9**(4), 393–400. http://dx.doi.org/10.1108/TG-07-2015-0029 (2015)
15. Bright, T.J., Wong, A., Dhurjati, R., Bristow, E., Bastian, L., Coeytaux, R.R., et al.: Effect of clinical decision-support systems: a systematic review. Ann. Intern. Med. **2012**(157), 29–43 (2012). doi:10.7326/0003-4819-157-1-201207030-00450
16. Yan, Z., Guo, X., Lee, M.K.O., Vogel, D.: A conceptual model of technology features and technostress in telemedicine communication. Inf. Technol. People **26**(3), 283–297 (2013)
17. Wei, X.: Hospital information system management and security maintenance. Comput. Intell. Syst. 418–421 (2011)
18. Dey, N., Mukhopadhyay, S., Das, A., Chaudhuri, S.S.: Analysis of P-QRS-T components modified by blind watermarking technique within the electrocardiogram signal for authentication in wireless telecardiology using DWT. Int. J. Image Graphics Signal Process. **4**(7), 33 (2012)
19. Nandi, S., Roy, S., Dansana, J., Karaa, W.B.A., Ray, R., Chowdhury, S.R., Chakraborty, S., Dey, N.: Cellular automata based encrypted ECG-hash Code generation: an application in inter human biometric authentication system. Int. J. Comput. Netw. Inf. Secur. **6**(11), 1 (2014)

20. Pal, A.K., Dey, N., Samanta, S., Das, A., Chaudhuri, S.S.: A hybrid reversible watermarking technique for color biomedical images. In: 2013 IEEE International Conference on Computational Intelligence and Computing Research (ICCIC), pp. 1–6. IEEE (2013)
21. Li, M., Yu, S., Zheng, Y., Ren, K., Lou, W.: Scalable and secure sharing of personal health records in cloud computing using attribute-based encryption. Parallel Distrib. Syst. IEEE Trans. **24**(1), 131–143 (2013)
22. Acharjee, S., Ray, R., Chakraborty, S., Nath, S., Dey, N.: Watermarking in motion vector for security enhancement of medical videos. In: 2014 International Conference on Control, Instrumentation, Communication and Computational Technologies (ICCICCT), pp. 532–537. IEEE (2014)
23. Biswas, S., Roy, A.B., Ghosh, K., Dey, N.: A biometric authentication based secured atm banking system. Int. J. Adv. Res. Comput. Sci. Softw. Eng. ISSN, 2277 (2012)
24. Bose, S., Acharjee, S., Chowdhury, S.R., Chakraborty, S., Dey, N.: Effect of watermarking in vector quantization based image compression. In: 2014 International Conference on Control, Instrumentation, Communication and Computational Technologies (ICCICCT), pp. 503–508. IEEEv
25. Imus, S.: Healthcare Cost Accounting: Strategies to Streamline Implementation and Quickly Achieve Measureable Results. http://www.oihealth.com/PDFs/Cost%20Accounting%20Implementation%20Strategies.pdf (2014)
26. Leardini, A., Belvedere, C., Ensini, A., Dedda, V., Giannini, S.: Accuracy of computer-assisted surgery. In: Knee Surgery using Computer Assisted Surgery and Robotics, pp. 3–20. Springer Berlin Heidelberg (2013)
27 Okamura, A.M., Mataric, M.J., Christensen, H.I. Medical and health-care robotics. Robotic. Automat. Mag. 17(3), 26–27 (2010).
28 Kenngott, H.G., Wagner, M., Nickel, F., Wekerle, A.L., Preukschas, A., Apitz, M., Termer, A. Computer-assisted abdominal surgery: new technologies. Langenbeck's Arch. Surg. 400(3), 273–281 (2015).

Author Biographies

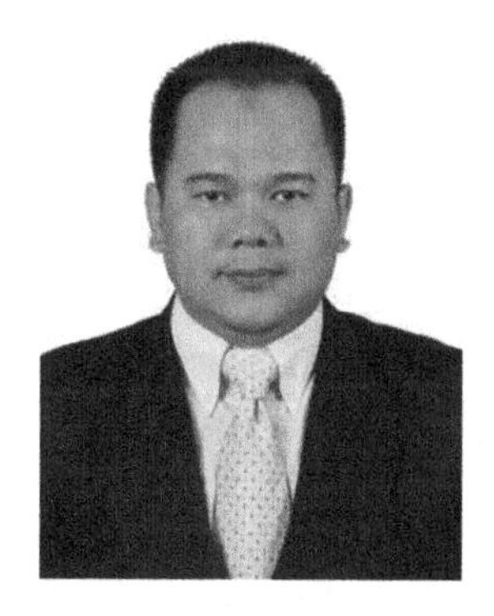

Heru Susanto currently as head of sub division and researcher at The Indonesian Institute of Sciences, Computational Science & IT Governance Research Group. Nowadays, he is also as Honorary Professor and Visiting Scholar at the Department of Information Management, College of Management, Tunghai University, Taichung, Taiwan. Heru had several careers and experience as IT professional, web division head and IT Strategic Management at Indomobil Group Corporation. He worked at Prince Muqrin Chair for Information Security Technologies, King Saud University. He received B.Sc.—Computer Science, from Bogor Agricultural University, MBA—Marketing Management, from School of Business and Management Indonesia, M.Sc.—Information System, from King Saud University, and Ph.D.—Information Security System, from University of Brunei and King Saud University. His research interests are in the areas of Information Security, IT Governance, Computational Sciences, Business Process Re-engineering, and e-Marketing.

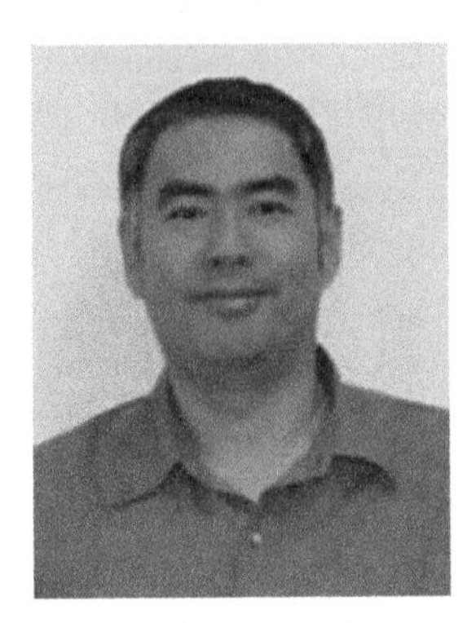

Chin Kang Chen is a Lecturer at Universiti Brunei Darussalam, where he teaches modules related to Business Information Systems and conducts research on topics related to cloud computing and e-government. He was a graduate of Royal Melbourne Institute of Technology with a Bachelors of Electrical Engineering in 1999 and completed his Master in Digital Communications in 2001 from Monash University. He recently completed another Master of Information Technology in 2011 from Queensland University of Technology. Before he started academic career, he worked in the private sector in the field of e-government and telecommunications deployment.

Health Informatics as a Service (HIaaS) for Developing Countries

Mridul Paul and Ajanta Das

Abstract With advancement of health monitoring systems and healthcare techniques, the reach of cheaper, sustainable and personalized healthcare is becoming a reality. Many developed countries have put forth standards and procedures that enable citizens to available medical services not only in designated hospitals or clinics, but also in their homes. Information and Communication Technology (ICT) has been leveraged to the fullest to achieve greater coherence in medical services. In developing countries, though there is a desire to increase reach of medical services, the infrastructure, policies and other factors create road blocks. The expectation in such countries can be met if there is a solution that is cheaper, reachable and easy to collaborate. Cloud computing paradigm can solve these issues. By leveraging cloud, developing countries can operationalize health informatics systems and enable all stakeholders to focus on refining of patient care services rather than worrying about the infrastructure for the solutions. But this requires a clear understanding of expectations from such solutions. This chapter aims at providing insights into the eHealth models that exist and challenges arising from those. The concept of HIaaS in cloud has been detailed out along with cloud based architecture for hosting eHealth services. It also illustrates application scenarios from developing countries where proposed architecture can be applied.

Keywords Cloud computing · eHealth · Health informatics · Health information technology

---

M. Paul · A. Das (✉)
Department of Computer Science & Engineering, Birla Institute of Technology, Mesra, Ranchi, 1582 Rajdanga Main Road, 4th Floor, Kolkata Campus, Kolkata 700107, India
e-mail: ajantdas@bitmesra.ac.in

M. Paul
e-mail: mridulpaul2000@yahoo.com

C. Bhatt et al. (eds.), *Internet of Things and Big Data Technologies for Next Generation Healthcare*, Studies in Big Data 23,
DOI 10.1007/978-3-319-49736-5_11

1 Introduction

Health Informatics is the field of Information Science focussed on managing healthcare data with the application of Information and Communication Technology (ICT). It's widely used synonyms are *Clinical Informatics* or *Medical Informatics* and *Biomedical Informatics*. The domain of health informatics is not limited to healthcare organizations and includes any entity directly or indirectly related to human health and wellbeing. Therefore governments and non-profit organizations, doctors, medical staffs, nurses, patients, diagnostic centres, clinics, medical disbursement stores and pharmaceutical companies fall under this domain.

As medical science is advancing, complexities involving these entities are increasing. In order to keep up the communication among different entities, regulatory authorities have been establishing standards. Standards such as Health Level-7 (HL7) [1], American Society of Testing and Materials (ASTM) [2], Clinical Document Architecture (CDA) and Continuity of Care Document (CCD) [3], Digital Imaging and Communication in Medicine (DICOM) [4] have been evolving with health innovations. There are various data sources for health informatics. Images coming out from medical systems such as Ultrasonography (U/S), Computed Tomography (CT), Magnetic Resonance Imaging (MRI) and Positron Emission Tomography (PET) [5] are highly valuable in assessing medical condition of patients. It is a rich source for health informatics. Medical equipment such as ElectroEncePhalogram (EEG) and ElectroCardioGram (ECG) [6] essentially consists of sensors that gather conditions from various organs of a human body.

In addition to sensors, there is a set of medical procedures to capture signals from biological sources within human body such as neurons and muscles [7]. Examples of such procedures include PhonoCardioGram (PCG), ElectroNeuroGram (ENG), ElectroMyoGram (EMG) and ElectroGastroGram (EGG). Genomic discoveries [8] for certain complex disorders or diseases such as cancer and research for personalized medicine, are sources for health informatics as well. Clinical notes [9] that contain clinical information from medical records on patient's health progress, contribute to health informatics. Such information is either sourced from data entry, transcription, or speech recognition applications. Besides, biomedical literature centred around biomedical and molecular biology domain (protein, gene, etc.) continue to provide inputs to health informatics.

Another interesting source for health informatics is social media that has emerged rapidly due to rise of usage of internet for wellbeing. Several social networking sites, blogs and forums contain public opinion on various aspects of healthcare. As health informatics is becoming vast due to increasing data sources, huge amount of data generated and complexity of interaction is increasing, technology needs to cope up and find better options to manage integration and enable medical systems on innovation. Another angle to this is the cost effectiveness of system infrastructure needs to increase.

Cloud computing has brought in a new paradigm on managing information and communication technology. The fundamentals are deeply rooted in service oriented architecture [10] that provides flexibility for creating services based on the need of the consumer. Cloud provides service models such as Infrastructure as a Service (IaaS), Platform as a Service (PaaS) and Software as a Service (SaaS) that allows consumers to choose from three distinct layers (hardware infrastructure or application platform or readymade softwares). IaaS enables users to access resources (computing power, storage, network, etc.) to host applications and does not need to configure or manage those resources. In other words, the user specifies the infrastructure requirement and rest is taken care by the IaaS provider. Additionally the user is benefited from the pay-as-you-go model with no upfront costs associated. PaaS model provide a development and deployment platform for running applications in the Cloud. The entire stack from infrastructure software platform is the responsibility of PaaS provider. SaaS model takes computing services to a level whereby users can use utilize readymade software for their business needs. SaaS providers own the entire stack of infrastructure to software applications and also provide tailoring on the software services, need be. The user is charged on usage basis and extremely beneficial for processes that are standard in nature.

National Institute of Standards and Technology (NIST) has promulgated the definition of cloud as a model for enabling universal, readily available, need based access to a common pool of configurable computing resources [11]. While the cloud platform provides unlimited computing and storage capacity, the solutions built on the platform can gain from the efficiencies brought by the cloud service provider. For instance, service providers engage dynamic scheduling of Virtual Machines (VMs) to ensure optimal utilization of computing resources. This ensures the high productivity of resources and lower cost to the service consumers. In the case of healthcare, the service consumers are the entities described in previous paragraph.

Healthcare organizations are steadily adopting Cloud based services for their computing and storage needs. These organizations have evaluated costly on premise solutions alongside cloud based solutions. Several organizations in developed countries, have leveraged cloud in health informatics such as HealthShare from InterSystems [12], Microsoft's HealthVault [13] and CareCloud [14] that have transgressed the boundaries of information technology domain to provide healthcare related services on cloud. These solutions or products provide several functionalities ranging from provide powerful utilities for data management and connecting different entities to analytical capabilities. The outcome of these efforts can certainly be extended to developing countries to uplift healthcare services in those countries as well. While there exists basic eHealth services in some developing countries (such as telemedicine in India [15] and Uganda [16]), however there is a room to implement health informatics for widen population. Not only the ICT enablers will help these countries but also formulation and revision of policies and governance framework to control and manage such initiatives. Despite the demographic and socio economic challenges that these countries have, world class cloud solutions for health informatics can be achieved through well-defined time bound roadmap for implementation. Thus in order to facilitate efficient implementation, it is necessary to derive flexible cloud based architecture. Such architecture must consider various healthcare entities, their interactions and requirements. This chapter attempts to propose such an architecture.

The structure of the chapter is organized as follows. Section 2 presents case studies on health informatics from developed countries. Section 3 covers various challenges present in developing countries for adopting health informatics. Cloud paradigm and service models are explained in Sect. 4. Section 5 focuses on computational Health Informatics and some of the existing models. Health Informatics as a Service (HIaaS) on cloud is dealt with in Sect. 6. Section 7 proposed HIaaS architecture in cloud for developing countries followed by detailed discussion and future direction in Sect. 8. Section 9 concludes the chapter.

2 Case Studies Related to Health Informatics

There has been several research work conducted by academicians, researchers, non-profit organizations and governments towards health informatics. The domain of health informatics is ever expanding with special thrust on leveraging technology. The researches have been focused on areas such as clinical guidelines and healthcare processes.

Clinical guidelines provide recommendation that are targeted towards patient care through systematic review of medical conditions [17]. These guidelines are generally focused on the various patient conditions. Several evaluation of clinical guidelines morbid conditions are been made, some of the recent ones such as, fetal disorders due to alcohol exposure [18] and hypertensive conditions in Andean and European countries [19]. However such research are limited to examination of guidelines for particular disease. An interesting research by Hughes et al. [20] on challenges faced by existing clinical guidelines for people having multi morbidity. The guidelines from National Institute of Health and Clinical Excellence (NICE), United Kingdom (UK) were examined to study the shortcomings. The results indicated that multi morbid conditions were not accounted in the guidelines which could cause considerable treatment burden and patient compliance issues. But this research does not account for the use of technology in order to update the guidelines to tackle this challenge.

Healthcare processes have evolved with complexities of discovering and defining sources of medical conditions. Bergman et al. [21] define five main processes from a citizen's perspective that may not appear in sequence. However it does no touch upon the involvement ICT that can engage citizens to improvement such processes. A notable work by Valdez et al. [22] elaborated on the healthcare processes that can leverage ICT to provide better connected patient welfare. It takes into account, patients' biomedical realities and personal skills and behaviours for designing Consumer Health Informatics (CHI) applications. The proposed patient work framework focusses on patients' health management in a larger processes and contexts of healthcare. Zheng et al. [23] researched on advance technology for acquisition of health related information through wearable devices and sensors. Use of body sensor network in capturing information of individuals on a daily basis enables early prediction and treatment major diseases. Shen et al. [24] explored use of clouds in managing eHealth monitoring systems. Since patients can be located in different geographies, the paper proposed to systems that can take advantage of geo distributed cloud in order to reduce service delays and increase privacy preservation.

Sultan et al. [25] explored the use of cloud computing in healthcare domain and derive benefits from the unique characteristics of cloud. The paper discusses the case study of Chelsea and West-minster Hospital (London) where UK funded health project was implemented on cloud IaaS and PaaS service models. Vilaplana et al. [26] take a dive in leveraging cloud computing for designing a system model that can be applied to eHealth. The system offers computing services and database servers to enable eHealth applications. The system model responds with better Quality of Service (QoS) in terms of averaged waiting times for applications.

Though these researches evaluated concepts of use of ICT in improving healthcare processes, the gap still exists in realizing benefits of implementing such processes from cloud service models. Service provisioning in cloud based on the available service and deployment models have been overlooked. The risks associated with cloud security have not been considered. Further, these implementation approaches have been designed for developed countries where sufficient infrastructure already established and may not work in developing countries. Hence it becomes critical to assess the current state and challenges of developing countries before these approaches are extended to such countries.

3 Challenges in Developing Countries

There has been considerable efforts and investment made by developed countries in embracing ICT in healthcare. European countries such as Netherlands and Switzerland are spending over 11 % of their Gross Domestic Product (GDP) in 2012, led by the United States of America (USA) which spent 17 % as per World Health Organization (WHO) report [27]. These developed nations have been investing on setting up policies, framework and infrastructure that promote inclusion of technology in delivery health services. With most of these countries are engaging researchers, entrepreneurs and business professionals to innovate technology solutions to solve healthcare problems. But when it comes to developing countries, there are certain challenges in implementing health informatics that can be broadly grouped as technology adoption, socio economic factors and healthcare policies. Before these challenges are discussed further in this section, the main elements of health informatics applications needs to be touched upon. These applications are driven by processes that transform information from sources into a standard format. These sources are already defined in Sect. 1. Information acquisition is the process of collating data from these sources that are available in various formats and ensure that relevant information is captured. The next process, information storage, triggers in as soon as new information is acquired from sources. Once the information is stored securely, information processing sets in for analysis that further refines and defines data set for stakeholders' use. The process of information transfer or display is triggered whenever request is placed by the stakeholders. These processes are further explored in Sect. 8 in context to future scope of the cloud based architecture proposed.

3.1 Technology Adoption

Most of the developing countries do not have clear vision of embracing ICT in their roadmap of healthcare services. Though there is spurt of technology awareness among medical fraternity happens to be urban cities, rural populations still utilizes age old health services. In many cases rural population has a limited access to hospitals. They have to travel a distance to avail medical facilities. But more often, the hospitals are not equipped with medical devices that can help doctors to diagnosis medical problems. Such scenarios demand technology infrastructure within hospitals to enable medical treatments. Besides, technology planning needs to be done to ensure patients don't have to wait till they are in hospitals to start diagnosis, but can connect from their homes as soon as they come across any problems.

Flexible and elaborate infrastructure is a precursor to a solid Health Information System (HIS). A solid HIS in turn is needed to improve health ecosystems of countries. Organizations can then introduce and plan new healthcare interventions that result in achieving better health goal [28]. Sophisticated medical devices, computers hardware and software is the need of the hour for developing countries. Computing and storage infrastructure enables smarter decisions based on the history of evidences that can be stored and retrieved any time. Basic internet technology has not penetrated in those countries which is one of the fundamental pillars for realizing eHealth services. Healthcare is all about of being real time where internet plays a major role. Not having internet means that healthcare providers cannot communicate and administer services to remote locations.

3.2 Socio Economic Factors

Healthcare investments are affected by macro economic situations of developing countries. In fact the technology investments by governments are based on the

	Health expenditure ratios[a]									
	Total expenditure on health as % of gross domestic product		General government expenditure on health as % of total expenditure on health[b]		Private expenditure on health as % of total expenditure on health[b]		General government expenditure on health as % of total government expenditure		External resources for health as % of total expenditure on health	
Member State	2000	2012	2000	2012	2000	2012	2000	2012	2000	2012
Egypt	5.4	4.9	40.5	39.0	59.5	61.0	7.3	5.8	1.0	0.4
Ghana[r]	3.0	5.2	50.0	68.3	50.0	31.7	7.8	10.6	14.8	11.8
India[n,t,t]	4.3	3.8	27.0	30.5	73.0	69.5	4.6	4.3	0.5	1.3
Iraq[n,v]	0.8	4.8	4.8	60.5	95.2	39.5	0.1	6.0	54.9	0.4
Kazakhstan	4.2	4.3	50.9	55.8	49.1	44.2	9.2	10.9	7.4	0.4
Kuwait	2.5	2.6	76.3	82.8	23.7	17.2	5.2	5.8	0	0
Libya[n]	3.4	4.3	48.7	70.3	51.3	29.7	6.0	7.9	0	0.1
Malaysia	3.0	4.0	55.8	55.2	44.2	44.8	5.3	5.7	0.7	0

Fig. 1 WHO statistics on health expenditure in developing countries [27]

percentage of Gross Domestic Product (GDP) which is quite low in developing countries. Governments focus on providing budget for basic medical facilities that may be the need of the hour, but need to consider the impact of technology on healthcare services. For instance, in India, the cost health services is estimated to be Indian Rupees 1.6 trillion over next 4 years [29]. While the government realizes the fiscal burden, it has initiated certain eHealth programmes (under "Digital India") in deeper penetration for economical healthcare services. The programme will leverage technology to build portals for citizens to maintain health records and book online appointments with hospitals using unique identifier Aadhaar [30] number. While such initiatives from government are going to impact the health fabric of the country, it is equally critical to look at the social factors that impact the effectiveness of such schemes. Figure 1 presents World Health Organization (WHO) statistics on health expenditure in developing countries.

It is a known fact that even modern systems will fail if they are not used by people. Awareness is critical factor in making a system successful. Technology investments need to focus on creating awareness among people. They need to understand details about the procedures and policies that govern HIS. Awareness programs that keep the user view in mind have to be developed to ensure that people can understand it usage and benefits. From the provider side, training programs are required for medical staffs in order to ensure correct usage of the system for disbursing medical facilities. Certain social factors such as job fear, illiteracy and ignorance to learning new technology come in way of effectiveness of such trainings. But such programs need to be complemented with awareness that can mitigate such factors. The governments also need to realize that a firm healthcare policy along with investments is a key to success for healthcare in their countries.

3.3 Healthcare Policies

Public health models in countries are driven by the healthcare policies that are envisaged and implemented. Most of the developing countries provide free access to health services. Policy advisors, officials and government representatives take into account the factors such as economic conditions, and demographics to ascertain key aspects pertaining to healthcare policies. While there are efforts made to amend policies in order to introduce technology in service management and disbursement, there are needs to be major focus on latest technology adoption in these policies. While several developing countries have made strides in introducing eHealth policies (Latin counties such as Brazil and Chile [31]), there are countries such as Congo and Cambodia where eHealth policies are non-existent as per WHO report [32].

Government policy towards eHealth requires a well-defined strategy in order to improve effectiveness of the medical services. The strategy needs to be focussed for a time period of 3, 6 and 10 years. During this period, government need to formulate, measure and monitor the impact and then reassess the details on the policy. There cycle of formulation monitoring and reassessment needs to be repetitive and followed during the entire period. The strategy should focus on four work streams —foundations, solutions, change and adoption and governance [33]. The foundations work stream should focus on establishing and strengthening the basic infrastructure nationwide. This will form the base for electronic sharing of information across the health sector. This basic infrastructure includes the following.

- The development of identification platform for uniquely recognizing the citizens and healthcare provider.
- The establishment of rules and protocols for information exchange among the healthcare providers, government agencies, medical clinics, doctors, patients, diagnostic centres.
- The implementation of underlying physical computing, storage and networking infrastructure for connecting different stakeholders mentioned in above point.

The solutions work stream should focus improving the capability of applications that deal with different medical processes. For instance, medical processes, such as patient admission and discharge in hospitals, need to be streamlined through use of standard softwares. These processes are basic and repetitive in nature and therefore right candidates for automation through softwares. The change and adoption work stream is where the government should formulate bodies that measure the effectiveness of the systems in place and provide recommendations based on their findings. Also these bodies need to collaborate with technology forums to pilot areas where latest technology can be tested and provide implementation models for adoption. The last work stream—governance, should focus on the imposing standards and policies, running awareness among the stakeholders about the benefits of

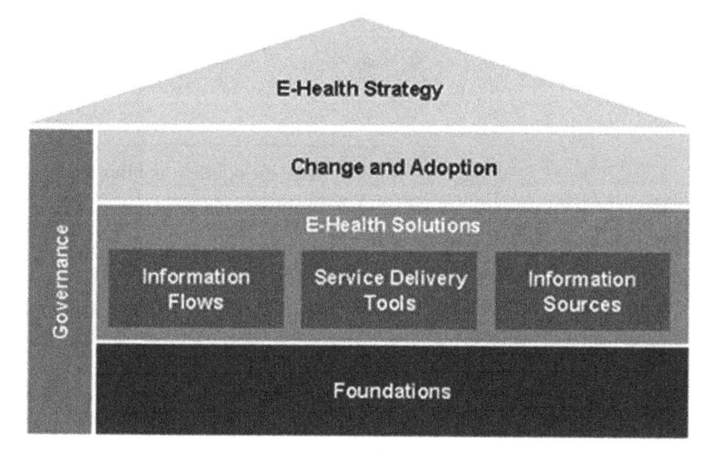

Fig. 2 eHealth strategic work streams [23]

the eHealth and ensure transparency, accountability and stakeholder involvement. Figure 2 summarizes strategy work streams for eHealth.

4 Cloud Service Models

Cloud computing has been a paradigm shift in the way computing services are being delivered to users. The key characteristics of cloud are scalability, agility, availability and reliability [34] that forms base for provisioning services. While healthcare providers do not have to worry about infrastructure, they can focus on building and deploying world class services. The cloud providers are responsible for scaling up and down underlying resources in short time. They ensure that underlying computing resources are available round the clock. The datacenters that power the cloud are located in different geographies and provide failover that ensure reliability. Service provisioning is a critical area for healthcare service providers. Hence it is important to understand cloud service and deployment models.

4.1 Service Provisioning Models

Cloud Computing provides three distinct layers for service provisioning—Infrastructure as a Service (IaaS), Platform as a Service (PaaS) and Software as a Service (SaaS). IaaS fast and almost unlimited processing capabilities and large and almost unlimited storage facilities [34]. The primary technique behind IaaS is the hardware virtualization. Several virtual machines (VMs) are configured and interconnected to define the distributed system. Each VM comprises of computing

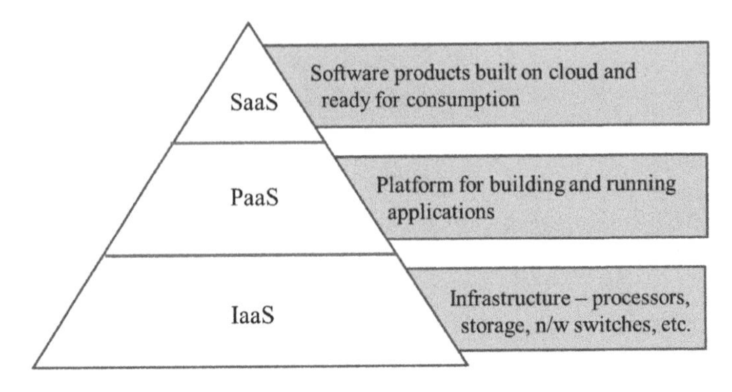

Fig. 3 Cloud service models [34]

components having specific characteristics: memory, number of processors, and disk storage. The users (also referred as consumers) can deploy applications on these VMs. Elastic Computing Cloud of Amazon (Amazon EC2) [35] and storage by Elastic Book Store (EBS) and Simple Storage Services (S3) are some of the existing IaaS platforms.

The next service provisioning model is PaaS that provides development tools and hosting options for consumers who want to create and manage their own applications [34]. It comprises of middleware which runs on top of the computing and storage infrastructure. The middleware creates a runtime environment without exposing the underlying infrastructure. Google AppEngine [36], one of the known PaaS offerings from Google, provides hosting platform for Web applications. The third service model—SaaS [34] enables access to applications through the Internet as Web based service. Such a service liberates consumers from worrying about the hardware and softwares required for running applications. All that is required for consumers is a Web browser through which they can access such service. One of the leading SaaS example is Salesforce.com that aims to facilitate creation, tracking and routing of customer cases within organizations. Figure 3 describes three distinct layers of service provisioning.

4.2 Service Deployment Models

The requirements from organizations and individual consumers drive the cloud deployment models. Essentially cloud provides four distinct deployment models that are described as follows.

- **Public cloud:** This deployment model is most dominant in current Cloud computing [37]. As the name suggest, public cloud is used by the general consumers who pay only for the duration of use (pay as you go model). Since the breadth of consumers is large, the scale bring down the cost for service provider that is passed on to consumers through reducing billing. The service provider takes full ownership of the public cloud, that is, the policies, profit, costing, and charging model are all managed by them. The examples of public clouds are Amazon Elastic Compute Cloud (EC2), Amazon Simple Storage Service (S3), Google AppEngine, and Force.com.

- **Private cloud:** As the name suggests, private cloud is operated solely dedicated to a single organization. This deployment model can be managed by the organization or a third party [37]. Organization choose such a model in order to maximize the utilization of in-house resources and limit security concerns (including data privacy and trust). Also for mission-critical engagements, organizations want a full control and dedicated cloud that reside behind their firewalls.
- **Community cloud**: This cloud is meant for organizations, belonging to an industry line (such as healthcare, manufacturing, etc.). Since these organizations share policies, requirements, values, and concerns, they jointly form a community to drive construction of cloud infrastructure. Such a community is beneficial in terms of economic scalability and democratic equilibrium. The cloud infrastructure could be hosted by a third-party vendor or within one of the organizations in the community.
- **Hybrid cloud:** Hybrid cloud, as the name denotes, is a combination of two or more clouds (private, community, or public) that exist as unique entities, but are connected to each other through standardized technology and protocols. Organizations, at times prefer such model when they have want to retain advantage of other cloud models. For instance, hospitals can deploy core systems on private cloud for processing financial transactions where as use public cloud for non core processes related to facilities management.

5 Computational Health Informatics

Traditional ways of medical treatments prevalent in both developed and developing countries, have limitations. For instances, medical emergencies are at times become fatal due to failure of timely reach of basic medical facilities available on the spot. Another case where elderly citizens have at times restricted mobility which causes physical trauma to reach to the medical centers for proper treatment. Even within hospitals and diagnostics centers, there are processes that sometimes take long waiting hours which is not beneficial for the patients. It is important now to get systems that can just not facilitate reach of medical assistance wherever and whenever it is required but also proactively monitors and predict any medical help that could be required.

With advancement of ICT, healthcare domain has benefited by adopting some of the recent trends in the field. Some of the models, that have been established over a decade to increase reach of medical treatment as well bring in efficiency in healthcare, are discussed as follows.

5.1 Electronic Health Record (EHR)

The volume of clinical information pertaining to individuals has been ever increasing. Diagnostic centers, hospitals, health camps, routine check-up, etc. have been generating information in the form of textual and visual information about the patient's condition. Thus EHR, a systematic collection and storage of this information with the use of ICT [38], has been major breakthrough in preserving and sharing of wide range of data that includes patients' biographical, demographical and medical information. Even detailed information such as clinical notes from physician's visits, laboratory test results, and vital signs are captured in the EHR. The information set is not limited to patient, but also details on visits and hospital records are also a part of EHR. The objective of EHR systems is to facilitate fast and easy access to patient's information to ensure right treatment is disbursed to the patient. The entire community of healthcare providers is benefited by adopting EHR. One of the major contributions of EHR systems has been the development of Natural Language Processing (NLP) [39]. NLP converts transcription of dictations to electronic format that supports searching, summarization, decision-support, or statistical analysis. Figure 4 represents a sample EHR for a patient.

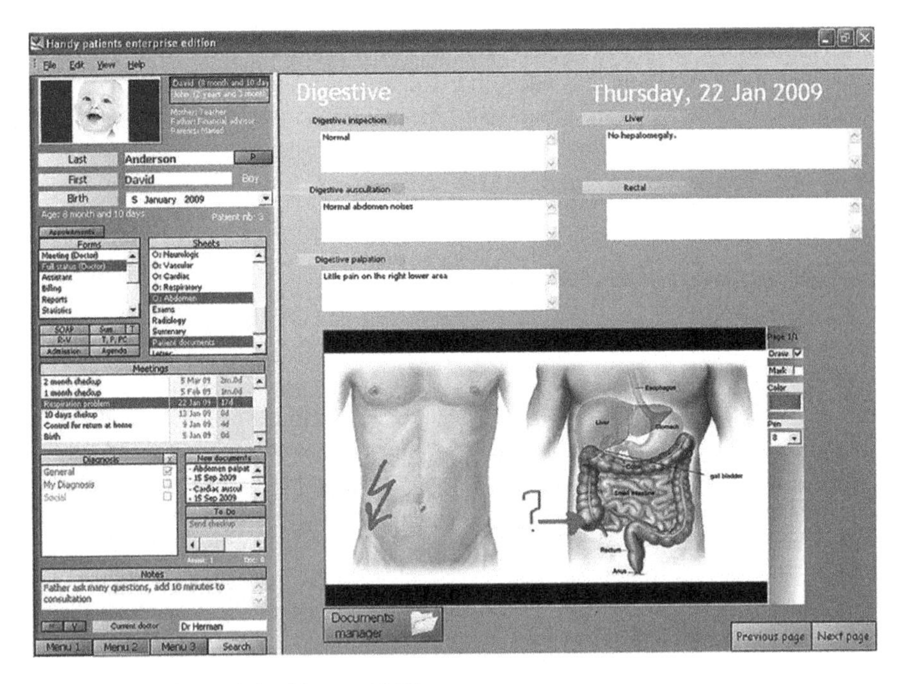

Fig. 4 Sample electronic health record [40]

5.2 Telemedicine

Tele-medicine [41] has been instrumental in bringing primary care and specialist referral services to remote patients. Use of interactive live video conferencing, sharing of diagnostic images, prescriptions, clinical notes and video clips is easily done through telecommunication equipment and standards. An important use case of remote patient monitoring can be addressed through these standards. Home bound patients can be monitored by sharing vital signs such as ECG and blood glucose with the doctor that can supplement use of visiting nurses. With increasing use of internet and wireless devices, patients can receive expert device through emails, discussion forums. Even doctors can provide references and collaborate through chat boards for critical care and also second opinions. Some of the successful implementations such as Apollo Telemedicine (India) and Tactive Telemedicine (Netherlands) [32] provide medical solutions for its rural population. Figure 5 depicts a view of telemedicine connecting remote hospitals with district hospitals for consultations with doctors.

5.3 Mobile Health (mHealth)

According to the International Telecommunication Union, in 2011, the mobile phone subscriptions globally stands close to 5 billion. Commercial wireless

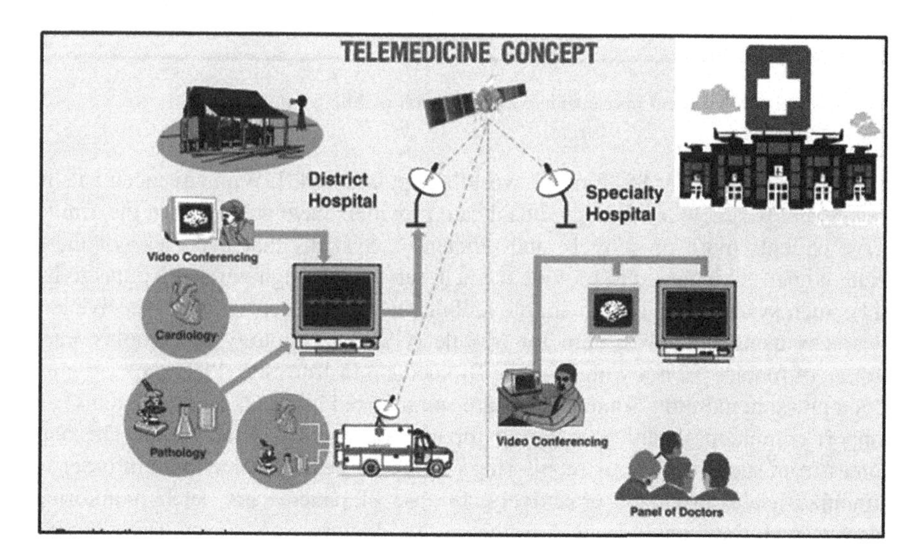

Fig. 5 Connecting remote hospitals using telemedicine [42]

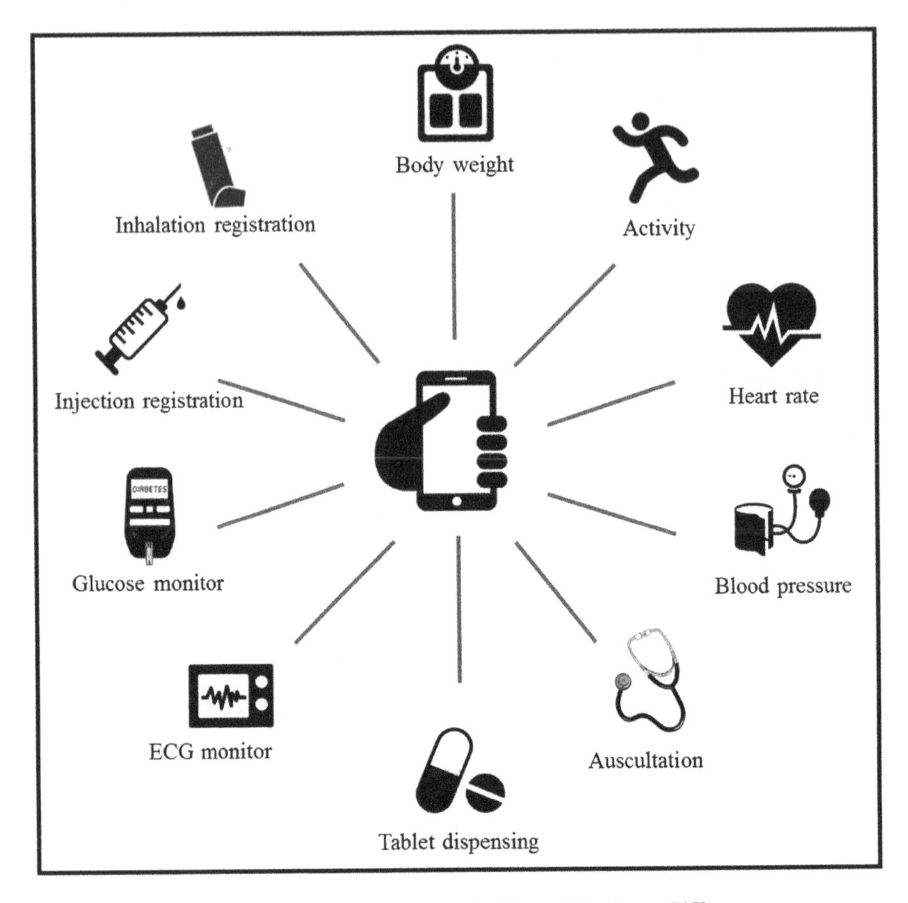

Fig. 6 Portable biomedical instruments connected with mobile phones [45]

technology covers over 85 % of the world's population [43]. With advancements in mobile and wearable technology, healthcare providers have got a shot in the arm to serve patients more proactively and efficiently. Systems that make use of these technologies are intended to provide medical services through wireless connectivity [44]. Such systems range from simple mobile phones that can send and receive test messages using Global System for Mobile (GSM) technology to complex integration of mobile phones with Portable Biomedical Instruments (PBI) such a digital blood pressure monitor. Some of PBIs are summarized in Fig. 6. These systems can support continuous health monitoring for individuals as well as group. The outcomes from such continuous monitoring can record healthy behaviours in order to minimize health problems proactively. In case of patient care, such monitoring ensures real time passing of information to doctors and nurses for effective observation. Smartphones and electronic body gears capture statistics pertaining to the patients while they are busy with their daily lives. The statistics collected by these smart devices help in diagnosis. mHealth applications are being developed and evaluated in a variety of domains, including diabetes, asthma, obesity, smoking cessation, stress management, and depression treatment. The mHealth has a tremendous potential given that mobiles have a deeper penetration among both developed and developing countries.

6 Health Informatics as a Service

The existing eHealth models leverage extensively ICT to enable services to the patients. These models have involved over the years from departmental functions to larger solutions at organization. The solution initially was implemented locally on standalone systems which over a time were interconnected with other peer systems to form integrated solution. With this the complexity of such solutions increased as the connections were more point to point. Also that propriety standards involved which made such solutions more rigid and complex. Some of these challenges are summarized in below section.

6.1 Challenges in Existing Health Information Systems

The existing Health Information Systems (HIS) pose challenges in terms of the setup and maintenance costs, limited connectivity, lack of regulations and standards. These factors are important for countries to realize the shortfalls and think upon avenues to address these problems. These factors are delved in more details as follows.

- **Implementation and Maintenance Overheads:** Setting up of HIS is a financial burden for healthcare organizations. It requires large scale investments for procuring software, hardware, technical infrastructure, and professionals to manage such systems. While large and medium sized organizations could plan for such investments, it becomes an entry barrier for small organizations to implement such systems. Even so, the implementations planning and schedule for such systems are longer and time consuming for healthcare professionals as they are already engaged patient duties. They need to share time and work extra hours to share their inputs for project implementation, which becomes an additional responsibility apart from pursuing important duties. The other aspect —maintenance for such systems are long drawn and need continued operational expenditure to manage, and upgrade.

- **Absence of Proper HIS Integration**: Healthcare organization usually have HIS in different departments in the form of small clinical or administrative systems. The challenge is with patient data that is in dispersed state existing in these systems. Such dispersed pockets of data make it difficult to integrate information together and share it across the organization or across different healthcare providers. Also the access restrictions on certain portions of this data within separate departmental systems come in the way of integrating these systems.
- **Lack of Regulations/Laws**: There needs to be a proper mandate for use and protection of electronic healthcare data capture and communication. Currently there are no well-established regulations mandating the electronic capture of patient data from different source systems. In addition to it, there isn't any stringent framework and laws that can deal with issues of protection and security of this data. For instance, there is no general law protecting the privacy of patients and the interchanges of their medical data between countries [36]. Each country has a different data protection standards and regulations. For example, in Europe, the directive on privacy and electronic communications [46] protects the personal information of patients while the Health Insurance Portability and Accountability Act (HIPAA) and in the United States, Subtitle D of the HIS for Economic and Clinical Health (HITECH) Act [37] enforces privacy and security standards for organizations covered by HIPAA.

6.2 Opportunities of Cloud in Health Informatics

Cloud computing brings in choices for healthcare providers to design and deploy world class health informatics services. While cloud takes care of infrastructure at the lowest level, it also provides ready to use platform and softwares that can be configured to build eHealth services. Thus it removes operational load from service provider's shoulder, enabling them to focus on the refining services. The service providers can leverage the scale of cloud infrastructure to increase the reach of their services. For instance, hospitals from different towns, cities, states and even countries can connect on the cloud platform and share services. The opportunities for cloud in healthcare services are elaborated as follows.

- **Improvement in Patient Care:** With the use of cloud computing, systems can offer a unified patient medical record containing patient details from all patient encounters in various entities within or outside healthcare organizations. Besides, healthcare providers can access these records anywhere and anytime. This will allow them to have a comprehensive view of the patient's history and provide the most suitable treatments accordingly. In emergency cases, real time integration is another aspect where healthcare providers can benefit from, by enabling immediate diagnosis and treatments.

- **Solve Resource Scarcity Issues:** In remote and rural areas, the communities living there face shortage of healthcare facilities due to lack of infrastructure [37]. The healthcare centers are equipped with minimal staffs and health experts are not always accessible in those centers. With use of cloud, these centers can access to large health repositories containing knowledge on case histories and notes on past cases. This can at least reduce some amount of dependency on the experts to be available.
- **Reduced Cost:** Cloud computing provides the feature to share environment and infrastructure resources, deployment models such as public cloud and community cloud enables cost sharing among organizations in the same fraternity. Thus the overhead costs can be minimized and the same benefit can be passed onto the patients. Also the pay per use model provides flexibility to only pay for actual resource utilization, thus bring down the cost further. Small and medium sized healthcare providers can benefit from these factors as often times the initial expenses on advanced IT infrastructures becomes an entry barrier.
- **Facilitate Research**: Large medical repositories can be build using cloud storage that can store millions of patients' cases. These repositories can serve as an integrated platform which can be uniformly and globally accessed. This integrated platform can be easily leveraged to create data mining models for discovering medical facts and conduct medical research to enhance medications, treatments and healthcare services. Also, pharmaceutical companies can utilize this platform for drug discovery.
- **Support National Security:** In order to detect disease outbreaks, monitoring systems can be setup in cloud that collate information from various sources and derive patterns on disease spread. Such systems can generate alert based on the patterns derived and notify medical agencies and professionals to undertake appropriate action.
- **Facilitate Strategic Planning:** Health Informatics on cloud can be a useful tool for decision makers that can process data for planning and budgeting for healthcare services. Even so, services can be configured in cloud that can integrate with existing data in order to help in forecast future healthcare service needs.
- **Support Financial Operations:** Financial and accounting applications are standard in nature. Healthcare providers can automate such operations in cloud that may not require human intervention. For instance, the payments process, that requires hospitals to settle expense of medical treatment and insurance companies to pay those expenses, can be placed in the cloud.
- **Support Clinical Trials:** Drug discovery is one of most complex areas in healthcare domain. Pharmaceutical companies and medical research institutions require immense collaboration during clinical trials for new medicines. Identification of trial patients need structured analysis of patient cases. Such activities can make use of cloud for analysis and processing of cases.

6.3 Security Issues in Health Informatics Cloud

With several opportunities brought by use of cloud in health informatics, there are certain challenges need to be considered while engaging cloud in health informatics. Patient's information is critical to healthcare industry and maintaining patient's privacy is of outmost importance. Therefore any transmission of such data needs to be secured and access to such data needs to be authenticated. A review work [44] indicated that, from user's perspective, techniques such as use of symmetric/asymmetric key and pseudo anonymity are common in EHRs. The preferred access control is role based and the systems must be capable of generating audit logs.

While cloud provides a novel way for storing EHRs and hosting eHealth services, data security is a major area that service providers are required to focus on. Data leakage during transmission and storage needs to be addressed from both user and providers' perspective. A survey by Agaku et al. [47] elaborates on the confidence of patients on the systems that secure their health records. The existing standards such as HIPAA, protocols such HTTPS and authentication techniques such as user credentials, lay out ground rules for securing health data, there are certain researches that are important to note in this area. Nandi et al. [45] leveraged ECG as unique identification for individuals to access data. Another useful technique based on watermarking ECG signals [46] and videos [48] can increase security levels. Biometric authentication based on retinal image [49] can generate unique bio keys that can be used for authenticating access. Further cryptographic solutions such as Searchable Symmetric Encryption (SSE), Threshold Secret Sharing (TSS), Identity-Based encryption (IBE) and Attribute-Based Encryption (ABE) can be deployed in cloud to enforce privacy [50]. SSE prevents information leakage by storing and indexing of encrypted documents. TSS can ensure that secret information is shared only among multiple entities that have privileged access. IBE, an asymmetric cryptographic solution, deploys public keys for accessing encrypted message with no prior key distribution. ABE enables fine grained access control to users through a set of attributes that define an access structure to encrypted data.

6.4 Expectations from HIaaS

The key consumers for medical services are the patients, hospitals, diagnostic centers, physicians and pharmacy stores, etc. Services designed in cloud, need to take into considerations the requirements from each of these actors. While existing eHealth systems would cater to some of those requirements in isolation, the eHealth services need to be designed based on the holistic view of the different entities and their interaction. Table 1 summarizes the requirements from different entities involved in healthcare.

Table 1 Healthcare entities and their requirements

Entities	Requirements
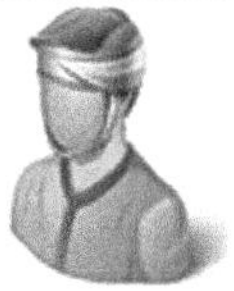 Patient	• Able to locate nearest hospitals, clinics and diagnostic centers • Able to book doctor appointments, • Get reminders on appointments • Able to view history of diagnosis, treatments • Get updates on the latest developments in medicine • During hospitalization, need seamless support with doctors, hospitals and insurance companies
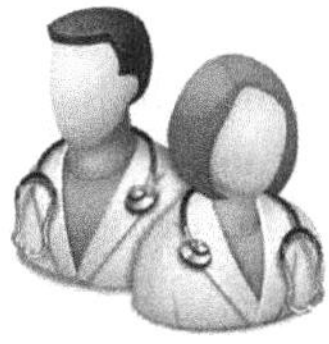 Doctor	• Able to view appointments • Able to enter prescriptions and diagnosis • View medical reports, clinical notes and history of ailments • Receive information on drug administration • View progressive medical evaluations and conditions
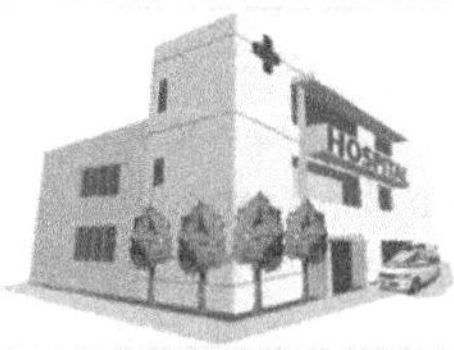 Hospital Administration	• Secure and fast storage and retrieval of patient records • Manage doctors availability and bookings • Seamless integration with Insurance companies • Receive information on disease outbreaks
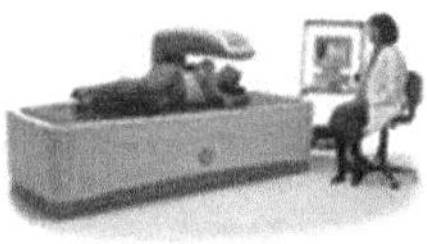 Diagnostic center/Clinic	• Access to relevant patient records and test recommendations • Upload test results and diagnostic reports • Seamless integration with Insurance companies
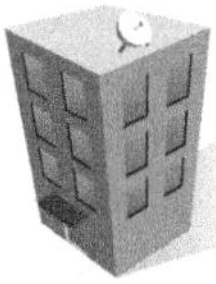 Insurance Company	• Access to relevant patient records and test recommendations • Seamless integration with Hospitals • Seamless co-operation with patient parties
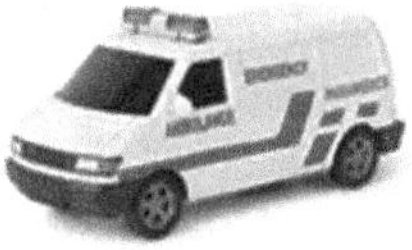 Mobile clinics	• Access to relevant patient records • Access channels to take appropriate assistance from doctors and hospitals • Store medical prescriptions
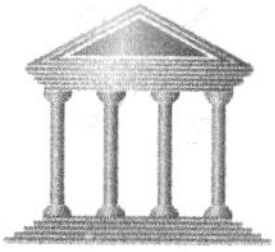 Government	• Access to citizen's health database at city and state level • Derive statistics on health information about the citizens for policy formations, change

7 Health Informatics Services for Developing Countries

In developing countries, there are various HIS initiatives taken based on the socio economic factors. Most of these are outcome of policies and efforts from the government and agencies. For instance, in India, National Rural Health Mission is aimed at using ICT to extend medical facilities in rural areas and also to collect health information of rural population [51]. A similar initiative in Brazil which is known as Saúde Health Information System [51] that is targeted at improving health status of poor population. This is been achieved through increasing efficiency in handling healthcare services and benefiting patients (by reducing wait times for appointments) and primary care units (by managing resources). Zambia is another example where SmartCare [52], an advanced HIS was established. The objective of this initiative was to ensure patient health records are available to the clinician. Healthcare professionals can make informed decisions about treatments when they are able to access complete case history through patient health record.

The initiatives such as above, can benefit from the use of cloud. The focus needs to be on utilizing existing infrastructure and build reusable core services. Core services such as data storage retrieval and analytics, can be composed and orchestrated to be used by variety of stakeholders. The next section proposes a cloud based architecture that can enable design and implementation of HIaaS for the benefit of developing countries.

7.1 Proposed Architecture in Cloud

The proposed healthcare architecture in cloud derives its fundamentals from basic tenet of cloud computing, that is, anything in cloud can be deployed as service (Everything as a Service, XaaS). In context of healthcare, various functions pertaining to health informatics can be simplified resulting in services provisioned in cloud. In other words, services that cater to the requirements of stakeholders (defined in Sect. 5.3) can be deployed in cloud, thus forming HIaaS in reality. This architecture considers that the services are deployed and managed in cloud leveraging IaaS and PaaS models. While IaaS provides underlying infrastructure for service deployments, PaaS provides platform for developing services. We propose a layered architecture that contains core services, orchestrates multiple services, manages users and device communication and can handle presentation logic for rendering services. Figure 7 summarizes this layered architecture. The description of each layer considered in the architecture is presented in the following.

1. ***Core services*** form the bottom most layer of the proposed layered architecture. This layer consists of Data Storage and Data Analytics services. Cloud provides data storage as service that can allow entities to store, update and retrieve textual and visual information.

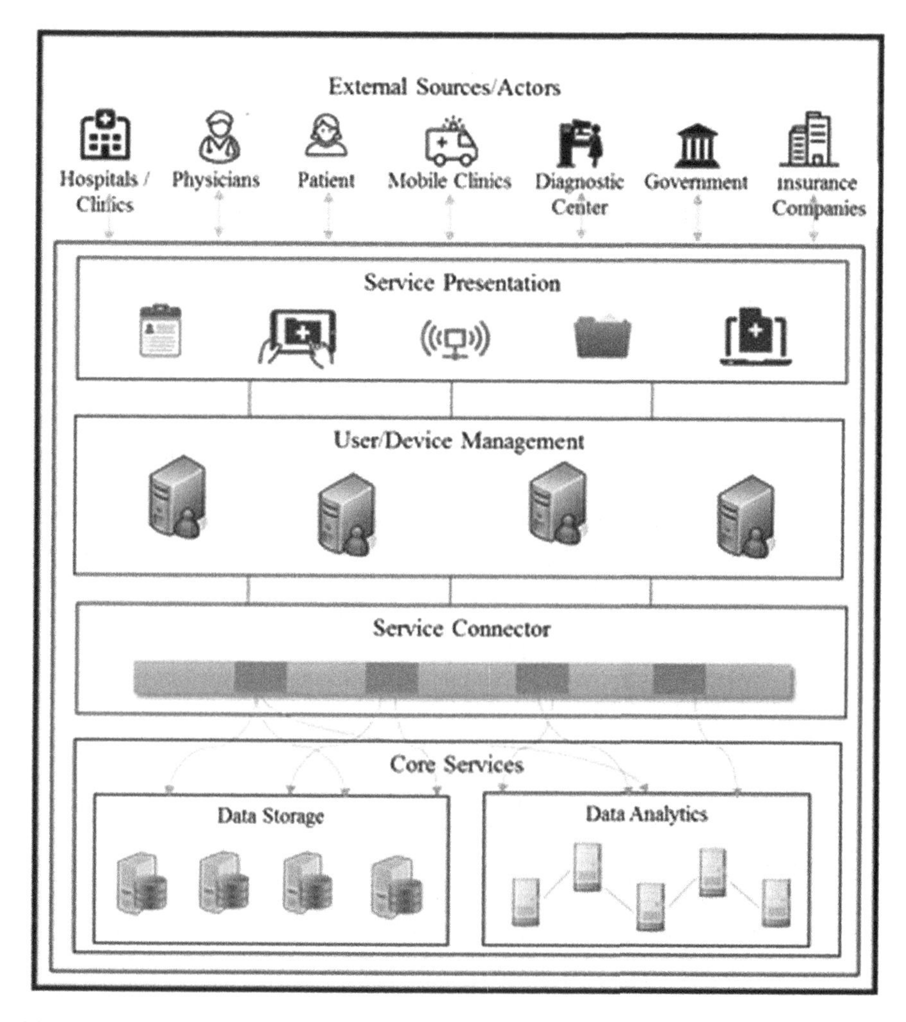

Fig. 7 Cloud based architecture for HIaaS

EHRs can be uploaded in the cloud storage. Both structured and unstructured data can be stored using NoSQL database instead of traditional ones [53]. In order to derive meaningful information from the data storage, data analytics services can be deployed that can provide pre-processing, analytics and visualization of data. Such analytics services can be utilized by healthcare providers (hospitals, clinics and physicians) in order to diagnose ailments and provide treatment options to the patients.

2. ***Service Bus*** forms the layer above core services. This layer handles that composition and orchestration of multiple core services based on the requirements of the external actors. For instance, a hospital may want to store EHRs of all

admitted patients and then analyze the top ten diagnosis and treatments that are done in last 6 months.
This would be required to forecast inventory of medical equipment and medicines that the hospital must keep in stock. In order to handle this scenario, appropriate Data Storage and Data Analytics services is required to be invoked. Service Connector handles such invocations and also manages inter communication among those services.
3. ***User/Device Management layer*** is located above Service Connector. This layer manages the communication with users (physicians, patients, hospital staffs, etc.) and devices (desktops, tablets, medical kiosks, automatic teller machines, etc.). When the user or device accesses first time, there are set of tasks for registering these actors. These actors can be uniquely identified through user ids and device ids and every time authenticated based on the unique identifiers. There can be user or device groups that could be created to grant appropriate access.
For instance, laboratory assistants should be allowed to upload clinical reports and should not have access to patient's diagnosis reports. A user group specific to this requirement can be created that has access to upload clinical reports only. Laboratory assistants can belong to this group and their access can be authorized based on the role. This layer provides most important feature, session management, where user sessions can be maintained through secured protocols such as Hyper Text Transfer Protocol (HTTPS) [54].
4. ***Service Presentation layer*** sites on top of User/Device Management. This layer acts as interface for different actors. While other layers are focused on service creation and composition, this layer manages service delivery. There are variety of channels that is required to deliver services.
For instance, hospitals would require File Transfer Protocol (FTP) to upload patient's information, physicians and patients may have desktops and mobile phones to access service and medical devices would require secure Internet of Things (IoT) protocols [55] to use the services.

The architecture provides seamless access to services and management of communication with different actors. While services essentially form the core of this architecture, the workflows are to be essentially managed through other layers. This architecture comes where advantages of adaptability and extensibility. The services that are considered here are Data Storage and Data Analytics. In case there are additional services that needs to be designed and offered to the users, this architecture allows such additions making it highly adaptable. Besides, this layered approach allows additional actors to be hooked onto the services without any change in the overall architecture, which makes it extensible.

While this layered architecture establishes an efficient way for provisioning services in cloud for smart medical treatment, it is important to validate applicability of this architecture on real scenarios where solutions can be derived based on the architecture.

7.2 Application Scenarios

In India, it's a common practice of citizens to undergo health insurance. There are several insurance companies that provide health insurance to masses. Though health insurance is not mandatory, individuals, based on the need and financial ability, can choose from variety of insurance policies available from the companies. However it is mandatory only at the beginning of the insurance to undergo medical test. The individuals request for insurance for a policy of interest along with medical reports. Once they are insured, they can claim medical expenses as per policy. However there is no mandatory check-ups or tests that are required during this period. The insured person can renew his or her insurance every year. One recommendation in this case is that there should be mechanism to enable health check-ups at regular interval during insurance period. For instance, the frequency of health check-ups can be one every year or every quarter. Both insured person and the insurance company will benefit by doing this practice. These check-ups can be done in hospitals and clinics, which in turn compile results and health summary that can be shared with that person as well as the insurance company. The person is benefited from such regular check-ups by taking advice for improving or maintaining health status. This process also benefits the insurance company by letting regular health update of the insured and reducing chances for bearing huge

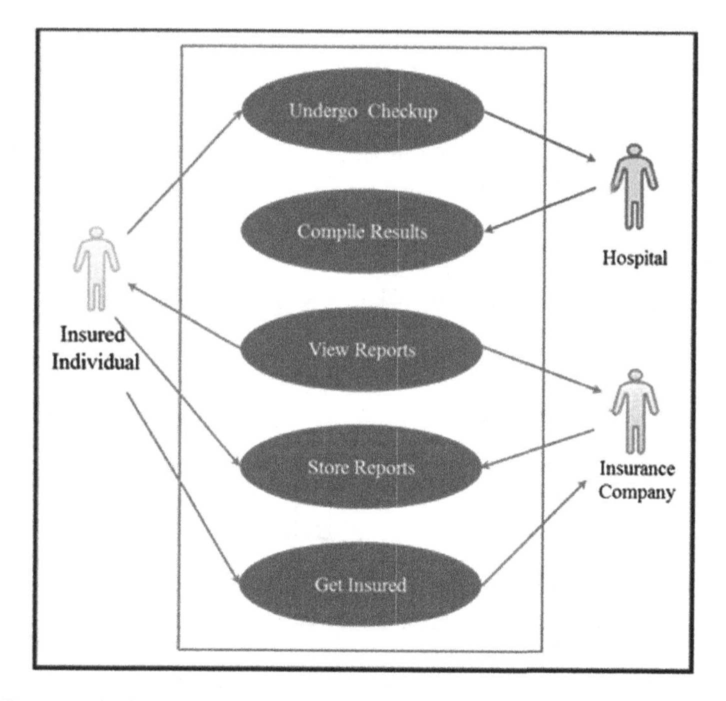

Fig. 8 Use cases for insured individual, hospital and insurance company

expenditure. Figure 8 summarizes the use cases from the above scenario. The solution to this scenario can leverage cloud using proposed architecture.

The solution comprises of set of services presented in Fig. 9 hosted in cloud. The individuals can book appointments through *Check-up Appointment Service* for health check-ups. They can choose from list of hospitals at nearby location and at convenient time. This service requires inputs from both insurance company (for instance, list of preferred hospitals which has tie up with this company) and hospitals for location and available checkup slots. Once the checkup is complete and results are ready, the hospital can use *Store Results Service* to upload diagnostic reports and health summary that can be later retrieved as required. *View Results Service* enables both individual and insurance company to view reports during the insurance period. The *Insurance Service* is established for individual and insurance company to accomplish tasks such as initiating new insurance, renewing insurance and access policy details at any given point of time.

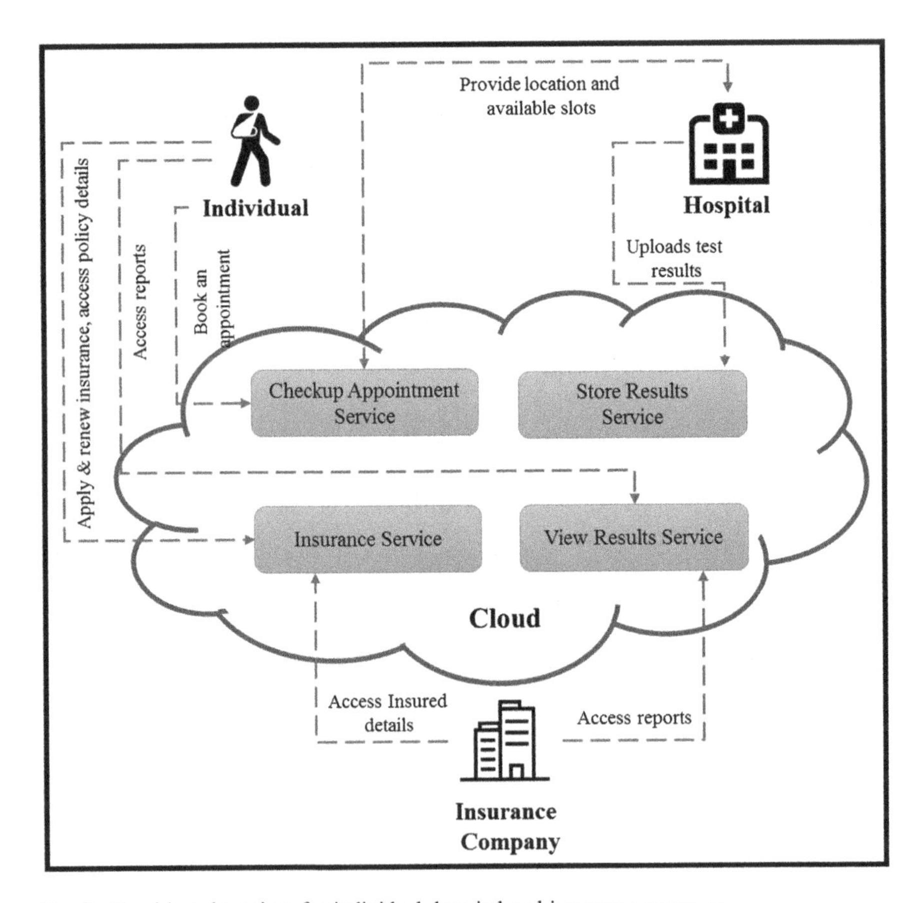

Fig. 9 Cloud based services for individual, hospital and insurance company

8 Discussion and Future Direction

The governments of developing countries are concerned about the citizens' health. Government agencies have joined hands with non-profit organizations and healthcare providers to increase reach of medical services, especially rural areas. Rapid urbanization in certain developing countries, has helped in extending infrastructure to connect remote areas. Governments of countries such as India have realized the importance of financially viable healthcare models. Viable lessons can be learned from implementation of health informatics models in those countries. At the same time, Chen et al. [56] maintained that up to 75 % of e-health programs fail during their operational stage. Hence it is important to envision the working business models that create value for healthcare provider as well as for the patient. Though initially eHealth programs need a sponsor till a breakeven point to incubate ideas, the thrust should be to use latest technologies to reduce operational costs. Cloud computing naturally comes as viable technology enabler that allows eHealth service providers to focus on services rather than on infrastructure that powers those services.

The layered architecture proposed in the previous section can handle elements of health informatics, which are, information, storage, processing and transfer or display. There are various channel that are considered in the architecture by which the sources can inject information to cloud. For instance, these sources can be smart medical devices that track health status of individuals, diagnostic centers that perform pathological tests on patients and physicians that write prescriptions for patients. The channels for that captures information are web, mobile and IoT. The information storage is on the of key core services. As soon as the information is transmitted in the cloud, the data storage services ensure that it is secularly stored and encrypted. Data analytics services further drive the processing that can transform, extract meaningful results and trends from the information stored. These services can execute based on the need basis from the stakeholders or be automated in background. Pandey et al. [57] tested cloud services that could perform ECG beat analysis on the information received from peoples' health data. The last important element in health informatics—information transfer or display connects stakeholders with health information in both raw and processed output using the same channels through the presentation layer of the proposed architecture that are used to capture information.

There are numerous possible application scenarios where health informatics in cloud can be of advantage. One such scenario is extending self health services to aging population [58]. Aged and elderly individuals are limited by age to access medical services. These individuals can not only leverage health services for monitoring health status regularly, but also engage with hospitals, clinics and physicians from their home. The entire process of capturing health status, diagnosis reports, prescriptions, etc. can be stored and accessed through services in cloud that can relieve individuals from keeping physical evidences. Another important scenario that can leverage cloud services is the administering first aid to emergency patients. Emergency cases such as cardiac arrest, where the patient requires dedicated medical attention from hospitals, the survivability of the patient diminishes with delay in administering treatment [59]. By accessing patient information history through cloud services, the preparation for administering appropriate treatment can start in hospitals even before the patient arrives in the compound.

The future scope of health informatics will need to access different application scenarios and extend cloud based architecture for deploying contextual and meaningful health informatics services. There will be avenues where government agencies, healthcare providers and research organizations have to collaborate further to tackle challenges pertaining to policy, technology and socio-economic hurdles as described in Sect. 3. While it is imperative for governments of developing countries to drive policy changes and update standards, the research organizations need to progressively evaluate cloud service models for realizing healthcare informatics for general population. The researchers have to focus on use cases for application scenarios, not limited to the ones referred in this chapter, and expand the architecture in cloud.

9 Conclusion

The area of Health Informatics has evolved with adoption of ICT. There has been major thrust on the research from developed countries to leverage ICT to build HIS. A variety of implementation models and associated paraphilia have been conceived across to benefit the healthcare stakeholders. However, there are issues prevailing in developing countries that requires attention and focus to get such models implemented. These challenges are quite evident in the statistics published by WHO and other organizations. The governments and other agencies can create an environment to foster modern medical services to reach to every corner of the nation. This chapter has delves into those issues and covered aspects such as technology adoption, socio-economic and policy factors. With right focus and open mind towards embracing innovations, developing countries can achieve health goals for their citizens.

The latest innovation that has changed the way people perceive about computing is cloud. Cloud computing, with its unique proposition of cost savings, XaaS and global reach, has created fervor amongst implementers. Healthcare providers can reduce their capital expenditure by deploying services in cloud. This chapter elaborates various service and deployment models available currently. The service providers can choose from IaaS, PaaS and SaaS models, based on their infrastructure requirements. They can further host services either in public, private, community and hybrid cloud based on financial capacities. The chapter discusses currently available models in health informatics that have leveraged ICT. These models have been implemented in several countries. However there are certain inherent challenges in the implementations such as cost implications, integration issues among car providers and lack of regulations are covered in the chapter. These challenges can be addressed by deploying services in cloud. The benefits of having cloud solutions for health informatics are elaborated here. Also the chapter elaborates on the requirements from HIaaS. Followed by that a cloud based architecture for HIaaS is proposed. In order to check the applicability, a real life scenario is considered. Associated use cases and solution in cloud in the lines of the architecture is examined.

References

1. Benson, T.: Principles of Health Interoperability HL7 and SNOMED. Springer Science & Business Media (2012)
2. Elkin, P.L. (ed.): Terminology and Terminological Systems. Springer Science & Business Media (2012)
3. Chronaki, C.E., Estelrich, A., Cangioli, G., Melgara, M., Kalra, D., Gonzaga, Z., Garber, L., Blechman, E., Ferguson, J., Kay, S.: Interoperability standards enabling cross-border patient summary ex-change, pp. 256–260. In: MIE (2014)
4. Silva, L.A.B., Costa, C., Oliveira, J.L.: DICOM relay over the cloud. Int. J. Comput. Assist. Radiol. Surg. **8**(3), 323–333 (2013)
5. Westwood, M., Joore, M., Grutters, J., Redekop, K., Armstrong, N., Lee, K., Gloy, V., Raatz, H., Misso, K., Severens, J., Kleijnen, J.: Contrast-enhanced ultrasound using SonoVue® (sulphur hexafluoride microbubbles) compared with contrast-enhanced computed tomography and contrast-enhanced magnetic resonance imaging for the characterisation of focal liver lesions and detection of liver metastases: a systematic review and cost-effectiveness analysis (2013)
6. Sanei, S., Chambers, J.A.: EEG Signal Processing. Wiley (2013)
7. Reddy, C.K., Aggarwal, C.C. (eds.): Healthcare Data Analytics, vol. 36. CRC Press (2015)
8. Bender, J.G., Verma, A., Schiffman, J.D.: Translating genomic discoveries to the clinic in pediatric oncology. Curr. Opin. Pediatr. **27**(1), 34–43 (2015)
9. LePendu, P., Iyer, S.V., Bauer-Mehren, A., Harpaz, R., Mortensen, J.M., Podchiyska, T., Ferris, T.A., Shah, N.H.: Pharmacovigilance using clinical notes. Clin. Pharmacol. Ther. **93** (6), 547–555 (2013)
10. Paul, M., Chowdhury, A.G., Das, A.: A ubiquitous E-learning architecture in cloud environment. Mater. Today: Proc. (2016).
11. National Institute of Standards and Technology. http://www.nist.gov/. Accessed 1 May 2016
12. HealthShare Overview. http://www.intersystems.com/our-products/healthshare/healthshare-overview/. Accessed 1 May 2016
13. What is HealthVault? https://www.healthvault.com/in/en. Accessed 15 May 2016
14. CareCloud. http://www.carecloud.com/. Accessed 15 May 2016
15. Jaroslawski, S., Saberwal, G.: In eHealth in India today, the nature of work, the challenges and the finances: an interview-based study. BMC Med. Inform. Decis. Mak. **14**(1), 1 (2014)
16. Mars, M.: Telemedicine and advances in urban and rural healthcare delivery in Africa. Prog. Cardiovasc. Dis. **56**(3), 326–335 (2013)
17. Consensus report, Institute of Medicine. Clinical practice guidelines we can trust. March 23, 2011. http://www.iom.edu/Reports/2011/Clinical-Practice-Guidelines-We-Can-Trust.aspx. Accessed 13 January 2012
18. Hoyme, H.E., Kalberg, W.O., Elliott, A.J., Blankenship, J., Buckley, D., Marais, A.S., Jewett, T., et al.: Updated Clinical Guidelines for Diagnosing Fetal Alcohol Spectrum Disorders. Pediatrics, e20154256 (2016)

19. Moreira, J., Jaramillo, E., Anselmi, M., Sempertegui, R., Ortiz, P., Mena, M.B., Tognoni, G.: Appraisal of five clinical guidelines for the management of hypertension in Andean Countries and Europe. World J. Cardiovasc. Dis. **4**(05), 211 (2014)
20. Hughes, L.D., McMurdo, M.E., Guthrie, B.: Guidelines for people not for diseases: the challenges of applying UK clinical guidelines to people with multimorbidity. Age Ageing **42** (1), 62–69 (2013)
21. Bergman, B., Neuhauser, D., Provost, L.: Five main processes in healthcare: a citizen perspective. BMJ Qual. Saf. **20**(Suppl 1), i41–i42 (2011)
22. Valdez, R.S., Holden, R.J., Novak, L.L., Veinot, T.C.: Transforming consumer health informatics through a patient work (2014)
23. Zheng, Y.L., Ding, X.R., Poon, C.C.Y., Lo, B.P.L., Zhang, H., Zhou, X.L., Zhang, Y.T.: Unobtrusive sensing and wearable devices for health informatics. IEEE Trans. Biomed. Eng. **61**(5), 1538–1554 (2014)
24. Shen, Q., Liang, X., Shen, X.S., Lin, X., Luo, H.Y.: Exploiting geo-distributed clouds for a e-health monitoring system with minimum service delay and privacy preservation. IEEE J. Biomed. Health Inf. **18**(2), 430–439 (2014)
25. Sultan, N.: Making use of cloud computing for healthcare provision: opportunities and challenges. Int. J. Inf. Manag. (IEEE) **34**(2), 177–184 (2014)
26. Vilaplana, J., Solsona, F., Abella, F., Filgueira, R., Rius, J.: The cloud paradigm applied to e-Health. BMC Med. Inform. Decis. Mak. **13**(1), 1 (2013)
27. World Health Statics 2015 (WHO). apps.who.int/iris/bitstream/10665/170250/1/9789240694439_eng.pdf. Accessed 31 May 2016
28. eHealth Exchange—Project Sequoia. http://sequoiaproject.org/wp-content/uploads/2016/05/eHealth-Exchange-Overview-Feb-2016-v2.pdf. Accessed 31 May 2016
29. Healthcare Industry in India. http://www.ibef.org/industry/healthcare-india.aspx. Accessed 3 June 2016
30. Aadhar Services—Resident Portal. https://resident.uidai.net.in/aadhaar-services. Accessed 3 June 2016
31. Jimenez-Marroquin, M.C., Deber, R., Jadad, A.R.: Information and communication technology (ICT) and eHealth policy in Latin America and the Caribbean: a review of national policies and assessment of socioeconomic context. Revista Panamericana de Salud Pública **35**(5–6), 329–336 (2014)
32. Kimble, C.: Business models for E-Health: evidence from ten case studies. Glob. Bus. Organ. Excellence **34**(4), 18–30 (2015)
33. Jolly, R.: The E Health Revolution: Easier Said Than Done. Parliamentary Library, Canberra (2011)
34. Paul, M., Das, A.: A review on provisioning of services in cloud computing. Int. J. Sci. Res. **3** (4), (2014)
35. Garfinkel, S.: An evaluation of amazon's grid computing services: EC2, S3, and SQS (2007)
36. Malawski, M., Kuzniar, M., Wojcik, P., Bubak, M.: How to use Google App engine for free computing. IEEE Internet Comput. **17**(1), 50–59 (2013)
37. Dillon, T., Wu, C., Chang, E.: Cloud computing: issues and challenges. In: 2010 24th IEEE International Conference on Advanced Information Networking and Applications, pp. 27–33. IEEE (2010)
38. Mantas, J.: Electronic health record. Stud. Health Technol. Inf. **65**, 250–257 (2001)
39. Meystre, S.M., Savova, G.K., Kipper-Schuler, K.C., Hurdle, J.F.: Extracting information from textual documents in the electronic health record: a review of recent research. Yearb. Med. Inf. **35**, 128–144 (2008)
40. Electronic Health Record—Wikipedia. https://en.wikipedia.org/wiki/Electronic_health_record. Accessed 3 June 2016
41. Hu, Y., Lu, F., Khan, I., Bai, G.: A cloud computing solution for sharing healthcare information (2012)
42. Telemedicine solutions. http://wwwvinamratech.com/products/telemedicine-solutions/. Accessed 3 June 2016

43. mHealth: New horizons for health through mobile technologies. http://www.who.int/goe/publications/goe_mhealth_web.pdf. Accessed 8 April 2016
44. Fernández-Alemán, J.L., Señor, I.C., Lozoya, P.Á.O., Toval, A.: Security and privacy in electronic health records: a systematic literature review. J. Biomed. Inform. **46**(3), 541–562 (2013)
45. Nandi, S., Roy, S., Dansana, J., Karaa, W.B.A., Ray, R., Chowdhury, S.R., Dey, N., et al.: Cellular automata based encrypted ECG-hash code generation: an application in inter human biometric authentication system. Int. J. Comput. Netw. Inf. Secur. **6**(11), 1 (2014)
46. Dey, N., Mukhopadhyay, S., Das, A., Chaudhuri, S.S.: Analysis of P-QRS-T components modified by blind watermarking technique within the electrocardiogram signal for authentication in wireless telecardiology using DWT. Int. J. Image Graph. Signal Process. **4**(7), 33 (2012)
47. Agaku, I.T., Adisa, A.O., Ayo-Yusuf, O.A., Connolly, G.N.: Concern about security and privacy, and perceived control over collection and use of health information are related to withholding of health information from healthcare providers. J. Am. Med. Inform. Assoc. **21** (2), 374–378 (2014)
48. Acharjee, S., Ray, R., Chakraborty, S., Nath, S., Dey, N.: Watermarking in motion vector for security enhancement of medical videos. In: 2014 International Conference on Control, Instrumentation, Communication and Computational Technologies (ICCICCT), pp. 532–537. IEEE (2014)
49. Biswas, S., Roy, A.B., Ghosh, K., Dey, N.: A biometric authentication based secured ATM banking system. Int. J. Adv. Res. Comput. Sci. Softw. Eng. ISSN 2277 (2012)
50. Tong, Y., Sun, J., Chow, S.S., Li, P.: Cloud-assisted mobile-access of health data with privacy and auditability. IEEE J. Biomed. Health Inf. **18**(2), 419–429 (2014)
51. Consulting VW, Health Information Systems in Developing Countries a Landscape Analysis
52. Mudenda, C., van Stam, G.: ICT Training in Rural Zambia, the case of LinkNet Information Technology Academy. In: International Conference on e-Infrastructure and e-Services for Developing Countries, pp. 228–238. Springer, Berlin (2012)
53. He, C., Fan, X., Li, Y.: Toward ubiquitous healthcare services with a novel efficient cloud platform. IEEE Trans. Biomed. Eng. **60**(1), 230–234 (2013)
54. De Ryck, P., Desmet, L., Piessens, F., Joosen, W.: Improving the Security of Session Management in Web Applications (2013)
55. Furht, B., Escalante, A.: Handbook of Cloud Computing, Vol. 3. Springer, New York (2010)
56. Chen, S., Cheng, A., Mehta, K.: A review of telemedicine business models. Telemed e-Health **19**(4), 287–297 (2013)
57. Pandey, S., Voorsluys, W., Niu, S., Khandoker, A., Buyya, R.: An autonomic cloud environment for hosting ECG data analysis services. Future Gen. Comput. Syst. **28**(1), 147–154 (2012)
58. Lin, Y.R., Lo, S.C.: The design of a cloud and mobile healthcare system. Int. J. Commun. Netw. Syst. Sci. **9**(05), 209 (2016)
59. Kao, J.H., Lai, F., Lin, B.C., Sun, W.Z., Chang, K.W., Chan, T.C.: Application of cloud computing for emergency medical services: a study of spatial analysis and data mining technology. In: Frontier Computing, pp. 899–915. Springer, Singapore (2016)

Analysis of Power Aware Protocols and Standards for Critical e-Health Applications

Monalisa Mishra, Sushruta Mishra, Brojo Kishore Mishra and Prasenjit Choudhury

Abstract There has been a constant surge of Electronic medical applications in this modern era developed to enhance the health care services. As a result, wireless technology has emerged as a prime medium in not only monitoring and coordinating various processes effectively in this domain but also ensuring real time data delivery in a precise and reliable way. The electronics miniaturization and information proliferation in healthcare for energy retention and energy scavenging, have made it feasible the application of wireless networks especially Wireless Body Area Networks (WBAN) into medical sector. These advances herald in a new era for patient monitoring, healthcare procedures and several other critical sectors in modern age healthcare. This chapter illustrates a detail architectural analysis of WBAN in healthcare domain. A hybrid combination of Privacy Preserving Scalar Product for Computation Protocol (PPSPC) with Cascading Information Retrieval by Controlling Access with Distributed Slot Assignment Protocol (CICADA) is studied along with its stages of operation to provide secure, reliable and energy efficient data transmission in wireless body area sensor networks. Its performance is evaluated in terms of some critical parameters and it has been demonstrated that it generates a reasonable throughput thereby proving to be efficient. Thus this chapter deals with discussion of WBASN and its implementation in health status monitoring of patients residing in remote areas at any time.

M. Mishra (✉) · S. Mishra
Department of Computer Science and Engineering,
C.V. Raman College of Engineering, Bhubaneswar, India
e-mail: monalisa.mishra85@gmail.com

S. Mishra
e-mail: mishra.sushruta@gmail.com

B.K. Mishra
Department of Information Technology, C.V. Raman College of Engineering,
Bhubaneswar, India
e-mail: brojokishoremishra@gmail.com

P. Choudhury
Department of Computer Applications, NIT, Durgapur, India
e-mail: prasenjit0007@yahoo.co.in

C. Bhatt et al. (eds.), *Internet of Things and Big Data Technologies for Next Generation Healthcare*, Studies in Big Data 23,
DOI 10.1007/978-3-319-49736-5_12

Keywords Wireless body area sensor networks (WBASN) · E-health · Privacy preserving scalar product for computation protocol (PPSPC) · Controlling access with distributed slot assignment protocol (CICADA) · Throughput · Message transfer ratio

1 Introduction

Health care is one of the most important information sensitive sectors and can benefit from the recent advances in communication and information technology. This digital revolution will have a great impact on how the patients and populations are treated by the physicians and healthcare delivery organizations. The term E-health is raw and an emerging field of medical informatics which characterizes a technical development and ensures that medical services and information are delivered with the help of Internet technology. E-health is now recognised as an economical and engaging way to deliver health care services. Electronic health applications help to increase the effectiveness in health self-management programmes and enhancing communication between patients and healthcare professionals. Thus, face-to-face contacts between the doctors and patients will decrease and the communication between the consumers and providers will increase gradually over the coming decade. The range of E-health applications spans from health education, disease detection to proper diagnosis of patients and conducting research. While there are potentially endless applications of E-health, the main supporting areas include:

- Effective storage, management and sharing of data.
- Support for medical Decision making information system.
- Delivery of professional experts and remote consumer care.

E-health has thus emerged as a new way of thinking, a commitment for global thinking leading to improvement in quality, care for all citizens, and avoidance of unnecessary cost to the public purse. Traditionally, the health care providers maintained paper records about the status and history of their patients. But the advancements in technology and the rising health care costs have given rise to the development of electronic tracking systems. The need for e-health has therefore grown out for improvement in documentation and proper tracking of patient's health. In this time of digital world the e-health consumers interact with medical experts to access data including clinical records, health status of patients and having a one to one interaction with others in the form of text, audio or video with the help of internet. Many mobile devices are also designed with Internet capabilities to download applications so that the users can access health information instantly. E-health plays a vital role in the rural and remote areas by providing consultations for patients linking them to urban-based specialists. This technology has been used by the emergency medical personnel for consultation during natural disasters and military battlefield situations. Similarly, automated computerized reminders help for recommended prevention interventions such as yearly physicals, mammograms, and prostate examinations. The physicians make use of computerized drug-ordering systems which reduces the risk of adverse drug events. Other benefits due to the advances in e-health include, the prescriptions could be ordered over the internet for delivery at home, hospitals or health care institutions can advertise about their expertise and services through web pages and the persons with disabilities can also communicate with the health care professionals through text, audio or video conferencing, etc. Thus E-health has benefitted both to the providers and consumers.

The main objectives of the E-health can be listed as follows:

- To increase the efficiency of health care thereby reducing the costs
- To enhance the quality of care by allowing comparisons between different providers
- To make the interventions as evidence based by scientific evaluation
- To empower the consumers and the patients by providing knowledge about medicines over the
- Internet
- To create a true relationship between a patient and a health care professional
- To educate the physicians as well as the consumers through various online sources
- To enable information exchange in a standard manner between health care units
- To make health care more equitable and extend the scope of health care beyond its boundaries

The major application areas of this technology are:

- **Electronic Health Records**: Storing the data electronically enables the patient's communication between different health care professionals
- **Clinical Decision Support**: Computer based patient's records facilitate clinical decision making and contribute towards the quality control of clinical processes
- **Telemedicine**: It enables a patient and a doctor to initiate an e-consult session using an appropriate client service media application
- **m-health**: It includes the use of mobile devices to collect patient data, provide information to health care researchers, real time monitoring of patients and suggesting medicines
- **Health Care Information Systems**: It provides software solutions for scheduling appointments, patient data management and other work schedule management.

One of the biggest challenges that the world is facing is to provide quality based medical facilities in a cost effective manner. Medical related costs will increase with the rise in chronic diseases. Thus there is a need of some drastic steps that is to be taken in medical field so as to reduce medical costs [1]. Developing medicines which are more preventive based rather than reactive are the expected modification in the clinical sector [2, 3]. In 2005, for the first time the modern computer technology was integrated with healthcare sector and it gave rise to a concept named the e-health revolution [4]. Usage of e-health may be helpful in decreasing the cost while increasing the effectiveness of treatment of patients. At the same time there is a rapid rise in wireless technologies with the availability of resources [5]. Several modern e-health applications with efficient medical services have successfully emerged with the advancement in digital electronics using wireless medium and smart sensors. Thus wireless technology has become a vital medium in not only controlling many operations dealing with e-health services but also in real-time data delivery maintaining a greater accuracy and reliability. Moreover, due to the rapid growth of information in medical sector, the miniaturization of electronic devices and the different methods of energy consumption have promoted the concept of Wireless Body Area Networks from theory to real practice. The development of low power sensing devices and advancements in wireless communication had given rise to mobile healthcare applications. Patients can either directly wear these devices on their body or can be placed in the medical equipments for continuous monitoring, data collection and aggregation and report generation. Thus, it takes us to that depth of information about the patient's health; it becomes sufficient for biometric identification of that individual. The electronics miniaturization and information proliferation in healthcare for energy retention and energy scavenging, have made it feasible the application of wireless networks especially Wireless Body Area Networks (WBAN) into medical sector. Due to improvement in low power wireless technology and sensing components many e-health applications are very well supported by wireless communication. It is helpful in areas like monitoring of patients status, diagnosis of outpatients and tracking of healthcare methodologies. It is important to secure he gathered data for transmission as well as storage. Proper protection of inappropriate access of wireless devices is very critical to avoid data falsification and impersonation. E-health applications provide mobility support functionality that give experts and healthcare centers provision to manage electronic records and healthcare billings so that patients are more aware of their well being. Information is required to be utilized properly so that patient safety and accountability may be taken care of. It is important to have integrated applications which are more acceptable to users. In order to develop a more robust, responsive and secure wireless system suitable for e-health applications several critical issues have to be addressed. Remote areas still lack direct access to healthcare experts since the clinical equipments cannot be interconnected to modern healthcare facilities. A patient data located at some office electronically may not be accessible from some other medical center. These issues may be handled with e-health services and standards that provide interoperability among medical records and communication standards. Common format based data or encrypted data responsible for error handling providing common addressing format id defined by standards. Commonly used standards that adhere to these architectures are:

- Focusing on higher interoperability
- Improvement in coordination of global e-health standards
- Enabling secure and private data communication
- Minimizing the standardization gap in modern world
- Taking advantage of existing methodologies like mobile technology and applications in social media.

This chapter discusses important e-health applications focusing on the state-of-the-art in wireless networking for e-Health applications while analyzing development and implementation in real world scenarios. Development of WBAN round human body is now feasible due to the rise of low power yet high performance sensor nodes. Since WBAN is very much efficient for e-health services like remote monitoring of patients so the entire medical community is very keen in this technology. Basically WBAN is body-centric consisting two kinds of nodes including in-body and on-body nodes. There is a coordinator arranged on human body. The nodes form a star topology while these nodes are responsible for data interchange with the coordinator in one-hop communication. With such a set up data collected from human body can be communicated to the coordinator for proper analysis and further display. These coordinators can also transmit data to remote centers in a wireless scenario. As such body information including human emotions and signals along with surrounding environment status can be aggregated without hampering human activities. The most critical thing that is to be considered in WBAN is energy retention since sensor nodes are battered operated and their lifetime is limited. Apart from this the latency and data rate transmission varies for different applications. The variations in different activities need to be regulated properly. Robustness of WBAN should be guaranteed against channel fading in WBAN due to power consumption and path interference due to surrounding environment.

2 Power Efficient Protocols for WBAN

There are many MAC and Physical layer power efficient protocols which are used in WBANs. Medical MAC is an energy efficient protocol which uses the TDMA method and follows Adaptive Guard Band Algorithm (AGBA) for maintaining clock synchronization. It is proved to be better than the IEEE 802.15.4 MAC. It only worked well for low data rate applications like respiration, pulse, etc. but did not work well with high data rate applications. Another protocol called EEMAC supports the centrally controlled sleep and wake up mechanisms for enhancing the power efficiency. It basically includes three methods: Link set-up, Wake-up procedure and Alarm generation. In this case, the issues like over hearing and idle listening are reduced. There is another TDMA based energy efficient MAC protocol termed BMAC using three different bandwidth management techniques: Burst bandwidth, Periodic bandwidth and Adjust bandwidth. These techniques help in enhancing the network stability and packet transmission thereby saving energy. HD-MAC for WBANs uses heartbeat rhythm information for maintaining synchronization among the nodes. Here, beacons with the heartbeat rhythm pattern has reduced the power consumption and increased network lifetime. Similarly, BLE is a physical layer protocol which operates in the frequency of 2400 MHz and uses the DSSS method. It helps in extending the battery life of the Bluetooth by consuming only 10 % of its power. It uses the sleep and wake up mechanism to send data when needed. But it suited well for only latency critical WBAN applications. WI-FI (IEEE 802.11 N) is another physical layer protocol used to connect electronic devices to each other, to the Internet and to the wired network with security, reliability and fast connectivity. But one of its disadvantages is, it cannot be used in small WBAN sensors around the human body because of its high energy consumption and probability of conflict with any other device working in the same frequency range. Zigbee (IEEE 802.15.4) is popularly known point-to-point protocol providing low power, wireless connectivity for various network applications focusing mainly on monitoring and control. It supports an indoor spread of 50 m and an outdoor spread of more than 500 m. It only works well with low data rate WBAN applications for which Zigbee Pro came into picture.

3 Problem Formulation

The MAC layer handles access control, error control, multiplexing, encoding and validation of frames. Similarly, the physical layer is responsible for signal detection, encryption and modulation and also carrier signal generation. They basically focused on the general parameters of network performance like throughput, delay and channel utilization, etc. But they lacked in ensuring energy efficiency, which is the most important factor in health care domain. Energy efficiency in health care is the key requirement where batteries are needed for years to go. For example, a pacemaker would require a lifetime of about 5–6 years. The main reasons for wastage of energy are collisions, idle listening, over-hearing and control packet overhead. Therefore, one of the most important characteristic of a health care protocol is the energy efficiency. A suitable MAC protocol should be designed to improve the quality of service and network capacity for WBAN communications. Properties like Long durations of sleeping nodes, degraded load/duty cycle and usage of power efficient protocols and techniques can all add to extension of battery life. In [6], Gopalan et al. made a comparison on four MAC protocols of WBANs which are, E^2MAC, Medical Mac, LDC-MAC, and B-MAC. They had also discussed about some of the open research issues in this paper. Barati has designed an effectual error control algorithm [7] to improve the lifespan of the network using a spare residue number system. Currently, the emerging protocols guarantee efficient delivery in variable and burst traffic as well as supports multitasking. Kutty et al. in [8], discussed the challenges in construction of MAC protocols and categorized the WBAN traffic into three types: energy reduction techniques, network configuration and frame formats. Generally, the IEEE 802.15.4 MAC operates in 3 bands: 2.4 GHz ISM band, 915 MHz ISM band and 868 MHz European band. It has two operational modes: the beacon enabled mode and the non-beacon enabled mode. In the beacon-enabled mode, the net coordinator controls and synchronizes the communication. A super-frame has active and inactive durations. The active duration consists of three parts: a beacon, a CAP using slotted CSMA/CA, and a CFP, which contains Guaranteed Time Slots. Ullah et al. [9] carried out a study showing the performance of different parameters between CSMA/CA and TDMA in WBANs. They concluded that TDMA has maximum bandwidth utilization and lower power consumption compared to CSMA/CA. In [10], the author presented an ultra-low power approach (WhMac) to work with Wake-Up Receiver (WUR) nodes. The Heartbeat MAC method (H-MAC) [9] that has been proposed by Ullah et al. uses the heartbeat rhythm to synchronize the nodes and results in improved power efficiency. In [11], the authors have presented a specially designed MAC protocol used for energy-harvesting WBANs. Different priorities are assigned to the nodes on the basis of the need of the data packets and the type of energy-acquiring source. In [12], Lee et al. have explained about a passive RFID system “A Wireless Sensor Enabled by Wireless power” (WPWS) which do not have power supply problem. Luis et al. [13] conducted a survey on various protocols of different layers which are used for health care applications. It mostly concentrated on energy efficient protocols for WBANs. He et al. [14] proposed a method to determine the special features of Medical Sensor Networks (MSNs) and analyze different node behaviors like rate of transfer, leaving period for detection of malicious nodes. He et al. [15] presented a Body Sensor Network which consists of biosensors and a local processing unit (LPU). Lim et al. [16] discussed a model to examine the changes in the anatomical complexity of various numerical arm models. Calculations for UWB signal propagation along a human are made and compared with the simulation results of various numerical arm models. Chiti et al. [17] developed a wireless communication system for critical applications, which helps in refining the process of data collection, extracting information as per the need and interrelating with on body sensed information. Fujii et al. [18] proposed an efficient FDTD model for a human body on the basis of accurate 2-pole Debye dispersion dielectric tissue characteristics. Alemdar et al. [19] proposed Pervasive Medicare Systems which continuously supervise, provide circumstantial information and use different mechanisms to alert against any abnormal conditions. Khalil et al. [20] presented various ways of devising the operations of WSNs by improving the battery and network life span. Gurjar et al. [21] proposed that shows the importance of gathering of physiological data and sensor networking for various health-related applications. Howlader et al. [22] developed an effective biomedical application which uses smart sensors to continuously monitor the patients in remote areas and systems for reconstruction. Here both surface and implanted sensors are considered for making comparison analysis. Al Ameen et al. [23] developed a WBAN which helps to supervise and track down humans with the use of wearable and non-wearable sensors. Phunchongharn et al. [24] presented a wireless communication system in health domain which had given rise to two critical issues:

First, the malfunctioning of biomedical devices due to the radio frequency transmission and second, the requirement of different quality of services for different e-health applications. The work in [25] describes the application of an Artificial Intelligence (AI) optimization technique to design Proportional-Integral-Derivative (PID) controller for Load Frequency Control (LFC) of single area re-heat thermal power system A comparison of the power system with/without non-linearity is performed. Moreover, robust analysis is carried out via varying the governor's time constants, turbine, re-heater and power system in about +50 to −50 % from its nominal value by the 25 % step. In [26] an application of bio-inspired flower pollination algorithm (FPA) for tuning proportional-integral-derivative (PID) controller in load frequency control (LFC) of multi-area interconnected power system is discussed. The supremacy performance of proposed algorithm for optimized PID controller is proved by comparing the results with genetic algorithm (GA) and particle swarm optimization (PSO)-based PID controller under the same investigated power system [27]. Presents the analysis of Automatic Generation Control (AGC)/Load Frequency Control (LFC) of conventional three area interconnected thermal power systems. The analysis established that Integral Time Absolute Error (ITAE) based conventional controller's yield better controlled response and good dynamic performance compared to other indices.

4 Problem Solution

4.1 A Wireless Flexible and Scalable Solution for E-Health Applications

Due to the advancement in wireless technologies, wireless body area sensor networks are practicable in which a set of communicating devices are attached to the human body [28]. The combination of wireless medium and modern information technology has been highly successful in creating a revolutionary trend in the field of medicine called as e-health [29]. This facilitates in providing medical help to distant places in a cheap way. The use of wireless body area sensor networks through biomedical and physical parameters may offer pervasive solution in monitoring of health of patients on a continuous basis. The health related reports are generated and are collected by these remote sensor systems which are later transmitted to a distant server where they can be stored and later analyzed by clinical experts [2, 3]. Once the data is present in server clinical professionals can access those data at any time as per the requirement. When such systems are integrated with machine learning based decision support systems equipped with expert knowledge they can perform health monitoring automatically at remote centers also. Many wireless standards like Bluetooth and Wi-Fi are chosen for implementing such scalable wireless body sensor networks. Certain vital parameters that evaluate the performance of wireless technologies include range, energy retention, security, robustness etc. as seen in the Fig. 1. It acts as an interface to medical providers, doctors and healthcare centers. There is also a provision of a mobile platform that act as a remote controlling center and another mobile platform is present so that medical experts can access the health status of patients.

Wireless Body Area Sensor Networks (WBASNs) are generally a category of wireless networks that implement biomedical sensors with three basic features [30]:

- Extremely low transmit power capable of coexisting with other clinical devices thereby providing energy efficient data transmission.
- Providing high rate of data transmission facilitating high QoS constraints.
- Highly feasible with low cost with minimum complexity and minimum size.

Such wireless body networks facilitate long term continuous monitoring of patients allowing ubiquitous accessing thereby generating warnings if the signal received does not match the predefined personalized ranges. A wireless body area sensor network is demonstrated in the following Fig. 2. It consists of various body area networks and a base station. Many sensors are attached to the patients that are responsible in monitoring and accessing various parameters. The sensors collect the information which is then aggregated and sent to the base station. A relay station receives this information passing through a backbone network and can be further accessed at monitoring stations connected to the network. This network offers a very flexible and real time responses which may be helpful in urgency cases [31–33]. The sensors that are integrated into human body are heterogeneous in nature. The quantity of biosensors depends on the health status of patient. Some

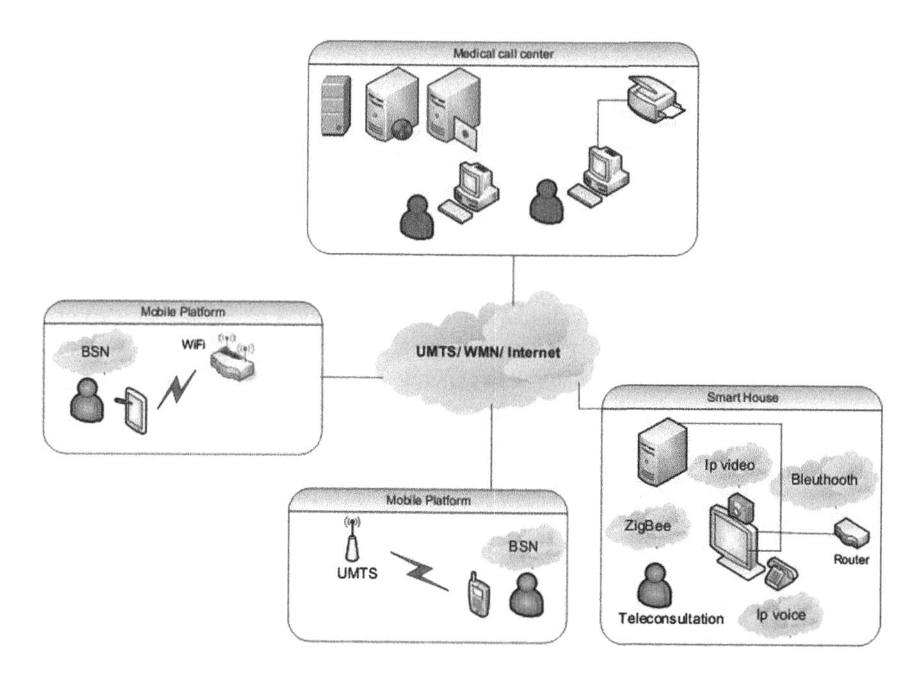

Fig. 1 Wireless flexible and scalable solution for e-health critical applications

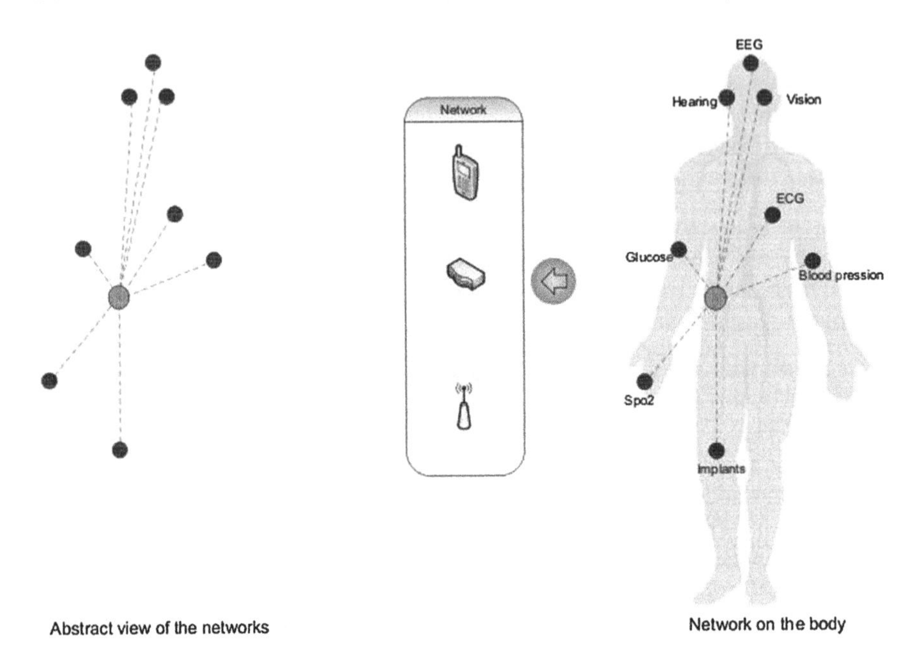

Fig. 2 Structure of a wireless body area sensor network

basic commonly used sensors include blood pressure, heart rate, glucose level, SpO2 "Oxymeter" to monitor the oxygen saturation in a patient's blood and to measure the body temperature, ECG to monitor the heart, EEG that is used to detect any brain disorders, and EMG to access the health of muscles and nerves [34, 35].

Table 1 shows various classifications of services provided by some commonly used bio-sensors.

Biosensor or a biological sensor is equipment consisting of a biological component like cell, enzyme, or an antibody and a physical component like a transducer or amplifier. The bio-component combines with the analyte to produce an electrical signal which can be detected by the transducer. A selected biological material like enzyme is used for typical methods like non covalent or covalent binding and physical or membrane entrapping. The material is associated with the transducer. The analyte combines with the biological material to generate a bound analyte. Sometimes it gets changed into a product which may be linked with the discharge of gases like oxygen,

Table 1 Classification of services based on physiological measures

Kind of sensor	Rate of data	Delay	Service type
EEG, EMG	Low	Low	Low rate in real-time
ECG	High	Low	High rate in real-time
Body temperature, glucose level monitoring, heart rate	Low	High	Low rate in non real-time
X-ray, MRI, healthcare images	High	High	Non real-time high rate

electrons or hydrogen ions and heat. Then the transducer converts the product into electrical responses which can be measured and amplified. In medical environment, biosensors help in analyzing physiological procedures and sends physiological data to a control device or a monitor. Traditionally, the data outputs collected from the devices were analog type and were aggregated in a manner that was not suitable for secondary or tertiary analysis. Biosensors play a vital role in monitoring, diagnosing and maintaining health. Moreover, the automatic data collection and analysis helps in proper management of chronic and incidental health conditions like diabetes, cardiac attack, etc. So care must be taken while synthesizing the data collected from a patient indoor or outdoor in critical situations. These are designed to react only with a particular substance and the result of this reaction comes in the form of messages that can be analyzed by a microprocessor. These biosensors can be considered as receptors or stimuli; communication systems based on sensors can display, stimulate, treat, or substitute human biophysics performance.

4.1.1 Methodology

A wireless body sensor network architecture implemented as a smart medical model comprises three vital features:

- Remote monitoring in real-time and long-term basis.
- Minimum complexity based small sized sensor.
- Easy integration with existing healthcare technology.

A scenario has been set up with various biosensors nodes being equipped to a patient body. Ns2 simulator with WPAN models is used [36]. Our experimental set up is being conducted with many topologies to validate the performance of wireless body area sensor network. The results are presented for a static network scenario due to the space constraints. The patient body is simulated with a set up of 2 m × 2 m area. The biosensor nodes are mounted over the human body. Each node is executed with a single biosensor ECG, blood pressure and glucose monitoring, SpO2, respiration with body temperature. The gateway node is also assumed to be static. The formation of transmission capability of devices is based on sensor nodes of body area network with real radio map. The simulation conducted using NS-2 determines the throughput and the delay of wireless body area network model. The deployment of WBASN using NS-2 simulator is shown in Fig. 3.

4.1.2 Results and Discussion

Analysis of throughput and message transfer ratio

Simulation is done on IEEE 802.15.4 network to identify the demerits of CSMA/CA. In our simulation a star topology was used where a slotted CSMA/CA enabled by beacon was selected and a PAN coordinator sent a beacon signal so that

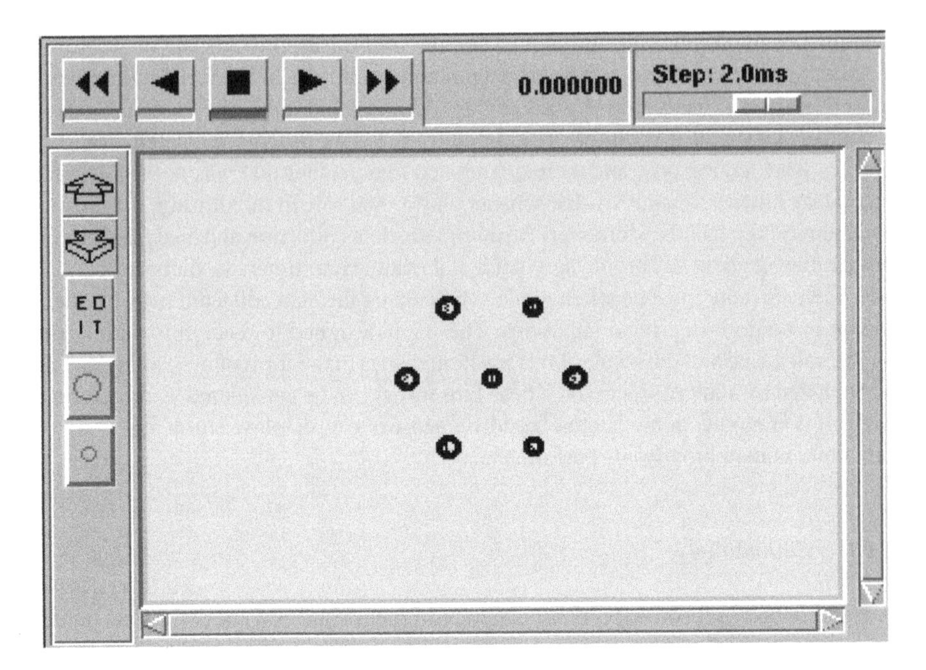

Fig. 3 NS2 implementation of WBASN

nodes will synchronize themselves with the beacon. Two cases were demonstrated to evaluate the performance of network. In the first scenario the cluster head receives data from a single node while in the second, 6 nodes were used to send data to the PAN coordinator or the cluster head. The network traffic was changed from 10 to 500 kbps. As shown in the Fig. 4 when the source is about 160 kbps the throughput achieved is optimum.

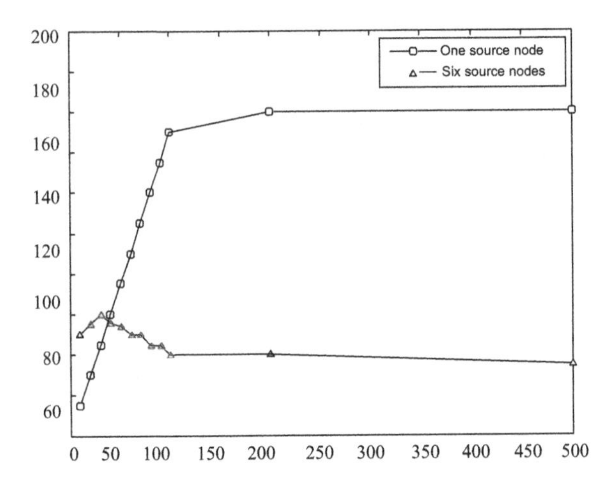

Fig. 4 Throughput of the patient monitoring system

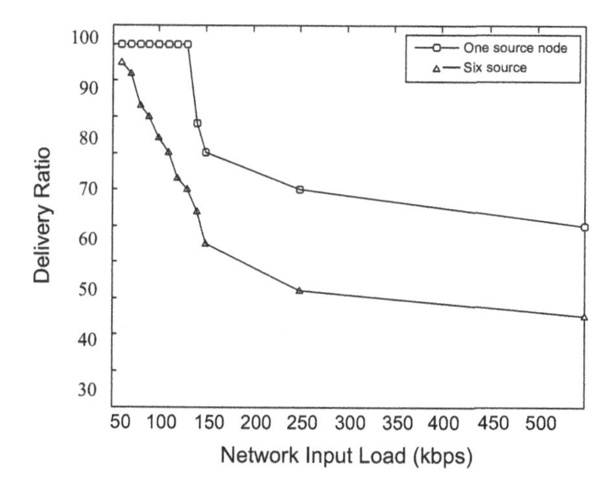

Fig. 5 A patient examining model in terms of message transfer ratio

As illustrated in Fig. 5 there is drastic fall in message transfer ratio when the data rate rises.

4.2 *A Secure, Reliable and Energy Efficient Hybrid Model for WBN in Healthcare Applications*

Some basic challenges of application of wireless network in medical domain are reliable transmission of data, rapid real time detection of events, in time data delivery, maximization of energy retention etc. The nodes in wireless network are capable of sensing, processing and communication data. Thus wireless body area networks in association with these nodes that can be used in monitoring of health of patients. This work presents a different approach formed due to a combination of privacy preserving scalar product for computation protocol (PPSPC) and cascading information retrieval by controlling access with distributed slot assignment protocol (CICADA). This hybrid protocol enables reliable, secure and power aware data transmission in wireless body sensor network (WBSN).

4.2.1 Methodology

The main motive of the developed protocol is to use wireless network for healthcare issues efficiently. This new proposed protocol addresses the three basic challenges of wireless sensor networks. PPSPC takes care of security while CICADA provides reliability and energy efficiency. Thus the combination of the two is able to meet the basic challenges of implementing WBAN in health care sector.

Phases in the Proposed System

Our new proposed protocol may be subdivided into five stages:

- Development of Network
- Hybrid Integration of PPSPC with CICADA Algorithm
- Generation of Protocol
- Optimization of Energy
- Evaluation of Performance.

Network development is the first step of this protocol. Here the entire network consisting of series of sensor nodes is partitioned into many clusters. Main task of sensor nodes are sensing the medium, gathering of information and forwarding them to its neighbor nodes. The second step basically deals with implementation of the algorithm. PPSPC protocol deals with the security issue by performing key generation algorithm. The energy efficient and reliable thing is taken care of by CICADA which in addition to this also is responsible of implementing a scheduling algorithm. The third step is concerned with generation of protocol. The information regarding data from sensor nodes are recorded various tasks are carried out on the data gathered to represent the relevant data in suitable format in the form of tables, figures and reports. The fourth step constitutes optimization of energy thereby minimizing the energy requirement during data transmission among nodes. Energy reduction is very vital in health applications while maintaining safety. The final step is associated with analysis of performance of the developed protocol. The steps are shown in Fig. 6. Some of the important metrics like throughput, message transfer ratio and end to end delay are considered while evaluating effectiveness of protocol. The entire set up is implemented in NS2 simulator software.

Phase 1: Network Development

In this step a network field of size 1500 m × 1500 m is taken in which 100 sensor nodes are randomly installed. The speed of the node is adjusted to 30 m/s. The nodes sense the medium and gather information and pass it to its neighbour nodes. According to the relay node the packet information is sent to the receiver node so that data information can be passed from the sender to receiver. The simulation is comprised of N base stations each having their respective nodes. Nodes are equipped with biosensors to facilitate communication among them. There are two fixed nodes that send beacon messages simultaneously on a periodical basis in the network. TDOA (Time Difference of Arrival) or TOA (Time of Arrival) methods are used to determine the gap between the sensor node and two fixed nodes. The neighbour nodes distance is calculated as:

$$d = \sqrt{(x_2 - x_1)^2 + (y_2 - y_1)^2} \quad (1)$$

where x_1, x_2, y_1 and y_2 denote the arbitrarily selected and allotted coordinates to every single node.

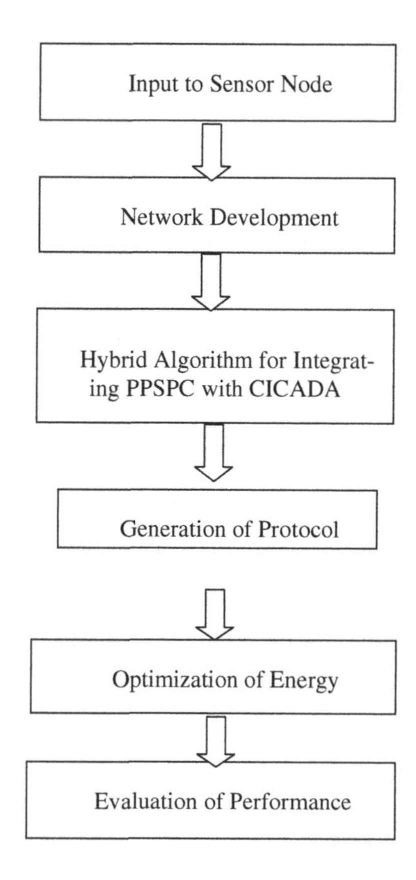

Fig. 6 Proposed system design

Phase 2: Hybrid Algorithm for Integrating PPSPC with CICADA

PPSPC protocol is responsible to provide security and it also performs key generation.

The algorithm involves,

$$\begin{aligned} \textbf{Input}: & \ a = (a_1, a_2, \ldots, a_n) \text{ denotes } U_0\text{'s binary vector} \\ & \ b = (b_1,\ b2, \ldots, b_n) \text{ denotes } U_j\text{'s binary vector} \\ \textbf{Output}: & \ \text{Vector dot product} \end{aligned}$$

Steps:

- The desired threshold value for several symptoms character is U_0
- The scalar product of Vector a.b $\geq$ th. U_j is assigned the current session key by U_0
- The raw PHI data send from U_0 can be decrypted and processed by U_0.

Reliability and Energy Efficiency is provided by CICADA protocol. A Distributed slot scheduling algorithm is used which identifies the links that will send data at any particular instant. A Schedule may be defined as a series of links activated at the same time. Each time slot is divided into two parts: a data transfer slot and a control slot. The delay is very less and it offers good resilience to mobility.

Steps:

Step 1 A "decision schedule" m is chosen, T denotes a control slot representing a set of links based on which state is changed wrt to its previous one

Step 2 Considering a link I in m (t) do

Step 3 Assuming that in its last data slot link, there is no active links in its conflict set N (i), three cases arise for I,

- probability (pi) = xi(t) = 1 with status active
- probability (1 − pi) = xi(t) = 0 with status inactive
- else link I is inactive = xi(t) = 0.

Both the protocols are incorporated using OLSR Protocol. While configuring OLSR, OTCL and C++ languages are used as frontend and backend respectively. Multipoint relays are a set of nodes which are arbitrarily chosen as intermediate nodes between source and destination.

Phase 3: Generation of Protocol

PPSPC and CICADA protocol are integrated together to provide security, reliability and energy efficiency. This protocol is designed for large scale accumulation of data in wireless sensor networks. AOMDV (Adhoc On demand Multipath Distance Vector routing Protocol) is used for the purpose of protocol generation.

Phase 4: Energy Optimization

Energy optimization is the most vital parameter taken into account while developing a protocol for wireless sensor networks. Minimizing energy requirement is crucial for maintaining health and safety in medical domain. Data aggregation helps in decreasing the traffic and the energy consumption in the network. Energy is denoted in joules. An initial energy level is set first and the energy value at every node is computed. The transmitted energy and received energy is determined at every round and is updated after every round.

$$\text{Energy} = \text{Power} * \text{Time} \tag{2}$$

Phase 5: Performance Analysis

Evaluation of performance is undertaken on AODV, Mod-AOMDV protocols using NS2 platform. Three common measures which include Average Latency, Packet Transfer Ratio and Throughput are used to determine the protocol performance. The average latency will be decreased while the throughput and packet transfer ratio will be increased. Latency is the average time elapsed between the sending of packets and delivery of packets. Packet transfer ratio represents the ratio of the information frames reaching the destination and the data packets introduced at the source node.

Throughput may be defined as the number of successful data transmissions performed in a given period of time.

4.2.2 Results and Discussion

Table 2 depicts the simulation metrics to be used in the experimental set up. The entire work is implemented using NS-2. In WBAN applications NS-2.34 simulator is widely used due to its support for wireless technology. The simulation domain consists of sensor nodes and a sink node. The sink node is located at a certain distance from the sensor nodes. The sensor nodes are unevenly spread in the entire sensing area. Total number of sensor nodes are taken as 100 as per the suitability of the network topology which is 1500 m × 1500 m area. Simulation time is chosen to be 200 s for successful completion of experiment. Since there are 100 nodes in our set up the initial energy set for each node is 20 J/node. Data packet size is taken as 1000 bits since the nodes are unevenly spread out in the topology and it has to span over a large network area. The data payload is set as 512 bytes per packet. The CBR traffic type is considered since the data packets is to be generated at a constant rate. When a base station collects data from all sensor nodes in the network, it completes one round of data transmission. Biosensors which are either implanted or non implanted devices are present with the nodes as well as for channels to communicate with each others. Two permanent nodes are responsible for simultaneous transfer of beacon frames in the network periodically.

The results illustrate the network formation phase, distance computation of neighbour node, configuration of OLSR protocol, generation of AOMDV protocol with calculation of energy consumption.

Figure 7 shows the network formation with 100 nodes scattered in the network with field area of 1500 m × 1500 m. The network comprises the simple and specific application oriented sensor nodes capable of sensing the medium, gathering data and forwarding them into the next hop neighbour nodes within a predefined time period. The estimation of distance between the moving node and the two permanent nodes are suitably done by using TOA (Time of Arrival) or TDOA (Time Difference of Arrival) approaches. Figure 8 shows the diagrammatic view of clinical usage of some vital wireless protocols. As it can be seen the modified

Table 2 Parameters for simulation

Parameters	Value
Simulator name	NS-2.34
No. of nodes	100
Simulation period	200 s
Sensing area	1500 m × 1500 m
Initial energy	20 J/node
Packet size	1000 bits
Data payload	512 bytes/packet
Traffic type	CBR

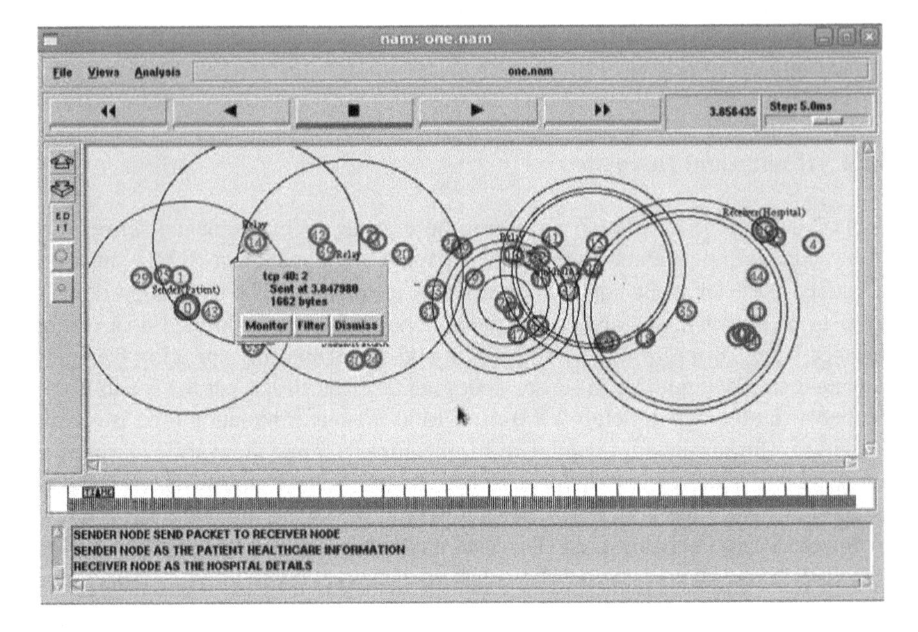

Fig. 7 Network formation

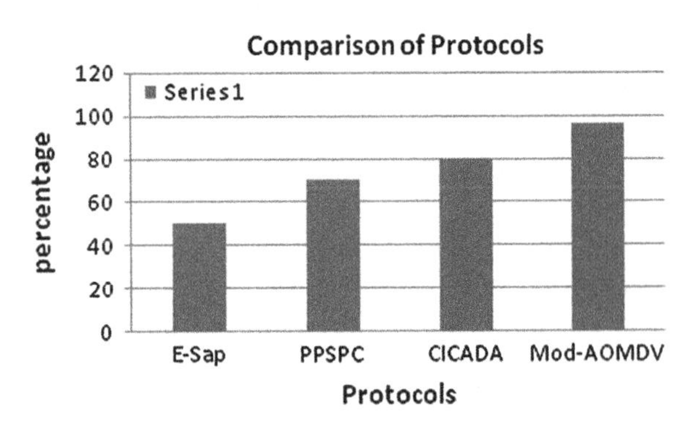

Fig. 8 Comparative analysis of wireless algorithms

AODV protocol is most popularly used in clinical applications while E-Sap is the least preferred used protocol.

Figure 9 depicts computation of distance between Neighbour Nodes. In such scenarios Nearest Neighbour Algorithm is implemented.

Figure 10 illustrates the architectural implementation of OLSR algorithm. Series of Neighbour nodes chosen in random way in the route between source and destination are referred as multipoint rays. The nodes represented by yellow color in the diagram denote the multipoint nodes. OLSR algorithm is used to combine two different algorithms into a single model.

Figure 11 shows the generation of AOMDV Protocol. It is designed for wireless technology used for large scale aggregation of data. In AOMDV protocol every node in the network have identical interfaces.

Neighbor Node Calculation

Node	Nb node	Node-Xpos	Node-Ypos	Nb-Xpos	Nb-Ypos	Distance(d)
0	1	117	122	105	187	66
0	14	117	122	272	261	208
0	16	117	122	387	186	277
0	25	117	122	63	194	90
0	29	117	122	16	185	119
0	33	117	122	259	39	164
0	36	117	122	377	97	261
0	38	117	122	278	132	153
0	43	117	122	173	113	56
1	0	105	187	117	122	66
1	14	105	187	272	261	182
1	16	105	187	387	186	282
1	25	105	187	63	194	42
1	29	105	187	16	185	89
1	33	105	187	259	39	213
1	36	105	187	377	97	286
1	38	105	187	278	132	173
1	43	105	187	173	113	100
2	6	516	282	530	267	20
2	7	516	282	474	135	152
2	9	516	282	740	181	245
2	14	516	282	272	261	244
2	16	516	282	387	186	160
2	17	516	282	467	196	98
2	19	516	282	715	247	202
2	20	516	282	591	236	87
2	21	516	282	697	260	182
2	23	516	282	663	158	192
2	24	516	282	522	8	274

Fig. 9 Neighbor node distance calculation

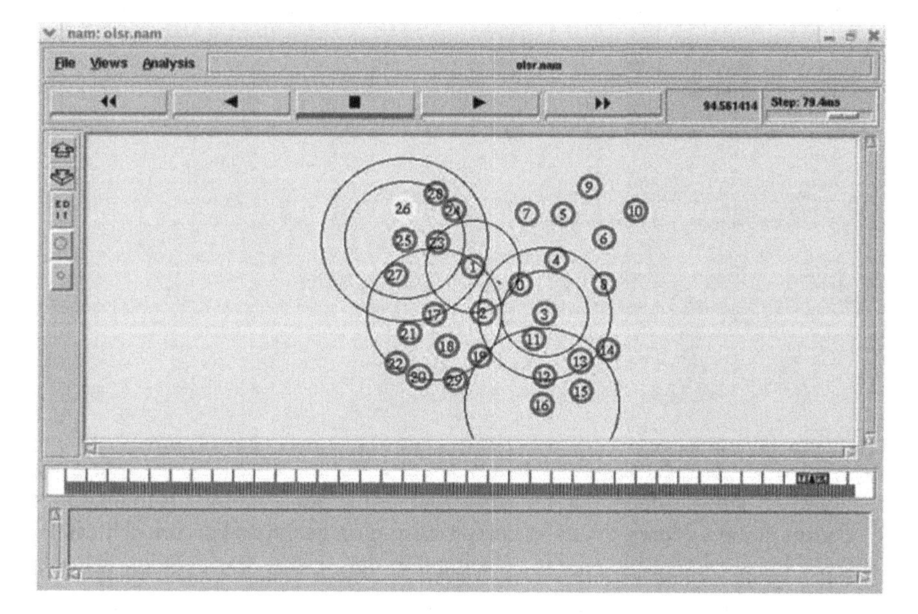

Fig. 10 OLSR protocol configuration

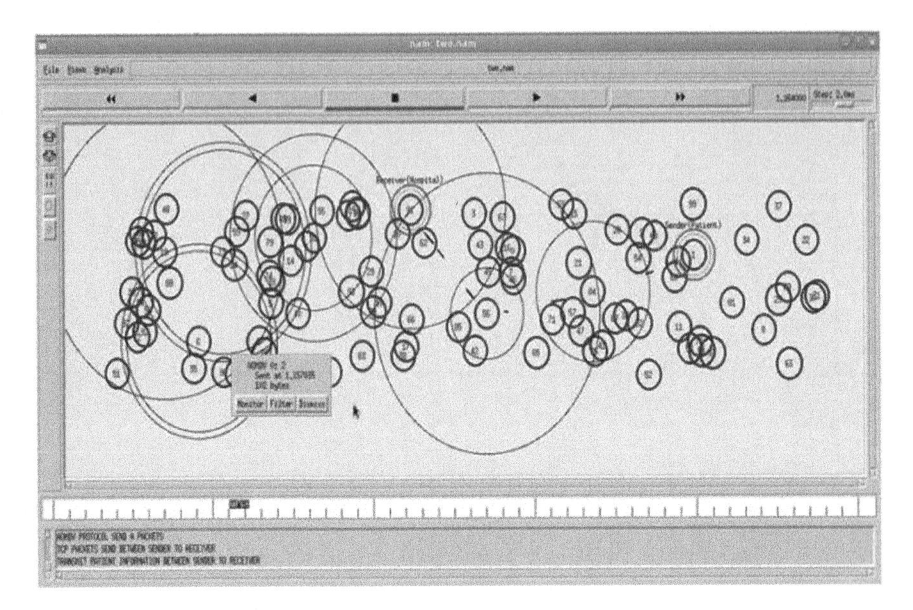

Fig. 11 AOMDV protocol generation

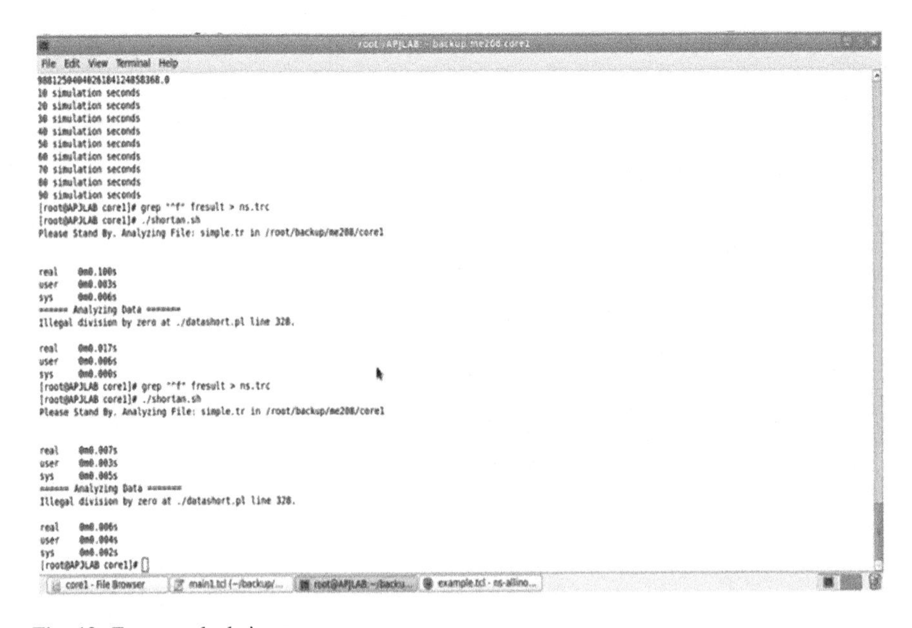

Fig. 12 Energy calculation

Figure 12 shows calculation of energy. One of the prime motives is to minimize the consumption of energy without compromising on health and security. It can be achieved by restricting the energy consumption during data transmission between the sensor nodes.

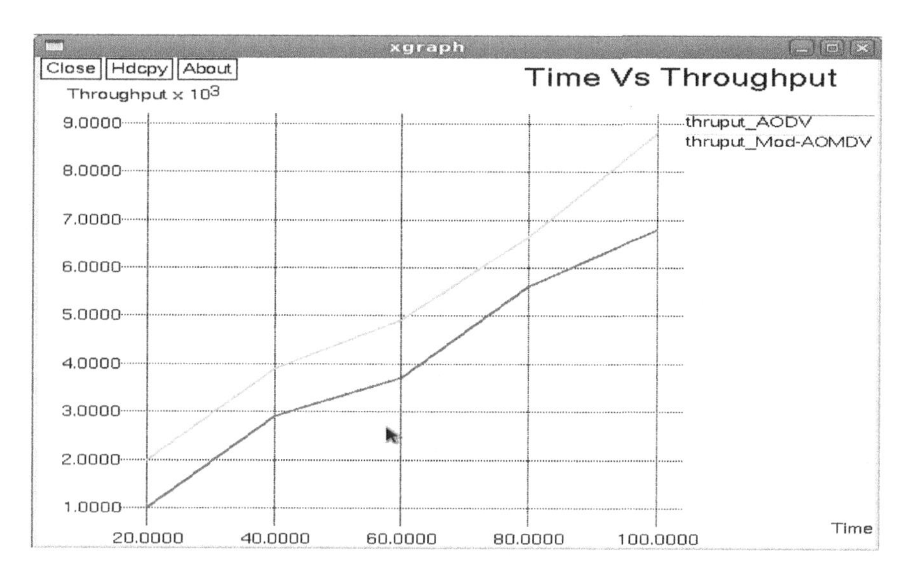

Fig. 13 Performance analysis of throughput

Figure 13 shows the throughput evaluation analysis. Throughput may be referred as the number of messages transferred to the destination node during data transfer period which is denoted by bits/bytes per second. It can be clearly observed that throughput is relatively more in AOMDV as compared to AODV protocol.

Figure 14 depicts the performance in terms of Message transfer ratio. It is referred as the proportion between messages sent to destination node and messages

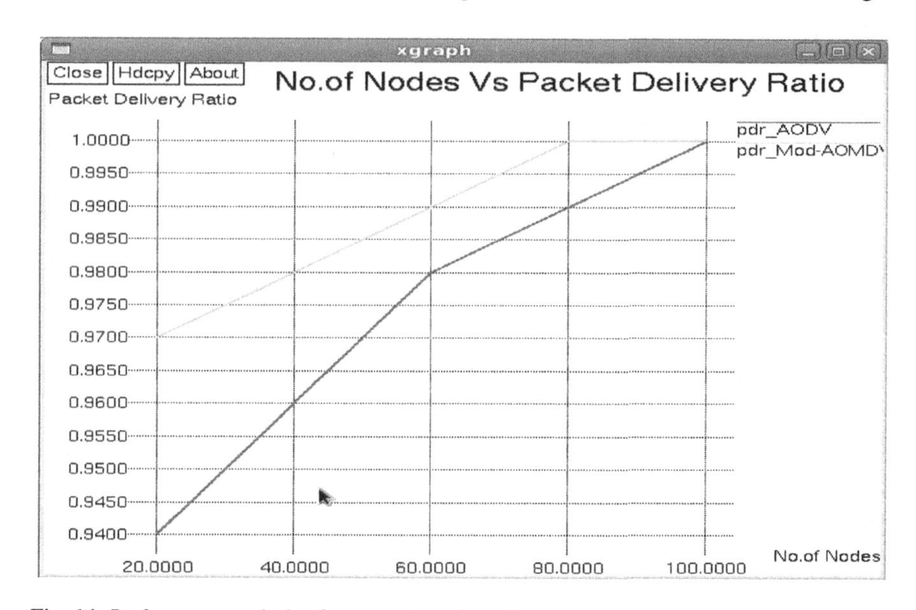

Fig. 14 Performance analysis of message transfer ratio

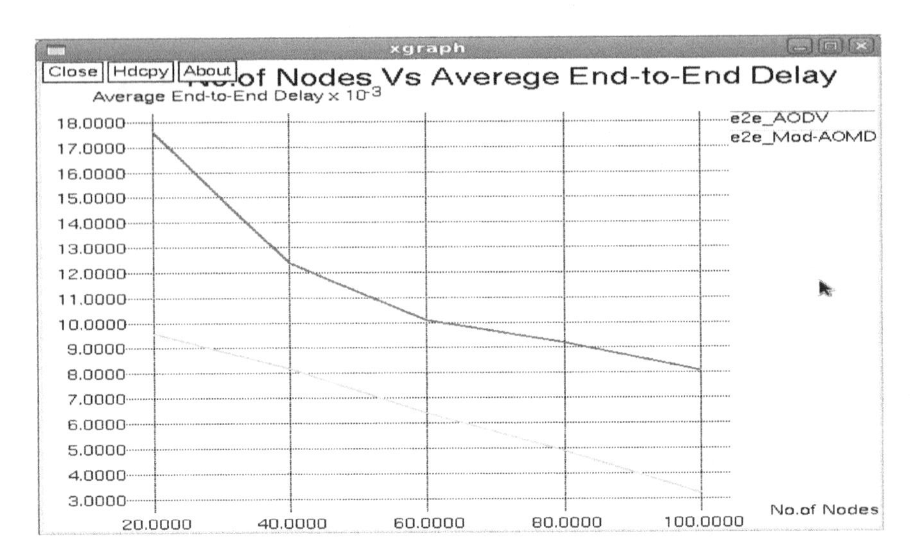

Fig. 15 Analysis of average end-to-end latency

produced by source node. AOMDV has a better message transfer ratio than AODV protocol.

Analysis of performance with respect to Average End-to-End Delay is denoted in Fig. 15. It is the average delay between packets sent and received.

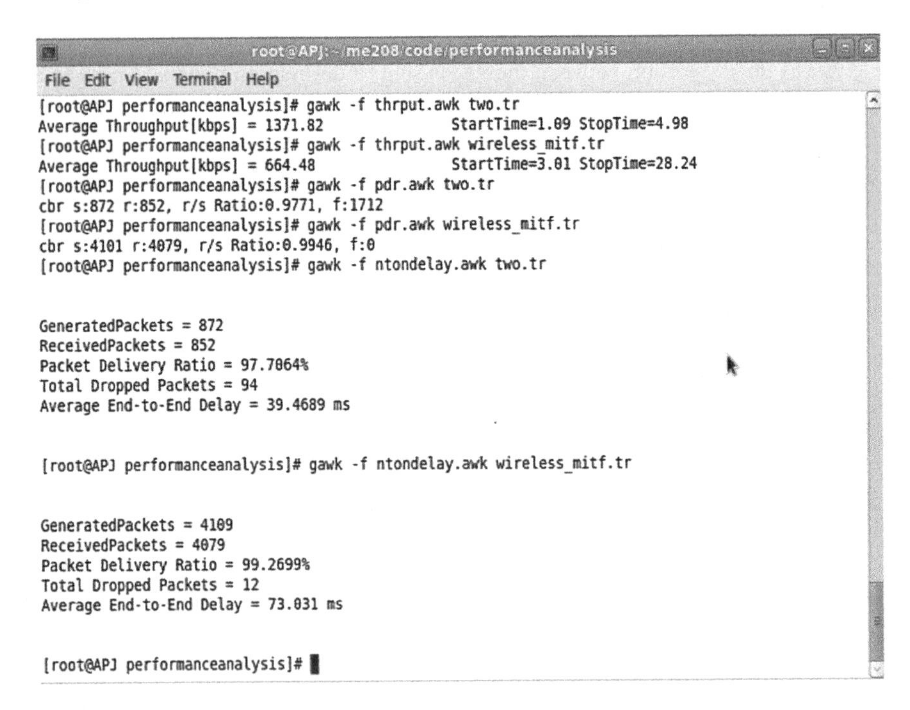

Fig. 16 Comparison of AODV and Mod-AOMDV protocol

Figure 16 illustrate comparative study of AODV and Mod-AOMDV protocol where analysis of message transfer ratio and Average End-to-End latency is done.

4.3 Conclusion

A good number of algorithms have contributed for reliable and energy efficient data transmissions for sensitive areas like that of healthcare applications. In modern era everything has become dynamic. To keep pace with this dynamism Wireless Body Sensor Networks (WBSN) is emerging as a feasible alternative to sense, process and communicate data efficiently. It can be viewed as a mobile solution in monitoring physiological activities and health status of patients anytime and at any place. In healthcare applications three crucial factors which include reliability, security and energy efficiency are absolute necessity for wireless networks. There are protocols which offer security alone while some provide reliable and energy efficient data transmission but achieving all three criteria is not seen in many protocols. In our chapter a hybrid combination of PPSPC protocol and CICADA protocol is proposed and the resultant model possesses three vital criteria thereby providing reliable, secure and a power constrained data transmission in wireless body sensor network. Based on the implementation with NS2 simulator three vital parameters like Message transfer ratio, Throughput and Average End-to-End Delay are analyzed to determine the protocol effectiveness. The basic objective of this chapter is to contribute towards wireless sensor networks and its application in healthcare sector for remote monitoring of patients. The reliability using IEEE 802.15.4 for both point-to point communication and multihop communication is demonstrated here. It is evaluated using throughput and packet error rate. The results demonstrate the usage of wireless body area network in remote areas for health status monitoring with good throughput. Future work includes development of complicated protocols which offer scalability and robustness features in wireless scenario without compromising lifetime of a network.

References

1. Fieldand, M., Lohr, K.: Guidelines for Clinical Practice: From Development to Use. Institute of Medicine, National Academy Press, Washington, DC (1992)
2. Tan, J.: E-Health Care Information Systems: An Introduction for Students and Professionals, 624 pp., Hardcover. ISBN: 978
3. Nee, O., Hein, A., Gorath, T., Hulsmann, N., Laleci, G.: SAPHIRE: intelligent healthcare monitoring based on semantic interoperability platform—pilot applications. In: IEE Proceedings Communications Special Issue on Telemedicine and e-Health Communication Systems
4. Mahar, M.: Money-driven medicine: the real reason health care costs so much. In: Harpercollins Trade Sales Department, 1st edn. (July 7, 2009)

5. Kohno, R., Hamaguchi, K., Li, H., Takizawa, K.: R&D and standardization of body area network (BAN) for medical healthcare. In: Proceedings of the IEEE International Conference On Ultra-Wideband (ICUWB 2008), Hannover, Germany, September 10–12, vol. 3, pp. 5–8 (2008)
6. Gopalan, S.A., Park, J.T.: Energy-efficient MAC protocols for wireless body area networks: survey, ICUMT (2010)
7. Barati, A., Movaghar, A., Modiri, S., Sabaei, M.: A reliable and energy efficient scheme for real time wireless sensor networks applications. J. Basic Appl. Sci. Res. **2**(10), 10150–10157 (2012)
8. Kutty, S., Laxminarayan, J.A.: Towards energy efficient protocols for wireless body area networks, ICII (2010)
9. Ullah, S., Shen, B., Riazul, S.M., Khan, P., Saleem, S., Kwak, K.S.: A study of MAC protocols for WBANs. In: Sensors, vol. 10, no. 1, pp. 128–145. View at Publisher · View at Google Scholar · View at Scopus (2010)
10. Marinkovic, S., Popovici, E.: Ultra low power signal oriented approach for wireless health monitoring. In: Sensors, vol. 12, no. 6, pp. 7917–7937. View at Publisher · View at Google Scholar ·View at Scopus (2012)
11. Ibarra, E., Antonopoulos, A., Kartsakli, E., Verikoukis, C.: HEH-BMAC: hybrid polling MAC protocol for wireless body area networks operated by human energy harvesting. Telecommun. Syst. **2015**(58), 111–124. doi:10.1007/s11235-014-9898-z. [Cross Ref]
12. Lee, D.-S., Liu, Y.-H., Lin, C.-R.: A wireless sensor enabled by wireless power. In: Sensors, vol. 12, no. 12, pp. 16116–16143. View at Publisher · View at Google Scholar · View at Scopus (2012)
13. Filipe, L., Riverola, F., Costa, N., Pereira, A.: Wireless body area networks for healthcare applications: protocol stack review. Int. J. Distrib. Sens. Netw. Article ID 213705, **2015** (2015)
14. He, D., Chen, H., Chan, S., Bu, J., Vasilakos, A.V.: A distributed trust evaluation model and its application scenarios for medical sensor networks. IEEE Trans. Inf. Theor. Biomed. **16**(6) (2012)
15. He, D., Chen, C., Chan, S., Bu, J., Zhang, P.: Secure and lightweight network admission and transmission protocol for body sensor networks. IEEE J. Biomed. Health Inform. **17**(3) (2013)
16. Lim, H.B., Baumann, D., Li, E.-P., Fellow, IEEE: A human body model for efficient numerical characterization of UWB signal propagation in wireless body area networks. IEEE Trans. Biomed. Eng. **58**(3) (2011)
17. Chiti, F., Member, IEEE, Fantacci, R., Fellow, IEEE, Archetti, F., Messina, E., Toscani, D.: An integrated communications framework for context aware continuous monitoring with body sensor networks. IEEE J. Sel. Areas Commun. **27**(4) (2009)
18. Fujii, M., Fujii, R., Yotsuki, R., Wuren, T., Takai, T., Sakkagami, I., Member, IEEE: Exploration of whole human body and UWB radiation interaction by efficient and accurate two-debye-pole tissue models. IEEE Trans. Antennas Propag. **58**(2) (2010)
19. Alemdar, H., Erosy, C.: Wireless sensor networks for healthcare: a survey. ELSEVIER J. Comput. Netw. **54**, 2688–2710 (2010)
20. Khalil, E.A., Bara'a, A.A.: Energy-aware evolutionary routing protocol for dynamic clustering of wireless sensor networks. ELSEVIER J. Swarm Evol. Comput. 195–203 (2011)
21. Gurjar, D., Alam, M.I., Tiwari, B., Pandey, G.N.: Wireless sensor network: an emerging entrant in healthcare. IOSR J. Comput. Eng. **4**(4), 43–48 (2012). ISSN:2278-0661
22. Howlader, M.M.R., Doyle, T.E.: Low temperature nanointegration for emerging biomedical applications. ELSEVIER J. Microelectr. Reliab. **52**, 361–374 (2011)
23. Al Ameen, M., Kwak, K.-S.: Social issues in wireless sensor networks with healthcare perspective. Int. Arab J. Inf. Technol. **8**(1) (2011)
24. Phunchongharn, P., Niyato, D., Member, IEEE, Hossain, E., Senior Member, IEEE, Camorlinga, S.: An EMI-aware prioritized wireless access scheme for E-health applications in hospital environments. IEEE Trans. Inf. Technol. Biomed. **14**(5) (2010)

25. Kaliannan et al.: Ant colony optimization algorithm based PID controller for LFC of single area power system with non-linearity and boiler dynamics. World J. Model. Simul. (2016)
26. Agatheesan et al.: Application of flower pollination algorithm in load frequency control of multi-area interconnected power system with nonlinearity. Neural Comput. Appl. (2016)
27. Kaliannan et al.: Particle swarm optimization based parameters optimization of PID controller for load frequency control of multi-area reheat thermal power systems. In: IEEE International Symposium on Applied Computational Intelligence and Informatics, May 12–14, 2016
28. Alasaarela, E., Nemana, R., DeMello, S.: Drivers and challenges of wireless solutions in future healthcare. In: International Conference on eHealth, Telemedicine, and Social Medicine (2009)
29. Nourizadeh, S., Song, Y., Thomesse, J.P., Deroussent, C.: A distributed elderly healthcare system. In: MobiHealth 2009, Porto, Portugal (2009)
30. Chehri, A., Hussein, M.: Performance analysis of UWB body sensor networks for medical applications. In: Zheng, J., Simplot-Ryl, D., Leung, V.C.M. (eds.) The book: Ad Hoc Networks. Lecture Notes of the Institute for Computer Sciences, Social Informatics and Telecommunications Engineering, vol. 49, Part 8, pp. 471–481 (2010)
31. Hongliang, R., Meng, M., Chen, X.: Physiological information acquisition through wireless biomedical sensor networks. In: Proceedings of the IEEE International Conference on Information Acquisition, June 27–July 3 (2005)[11] Blount, M.: Remote health-care monitoring using personal care connect. IBM Syst. J. **46**(1) (2007)
32. Baker, R., et al.: Wireless sensor networks for home health care. In: 21st International Conference on Advanced Information Networking and Applications Workshops (AINAW 2007). IEEE, Los Alamitos (2007)
33. Ben Slimane, J., Song, Y.O., Koubaa, A., Frikha, M.: A three-tiered architecture for large-scale wireless hospital sensor networks. In: MobiHealthInf 2009, pp. 20–31 (2009)
34. Gyselinckx, B., Van Hoof, C., Donnay, S.: Body area networks: the ascent of autonomous wireless Microsystems, pp. 73–83. Springer, Heidelberg (2006)
35. www.isi.edu/nsnam/ns/
36. Lee, C., Kim, J., Lee, H., Kim, J.: Physical layer designs for WBAN systems in IEEE 802.15.6 proposals. In: 9th International Symposium on Communication and Information Technology, Incheon (September 28–30, 2009)
37. Wireless Medium Access Control (MAC) and Physical Layer (PHY) Specifications for Low Data Rate Wireless Personal Area Networks (WPAN) IEEE. Piscataway, NJ, USA. IEEE Std.802.15.4 (2006)

Part IV
General Applications

Social Network Analysis in Healthcare

Kiran Baktha, Mukul Dev, Himanshu Gupta, Aman Agarwal and B. Balamurugan

Abstract Ever since the launch of Facebook and Twitter Social Networking has been booming. Healthcare is improving mainly due to services provided by social media websites such as Sermo, Ozmosis and MomMD. This chapter's main objective is to broaden the understanding of healthcare services provided by social media. The reader will be able to understand the means by which medical information is exchanged online and how to interpret this information with some specific examples. In addition to describing the architecture behind social media further insights to mobile applications has been given. Big data in healthcare and risks involved in using social media for healthcare have been discussed to caution its usage.

Keywords Social media · Social media analytics · Mobile Health · Big Data in Healthcare · Extracting information from Social media · Keeping up to date in Medicine

K. Baktha (✉)
SENSE, VIT University, Vellore, India
e-mail: sundarambaktha@hotmail.com

M. Dev · B. Balamurugan
SITE, VIT University, Vellore, India
e-mail: mukul.dev@outlook.com

B. Balamurugan
e-mail: balamuruganb@vit.ac.in

H. Gupta · A. Agarwal
SCOPE, VIT University, Vellore, India
e-mail: himanshu199586@gmail.com

A. Agarwal
e-mail: aman9425307728@gmail.com

C. Bhatt et al. (eds.), *Internet of Things and Big Data Technologies for Next Generation Healthcare*, Studies in Big Data 23,
DOI 10.1007/978-3-319-49736-5_13

1 Introduction

Social media is an online medium of communication that allows users to share information, interact and collaborate with each other. Most prominent examples include Facebook, Twitter, Snapchat and so on. It has evolved from just being a tool for individuals to share their private pictures to fostering significant discussions on health, business and technology. Social media is such a vital part of our day-to-day lives that it comes as no surprise how effective health communication can be done through social networks. It tends to be mutually beneficial to both the healthcare service providers and the patients. Medicine alone is insufficient to combat illness. Social support tends to boost mental and other health outcomes. Social media is ensuring that people rely more on the information available online and rely less on advertising in making purchasing decisions. In healthcare, this has become increasingly important as the public has access to quality and cost ratings. The various roles played by social networking in Healthcare are:

(a) **Marketing:** Marketing is a very important skill for many healthcare agencies in this highly competitive world. Social Networking can be used as medium to express an organization's mission and culture and gain patient loyalty. Related work in this field include Mayo Clinic, Go Ask Alice and many others which can be referred here [15].
(b) **Information Exchange:** Exchange of unbiased information among users is the most essential role of any social networking platform. Most widely discussed topics include tips for a preventive measure, updates on latest practices and so on. One important factor to be kept in mind is that patient specific information cannot be disclosed by any organization without the patient's consent. Healthranker is an example of a website dedicated to spread the latest health updates to its users.
(c) **Research Purposes:** Certain social networking sites such as HealthMap aid healthcare researchers in analyzing a particular disease. There are websites dedicated to serve doctors, nurses or medical students in order to provide a professional connection which can aid in medical developments.
(d) **Patient Support:** Social networking sites such as DailyStrength have been developed to support to caregivers and survivors. They enable patients to discuss daily struggles and experiences and help provide emotional support.

In addition, we need to be well aware of the data analysis techniques used in Social media. Once raw data has been obtained we should be able to analyse and extract useful patterns from that data. This process is termed as Social Media Mining. The various data mining techniques used to analyse social media include Opinion Analysis, Sentiment Orientation, Unsupervised Classification. Note that this list is not exhaustive and there are various other techniques that could be used as well [16].

2 Social Media in Healthcare

The healthcare industry is rapidly evolving with an incredible speed and the major contributors to this change are the dramatic upsurge in healthcare communication is brought about by social media. It offers an opportunity of communicating with consumers quickly and inexpensively by helping in promoting new wellness programs, marketing new services and announcing the latest developments in patient care. An interesting project undertaken to improve social media in health care is "Healthcare Hash-tag Project" which has made Twitter more accessible for the healthcare community as a whole by searching and capturing hash-tags related to healthcare. Social media for healthcare application can be used briefly for two major purposes as given in Table 1. Social media helps patients become more aware about the various health options available thereby taking more control of their health. Very soon companies may have to embrace social media in a better way not by just giving away information but by improving their ability to listen to patients needs. It helps patients in self-diagnosis and in some cases visiting the doctor is curtailed. Let's look at some statistics [14] about social media in health care:

1. 90 % of respondents between the ages of 18–24 said they would trust medical information shared by others on their social media sites.
2. 31 % of healthcare firms have specific social media guidelines in written form.
3. 19 % of Smartphone owners have at least one health app phone with the most popular being Exercise and diet apps.
4. 41 % of the people said social media would affect their choice of a specific doctor or hospital.
5. Parents are more likely to seek medical advice from social media.

These statistics show us how important social media is gaining importance in healthcare. Once a hospital enters into social media for promotion it cannot back off as inactive hospitals online spread a negative awareness among people. Health 2.0 and Androctor Anna (Artificial Intelligence Doctor) are a few examples of emerging technologies in online healthcare.

Table 1 Purposes for social media in healthcare

Purpose	Who	Information required
Marketing/business purpose	Pharma and medical agencies	Drug or service feedback
Health related purpose	Medical professionals, patients or researchers	Disease/treatment information

3 Social Media Analytics

Social media analytics is the process of taking social media data and applying analytical tools to help us make better business decisions. The key to gain a successful social media strategy is to carefully analyze the information being exchanged whether positive or negative and craft people's needs and desires. This is where the proper utilization of social media analytical tools come into picture. Depending on the source of the social media, the analytical tools can be chosen to get accurate results. Iconosquare is an effective tool for Instagram, Followerwonk for Twitter, Quintly for Facebook, YouTube, etc. are a few examples. Most of these are free of cost but they have certain restrictions example in the free version of Quintly, you can access analytics for only up to three Facebook pages [35]. An example of how Iconosqare analysis is given in Fig. 1. Many Social networking websites actively encourage researches to focus on analytics. Twitter for example has an API (Advanced Programming Interface) that allows developers building social media analytical tools to access tweets to analyze the anonymized data. This

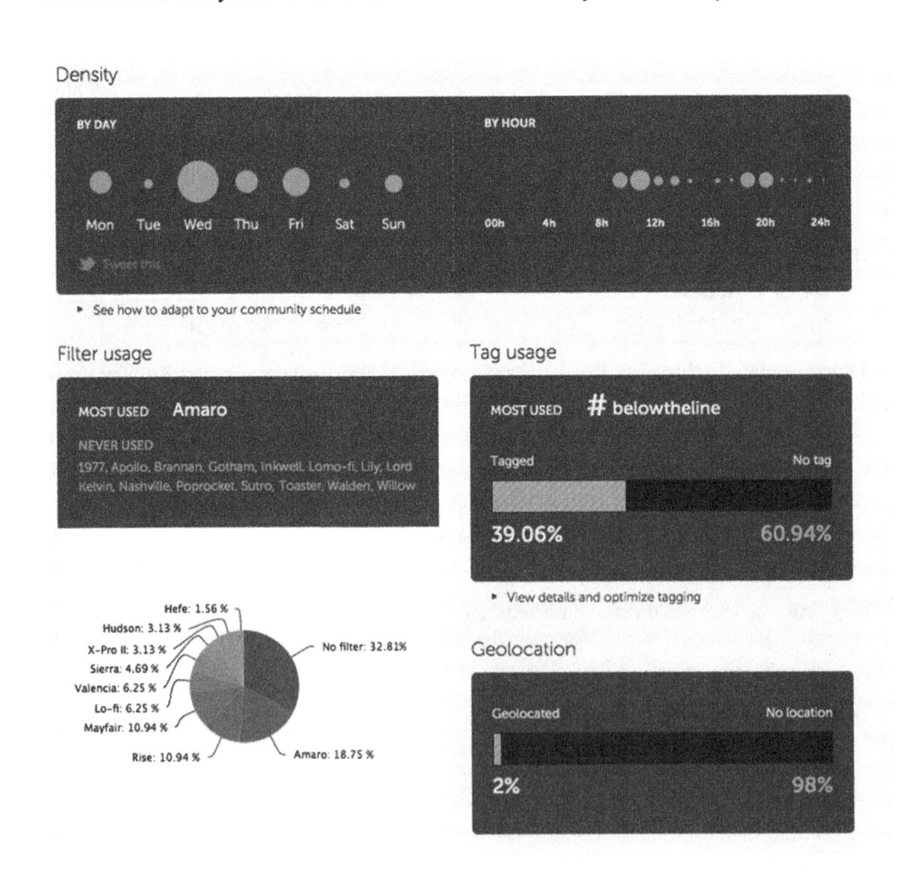

Fig. 1 Iconosquare analysis

is extremely beneficial because if a particular drug for example is becoming more and more infamous due to criticizing tweets, being able to extract that information could help pharmacists rectify the flaw easily.

Analyzing social media tends to have a myriad amount of advantages for a firm. Reviews shared online tend to be honest and by monitoring for mentions of corporate and brand names, analysts can learn what people really think about a firm. It becomes relatively easy to make improvements when you clearly know how people feel about a particular product or service. Analytical tools help to identify the target audience more easily. A good example is Trichology (branch of dermatology that deals with the study of hair and scalp). Trichologists are not found in majority of the hospitals and they tend to treat in clinics. Therefore, not many people would be aware of their existence and social media analytics could help them reach the target audience (like patients suffering from hair loss) by analyzing and filtering the discussions related to hair or scalp.

One of the major threats to any pharmaceutical company is the potential reporting of adverse events. They tend to harm the company's reputation as the whole world is exposed to their dangers. Every country has an agency that keeps a track of the adverse effects and medication error reports. In the United States it is the job of the Food and Drug Administration (FDA). In Canada, it is done by Health Canada. In a survey of 500 random healthcare related messages on social networks as shown in Fig. 2, only 1 met all the 4 criteria for being a reportable Adverse Event (AE) [34].

3.1 Steps Involved in Social Media Analytics

Generally, there are three steps involved in social media analytics, the steps include capture, understand and present [6].

Capture: The first of the three steps is Capture where an organization identifies the information related to their brand, services, reviews, products etc. leveraging the social media platforms like Facebook, Twitter, YouTube and other blogs. From a single platform alone a company can acquire huge amount of data. In order to move on to next step various operations on the collected data are to be performed such as capturing and linking data from different sources and storing the compiled data in a single data mart, creating some type of data model, highlighting and extracting out specific highlights from the data, removal of useless data, noise and other inconsistencies in the available data to obtain more meaningful analysis and performing other different types of operations on the data that will support the analytics on the acquired data.

Understand: Once the data is acquired and processed in a single mart the actual analytics of data begins. Understand is the main part of the entire social network analytics process. The analysis of collected data in this stage will provide organization the information about client's feelings which states that how customer base feels about the organization and its products or services. After analytics of certain

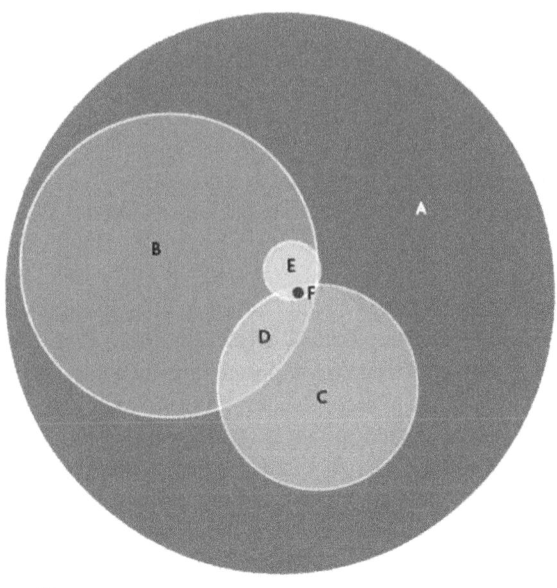

Fig. 2 Adverse effects analysis

clusters and metrics we can understand and predict about the likelihood of customer to purchase and use the product or services of the physician or organization after seeing an ad campaign. Many useful clusters and metrics and trends about users are formed during analytics at this stage. Example of clustering and other metrics for better analytics of social media could be volume, how many people participating in the conversation about the brand, services, product etc. Engagement can be other metric where clusters can be formed to analyse how people on social media are engaging on the activities related to the conversation and recommendation of the organization's product and services. The results of understanding the data and metrics will have a major effect on the next step, present.

Present: This is the last step where the results of the analytics on previous steps are evaluated, summarized and presented to the organization or pharmacist in the format they can understand. Various virtualization techniques are used such as

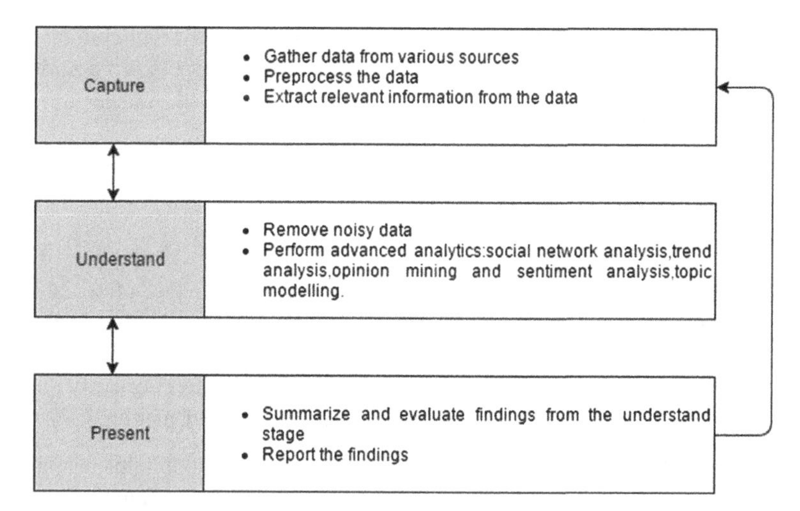

Fig. 3 Steps involved in social media analysis

visual dashboard which can present the summarized information from various different sources which includes different types of graphs etc. (Fig. 3).

3.2 Architectural Framework

The architectural framework for big data analysis project in healthcare is almost similar to that of a traditional report on healthcare analytics or healthcare informatics. The process of execution is the key between the big data analytics and traditional analysis. In a traditional healthcare analytics project a stand-alone system is sufficient, installed with business intelligence tools which can perform the analytics on the acquired data from the social networks; the stand-alone system can be laptop or desktop. As we know that big data is very large by nature hence processing is distributed and executed across multiple systems called nodes. Healthcare provides with the large data repositories to perform better decision making hence the problem of analysing very large datasets arises. Open source platforms such as Hadoop and MapReduce are used to analyse big data related to healthcare collected from the social media. These days these open source platforms are also available on cloud which encourages the application of big data analytic in healthcare industry [4, 5].

The user interfaces and hence user experience of both traditional analytics tools and big data analytics tools are entirely different but the models and algorithms are quite similar. These days the traditional analytics tools in healthcare industry have become very user friendly and quite transparent but the analytics tools available for big data analysis now are very complex and programming intensive and the operator of these tools is required to be skilled with required programming skills, therefore these tools lack the user friendliness and support. As Fig. 13 descript that the complexity begins at very beginning with the data itself [4, 5].

3.3 Metrics in Social Media Analytics

Social media metrics are the metrics used to estimate the impact of social media activity on an organization. There a hundreds of metrics that could be used but the real challenge lies in choosing the ones that matter the most. It is very essential for healthcare marketers to actively monitor the social landscape to effectively compute the value of their brand. Here is a list of few commonly used metrics [27]:

(a) **Volume:** One of the easiest metrics to measure is volume. It helps in analyzing the number of messages of a particular brand as well as the number of people who post these messages and how these change over time.
(b) **Reach:** It helps in measuring the spread of a social media activity. Reach has to be combined with other metrics to be very powerful and is used as the denominator in social measurement equations.
(c) **Engagement:** Engagement helps in informing how interesting a particular social activity is? It measures the activity level of people and the measures taken to spread the activity or engage in it.
(d) **Influence:** Next we need to be able to judge the effectiveness of various people in the activity. Some are very influential while others are not. This type of information helps in deciding on who to approach to disseminate a particular activity.
(e) **Share of Voice:** It order to excel you must always be ahead of your competitors. This metric focuses on the related to a brand compared to its main competitors.

Demographics Pro [28] is a tool which helps marketers to get the essential social media metrics from their social activities in popular websites such as Facebook, Twitter and so on. Figure 4 shows the technologies page from the audience profile of Signature HealthCare's feed using Demographics Pro [29]. This type of visualization can help marketers determine which platforms to target for maximum benefit.

3.4 Architecture Capabilities for Social Media Analysis

There are many different varieties and sheer volume of social media data available that can make analysis a tedious task but healthcare companies need not complain. What they need to do is adopt a data-driven marketing strategy which involves

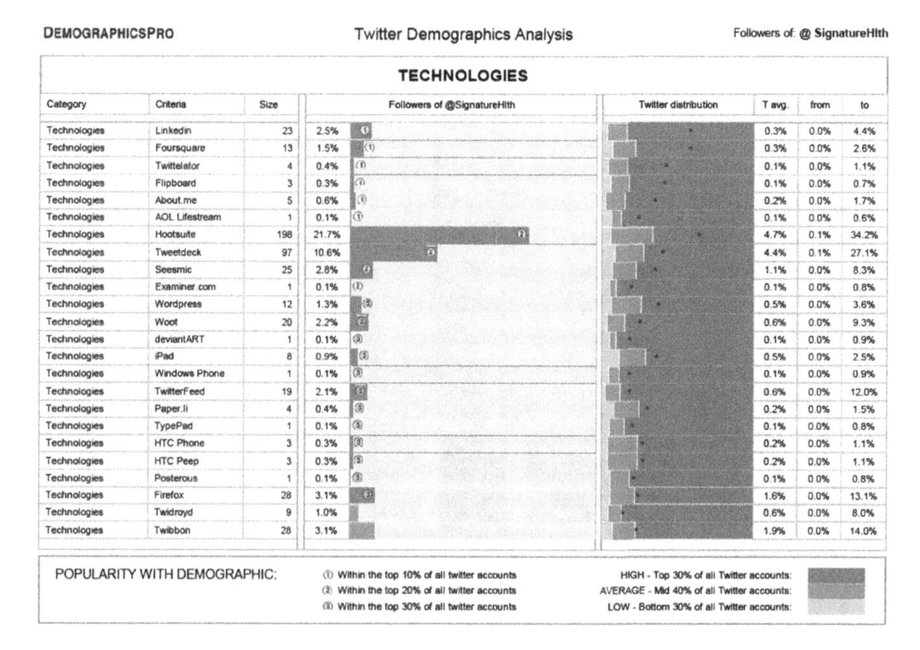

Category	Criteria	Size	Followers of @SignatureHlth	T avg.	from	to
Technologies	Linkedin	23	2.5%	0.3%	0.0%	4.4%
Technologies	Foursquare	13	1.5%	0.3%	0.0%	2.6%
Technologies	Twittelator	4	0.4%	0.1%	0.0%	1.1%
Technologies	Flipboard	3	0.3%	0.1%	0.0%	0.7%
Technologies	About.me	5	0.6%	0.2%	0.0%	1.7%
Technologies	AOL Lifestream	1	0.1%	0.1%	0.0%	0.6%
Technologies	Hootsuite	198	21.7%	4.7%	0.1%	34.2%
Technologies	Tweetdeck	97	10.6%	4.4%	0.1%	27.1%
Technologies	Seesmic	25	2.8%	1.1%	0.0%	8.3%
Technologies	Examiner.com	1	0.1%	0.1%	0.0%	0.8%
Technologies	Wordpress	12	1.3%	0.5%	0.0%	3.6%
Technologies	Woot	20	2.2%	0.6%	0.0%	9.3%
Technologies	deviantART	1	0.1%	0.1%	0.0%	0.9%
Technologies	iPad	8	0.9%	0.5%	0.0%	2.5%
Technologies	Windows Phone	1	0.1%	0.1%	0.0%	0.9%
Technologies	TwitterFeed	19	2.1%	0.6%	0.0%	12.0%
Technologies	Paper.li	4	0.4%	0.2%	0.0%	1.5%
Technologies	TypePad	1	0.1%	0.1%	0.0%	0.8%
Technologies	HTC Phone	3	0.3%	0.2%	0.0%	1.1%
Technologies	HTC Peep	3	0.3%	0.2%	0.0%	1.1%
Technologies	Posterous	1	0.1%	0.1%	0.0%	0.8%
Technologies	Firefox	28	3.1%	1.6%	0.0%	13.1%
Technologies	Twidroyd	9	1.0%	0.6%	0.0%	8.0%
Technologies	Twibbon	28	3.1%	1.9%	0.0%	14.0%

Fig. 4 Technology analysis using demographic pro

recognizing and integrating deep behavioral analytics. This helps to deliver the best possible real-time communication possible to patients. In order to have an effective data-driven marketing strategy the final architecture should enable three core capabilities [13]:

1. *Marketing analytics and data management:*

Due to the vast number of data out there the initial step should be to collect, connect and understand the data being provided by patients and members. A data warehouse would help improve the patient and member communications. The data warehouse should be capable of supporting integrated and shared data environments that deliver smart and functional analytics. Adoption of rapid discovery analytics is very much necessary to unlock big data insights through iterative exploration.

2. *Integrated marketing management:*

Integrated marketing management is going to improve the efficiency of social media campaigns by managing resources and content to help in the delivery of right messages to the right audience in the right time. Gartner, a technology research firm predicts that using an integration marketing strategy is going to lead to a 50 % greater ROMI (Return On Marketing Investment).

3. *Marketing resource management:*

What is the use of marketing analytics and integrated marketing management if one cannot measure the success of a marketing campaign? Marketing resource

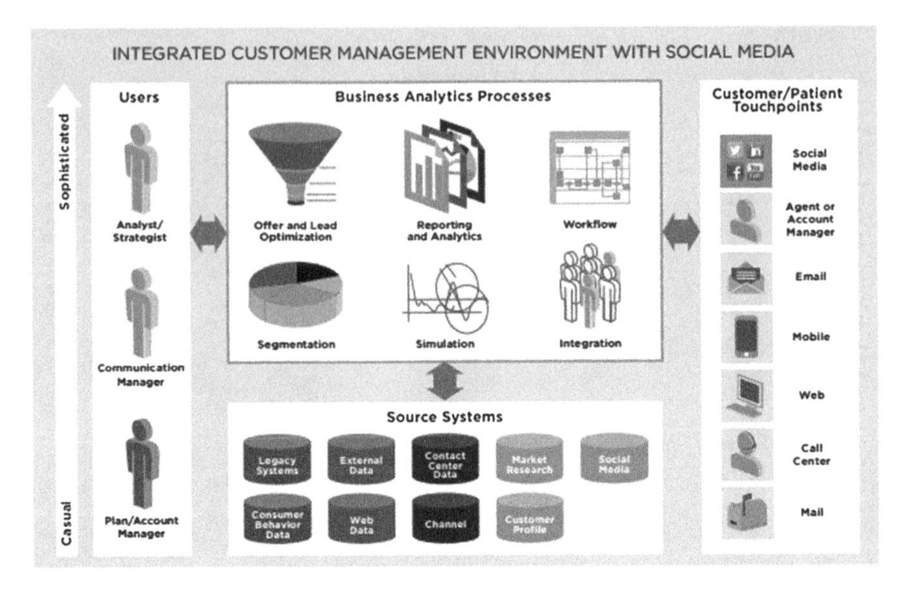

Fig. 5 Integrated customer management environment

management can prove how your social media efforts are paying off by connecting campaign results with internal operations and spend.

It is essential to remember that social media is just one of the many channels healthcare agencies need to use to strengthen patient and member engagement. The important key is to have an integrated customer management environment (Fig. 5) that uses and analyzes key data in the organization and allows for smooth engagement across each channel. By having a data-driven marketing approach healthcare companies are in the right position to enhance satisfaction, bring in more patients and members and ultimately create a healthier population.

4 Social Media in Clinical Care

The most important goal of Clinical care is to bring a sense of wellbeing in a patient. Clinical Care generally consists of any salubrious activity that causes this to happen, ranging from medication to clinical trials to investigations. There exists an interaction involved between the patient and the caregiver whenever a clinical care is administered. Social media platforms are now being extensively used for the advantages they offer. They make activities happen in extremely quick time. Heath camps are very much benefited when a massive awareness is created among people. One very good example would be the polio vaccination camps whose success can be clearly seen by the massive suppression of the disease [41].

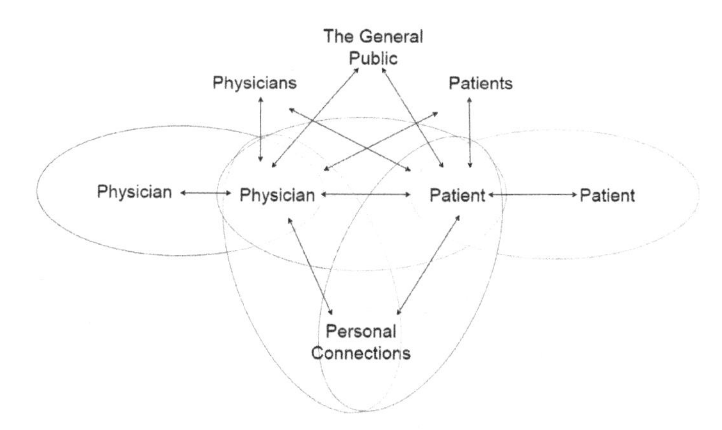

Fig. 6 Key social media interactions among patients, physicians and the public

By offering a public reservoir of information, social media can help serve as a source of patient information in times of need. One report in literature describes how physicians were able to contact the relative of a patient affected by amnesia using Facebook when all other traditional sources applicable failed. Some physicians also try to connect with patients using social media to seem more approachable. Face to face visits are very time consuming and as video chatting becomes more common, this type of communication is emerging as a way for patients to consult with physicians about non-urgent issues such as follow up questions or to connect with patients in geographically dispersed locations that may not have nearby access to specialists. Figure 6 shown above illustrates the key social media interactions among patients, physicians and the public. The solid lines indicate secure interactions and the dotted lines indicate personal networking interactions [2].

Due to the vast data collection capability, healthcare providers would require aid in analyzing the data. Visualization of data is very crucial and it is important to get an overview on the changes of health status. Hospitals have long recognized the power of social media as a tool for marketing and engagement of their patient base. To increase the social media utilization many health care agencies are employing social media experts. For example, Detroit Medical Center has a social media manager post, MedStar Health has a similar post but it is called as a social media coordinator and so on. Data privacy and security issues are also necessary. The data obtained should be accessed only by the relevant people involved in the treatment of the process. Healthcare providers are required to comply with mandates such as HIPAA (Health Insurance Portability and Accountability Act) or HITECH (Health Information Technology for Economic and Clinical Health). The various risks of improper security measures include Identity theft, Unauthorized disclosure, Trademark infringement and so on. Patients too must be wary about their posts. They should maintain a balance between anonymity and transparency and this balance involves sharing personal information whilst reading the terms and conditions to participate [17, 18]. Several research has been carried out in improving data privacy in healthcare. Electrocardiogram (ECG) hash code was tested as a biometric feature due to its uniqueness [19]. Crypto-Biometric authentication scheme in ATM banking systems was developed [20]. Effects of Watermarking in Vector quantization based Image Compression for quick and direct transmission of images were analyzed [21]. A comprehensive study for the behavior of some well-established watermarking algorithms in frequency domain for the preservation of stroke-based diagnostic parameters was conducted [22]. A reversible watermarking method called the Odd-Even Method was used for watermark insertion and extraction in a bio medical image with large data hiding capacity, security as well as high watermarked quality [23]. Application of Watermarking in motion vector for security enhancement in Medical Videos [24].

There are certain ethical and professional implications of physician use of social media for the health care purposes. The American Medical Association (AMA) serves as a frame work for these implications. For more in-depth understanding of these implications please refer the 9 principles of medical ethics by the AWA [30]. SERMO is one of the leading social networking sites for doctors only discussing about real world medicine.

5 Keeping Up-to-Date in Medicine

Technology is changing medicine rapidly and it is very important to be up to date with medicine. While this is most crucial for doctors it would be beneficial if patients are also briefly aware of what is happening. In the United Kingdom keeping up to date is compulsory. It is called as *revalidation* introduced by the General Medical Council (GMC). It is applicable to nurses and midwives as well and it is to ensure that their skills are up to date and they remain highly capable to practice medicine. It improves the confidence a patient has on the doctor. While doctors need to undergo revalidation every 5 years, nurses and midwives need to revalidate every 3 years. Revalidation involves lot of steps including Appraisal, Patient feedback and Colleague feedback. Detailed procedures are mentioned in the GMC official website.

Keeping up to date with medical literature is challenging. For example, in May 2016, there were around 40,000 systematic reviews that were added to the PubMed database [37]. PubMed is a search engine that accesses the MEDLINE (Medical Literature Analysis and Retrieval System Online) database. The best method to be used for keeping updated depends on the learning requirement as well as individual preferences and available time. It is generally recommended that a mix of formal and informal methods be used.

RSS (Really Simple Syndication) is a technology that is being used by a lot of people around the world to keep a track of their favorite websites. First you need to have a RSS feed reader such as Netvibes or freely. Figure 7 below shows the user interface of Netvibes.

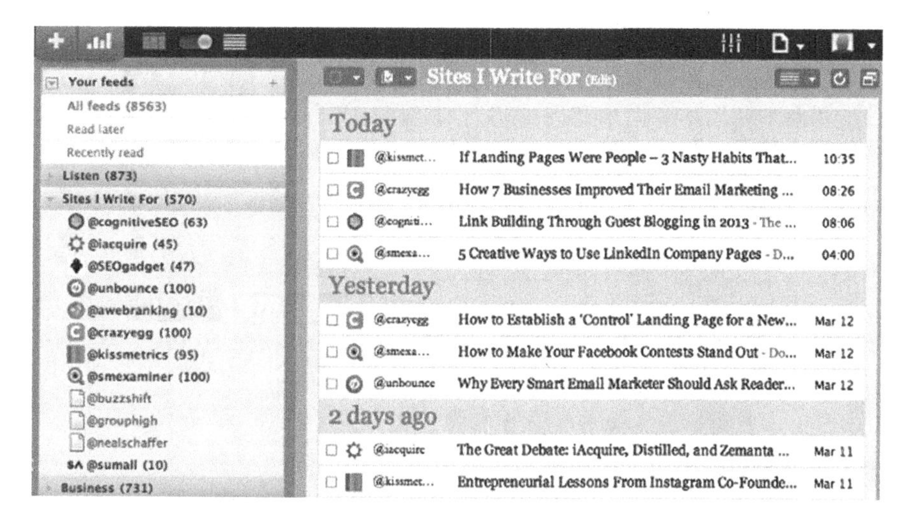

Fig. 7 Netvibes user interface

Feed readers generally work like email. When you subscribe to a feed, all the unread articles from the site you are tracking will be marked as bold. RSS feeds generally get you are range of information from News sites, Web search results, Papers from peer-reviewed journals, updates from clinical guidelines and many more.

The second thing that you need to do is subscribe. Now there are 2 places you can look for the site's feed to subscribe:

(a) *On site Subscription*—These come in the form of little buttons and widgets that appear on many sites and blogs having words like RSS, XML, ATOM, etc. written on them. Figure 8 shows the common widgets you can come across.
(b) *Browser Subscription*—Rather than trying to look for a widget many internet browsers have subscribe to RSS feeds built right into them. They are located on the address bar where you type the URL. To subscribe you simply click on the feed icon and by default they will subscribe you using the in-browser reader. Figure 9 shows how the icon appears in your browser. The orange icon in the right is the standard icon for RSS.

Many social media platforms make the RSS feed of the channel available automatically. One thing that is very important is that you must know how to search for things on the internet. Get to know which sites are the best for the illness you are looking for. Table 2 gives a list of some famous disease specific sites you can visit. In addition, there some top sites on general health issues like MayoClinic.com and Medlineplus.gov.

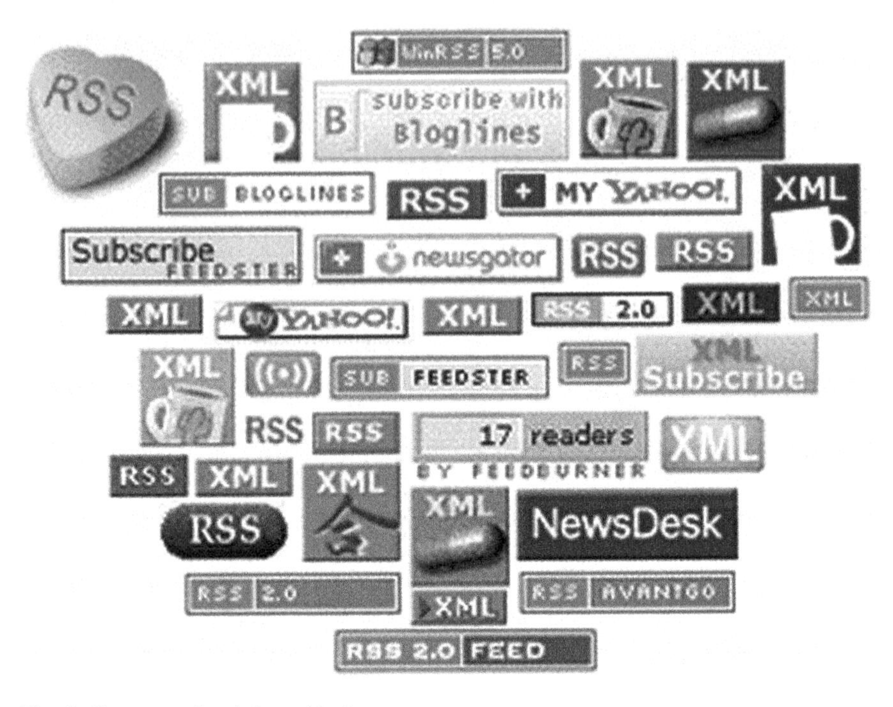

Fig. 8 Common subscription widgets

Fig. 9 Browser subscription icon

http://www.problogger.net/

Table 2 Top rated disease specific sites

Disease	Websites
Cancer	(i) American Cancer Institute (www.cancer.org) (ii) National Cancer Institute (www.cancer.gov) (iii) Cancer Care (www.cancercare.org)
Heart disease	(i) American Heart Association (www.americanheart.org) (ii) National Heart, Lung and Blood Institute (www.nhlbi.nih.gov) (iii) Congenital Heart Information Network (www.tchin.org)

(continued)

Table 2 (continued)

Disease	Websites
Diabetes	(i) American Diabetes Association (www.diabetes.org) (ii) Diabetes Monitor (www.diabetesmonitor.com) (iii) National Diabetes Education Program (www.ndep.nih.gov)
Alzheimer's disease	(i) Alzheimer's association (www.alz.org) (ii) Fisher Center for Alzheimer's Research (www.alzinfo.org)

Another convenient way to keep you updated is to download apps that you can read on the go. Docphin, Read by QXMD, Browzine and DocNews are great apps that help you read medical journals on your tablet or Smartphone.

6 Extracting Information from Social Media

Data about diseases and outbreaks are disseminated throughout the internet through online announcements by government agencies and informal channels. In order to allow for a smooth processing, we need to not only extract the relevant information but also represent it in an adequate manner. There are various sources while provide insight to a variety of health issues all over the world (Refer Table 3). There are also various challenges that make information extraction more complex. The most common challenges are:

(a) The posted texts are generally noisy and written in an informal text. They include misspellings and lack of punctuation and capitalisation.

Table 3 Main sources of information for health personalization in Social Web

Sources	Examples of information that can be extracted
Personal health records	Personal health, demographic and genetic information
Online user profiles	Health risk behaviours (like smoking), demographic information and user preferences
Forum posts and comments	Personal health information, emotional or mental state of users and type of content (like informational or controversial)
Search queries	User interests
Facial photos	Emotions, gender and age
Videos	Diagnosis and characteristics of videos
Ratings	User preferences and similarities
Web usage data	Navigational data classification of users

(b) Some messages are very short like the ones posted on twitter because of a post length limit.
(c) Not every information available is trustworthy. Sometimes many conflicts occur between users regarding the same matter.

Regardless of these developments, technological advancements help using in getting the information we need. The MetaMap System which is operated by the National Library of Medicine is a tool designed to map the biomedical text to the UMLS Metathesaurus. The UMLS (Unified Medical Language System) Metathesaurus is a huge, multi-lingual and multi-purpose thesaurus that has several biomedical and health related concepts including their synonyms and their relationships. MetaMap works in 5 steps. First the arbitrary text is parsed into simple noun phrases thereby making the mapping effort more tractable. In the second step variants are generated using the knowledge in the SPECIALIST lexicon (refer National Language Processing for more details) and a supplementary database of synonyms. The variant generation of MetaMap before the inflections and spelling variations are computed are given in Fig. 10. In the third step candidate retrieval of all the Metathesaurus containing at least one of the variants is retrieved. In the fourth step each candidate is evaluated against the input text by mapping from the phrase words to the candidate's words and then estimating the strength of the mapping using linguistically principled evaluation. In the final step the construction of mapping takes place. These mappings are done by joining candidates involved in disjoint parts of the phrase [38].

In a qualitative study conducted by Denecke [1], the average accuracy that was achievable by Metamap was only 64.89 % while cTakes gave an average accuracy of 94.28 %. cTakes is a natural language processing system for extraction of information from electronica medical record clinical free-text. It was built using the Apache UIMA (Unstructured Information Management Architecture).

Another interesting tool is HealthMap. It mines public data in 15 different languages, including news reports, tweets, information from the government and public health groups. The data obtained is geocoded (converting normal address in

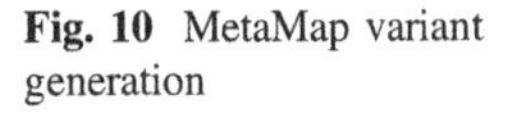
Fig. 10 MetaMap variant generation

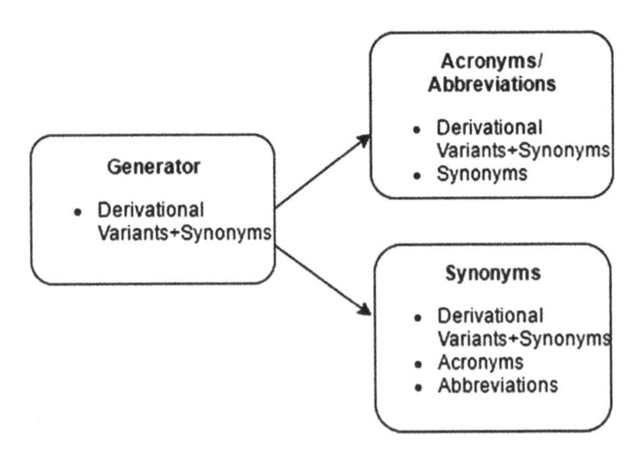

terms of latitude and longitude) and is presented on HealthMap's map based visual display. Let us see an example of how HealthMap was used to map the Ebola outbreak that happened a few years ago all around the world especially in Africa. HealthMap caught the world's attention when it detected the Ebola outbreak 9 days before it actually occurred [36].

Ebola is a very dangerous disease caused by the Ebola Virus. Patients bleed internally and externally mostly leading to death. It is considered to have an average survival rate of 50 %. The outbreak ended in late 2015 and on 29 March 2016, it was no longer declared as emergency. In March 2014 when eight people got the mysterious disease, it raised curiosity in the Healthcare industry. HealthMap started working on it and developed a machine learning algorithm to map the disease. The final outcome can be seen in Fig. 11. The algorithm worked by analyzing the RSS feeds and APIs looking for texts and geographical location of the information by continuously removing noise.

Genetic research is an important branch of medical science. It helps identify the changes in chromosomes, genes or proteins. It helps to determine whether a person is bound to be affected by genetic disorders. GenePath is a web based software developed using the Prolig logic cased programming language. With advancing technology that has facilitated higher experiment rates and huge data gathering manual approaches in genomics became highly error prone. GenePath uses genetic patterns to determine which genes influence the outcome and which genes block or don't block the other genes.

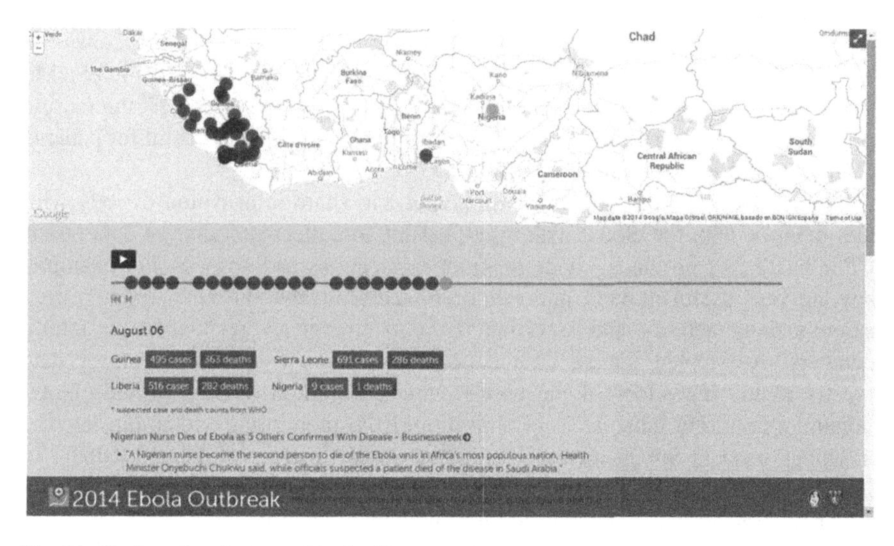

Fig. 11 Ebola outbreak mapped by healthmap

7 Social Media in Mobile Health and Internet of Things (IoT)

With the rapid increase in online patient communities who use social media as a platform to exchange information there has been a great concern for improving mobile apps to further enhance this experience. Demand for apps and wearable devices have increased drastically. Most leading pharmaceutical companies have started focussing on app development and from 2013 to 2014 alone there was a 63 % increase in the number of unique apps (An app available on both iOS and Android is counted as a unique app) published by pharmaceutical companies. There are 3 main reasons why apps and wearables are very important [3]:

- Wearables work well only in conjunction with software such as apps
- There is a clear demand for the need for monitoring devices that are very simple to use and do not interfere with our normal life
- A large number of small companies design and develop wearable devices leaving the market highly fragmented.

PatientsLikeMe is an online community that helps patients find clinical trials that suit them and the companies find patients who suit their trial. Their app has made a huge success in the market. It collects the data reported by the users about real world nature of diseases to help other users, researchers, pharmaceutical companies and other non-profit organizations. The moral health of a patient is improved when patients who have the same disease or condition share their own experiences and bond with each other. This is the main objective of PatientsLikeMe. There are about more than 400,000 members who connect with each other. Figure 12 shows the details collected and displayed about a drug called Baclofen in the PatientsLikeMe App. Baclofen is a muscle relaxer and an antispastic agent used to treat the muscle symptoms caused by multiple sclerosis. Such information is very useful for patients to understand the treatment in a better way.

Internet of things enable devices to gather and share information directly with each other or with the cloud, making it possible to collect and analyse data faster. IoT in healthcare provides a wide range of applications and services. For example, they are very useful in early intervention of a disease by constantly monitoring a patient's daily activity and reporting them to emergency responders or family members. Automated patient data collection systems collect and transfer data directly to the repository of the user's choice. Common devices provide blood pressure monitoring, glucose level indication, ECG monitoring and so on. Internet of Things used in Social media is called as Social Internet of Things (SIoT). In SIoT, a social relationship can be established between all smart objects. In particular SIoT is very advantageous to the marketers to identify and take advantage of new emerging trends and customer data collection becomes much simpler [25, 26].

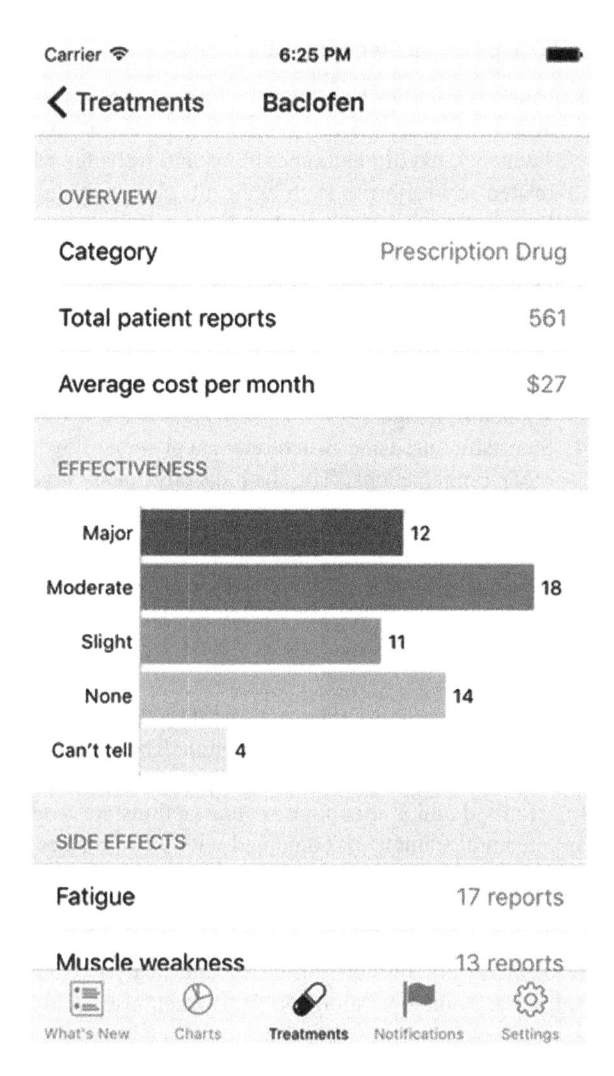

Fig. 12 PatientsLikeMe App interface

8 Sources of Big Data in Healthcare

In healthcare industry big data can come from many sources such as internal sources, external sources etc. and the acquired data is often in multiple formats such as flat files, relational tables, csv, text etc. The above mentioned internal sources includes electronic health records and clinical decision support systems and external sources includes government sources, pharmacies, laboratories and data collected from insurance companies etc.

Data is distributed across the various different geographic locations hence the distributed data and processing concepts id used because sometimes it's not possible to collect the data at one place and apply analytics.

Sources of data types include [7]:

1. Data collected from social media and other web sites such as people's interaction and communication data from social networking sites such as Facebook, Twitter, LinkedIn and other blogs and websites which can also include websites related to healthcare such as health plan websites and apps etc.
2. Structured, semi-structured and unstructured data available from billing records and other healthcare related claims.
3. Data collected using IOT devices and other sensors such as vital sign devices and other health related sensors. Some sensors include biometric sensors which results in biometric data such as data collected from finger prints, retinal scans, X-ray scans and other bold pressure, pulse-oximetry readings and other medical scans and images.
4. Semi-structured and structured data generated by humans such as physicians and other organizations. This include physicians notes i.e. email and paper documents, EMR's etc.

8.1 Transforming 'Raw' Data

For the purpose of big data analysis this data has to be acquired and pre-processed in a single data mart or other collection. The data currently is in 'raw' state because the data is in different formats this raw data is required to be processed and transformed and at this point several options are available such as service-oriented architectural framework combined with web services acting as middleware [8] here data remains raw and web services are used to retrieve and process data whenever required i.e. data is distributed across the web, other services can also be used such as data warehousing here the data is stored and aggregated and pre-processed and made ready for further processing and analytics although data is not available in real time. Some operations on data warehouse include extract, transform and load.

8.2 Big Data Platforms and Tools

The most popular and widely used platform for big data analytics is Hadoop. Hadoop is an open-source distributed big data analytics platform which uses apache platform. Initially Hadoop was developed for aggregating the distributed web search indexes. It belongs to "NoSQL" technology family some other members include MongoDB and CouchDB. These databases do not use SQL and relational schema to store the data in the secondary storage devices. Hadoop can process extremely large amounts of data mainly by leveraging the concept of distributed processing i.e. by distributing the data to other servers and nodes each of which have responsibility of operating numerous operations on their part of data

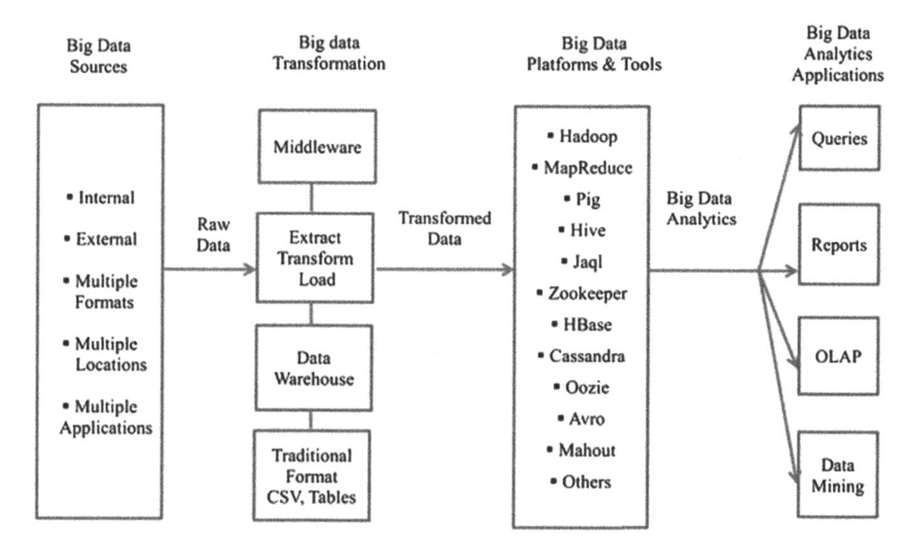

Fig. 13 An applied conceptual architecture of big data analytics

and then data is integrated and final result is integrated and analyzed [9–12]. The basic architectural framework for big data analytics along with various platforms and tools is mentioned in Fig. 13 [4].

8.3 *Big Data and Social Media*

In the last decade, the world has become more connected via the social platform than it's ever been. The most basic concept in understanding Big Data's impact on social media is that the social media is part of big data. Big data from the social media is the vast set of information which is gathered by researchers at various social-tech giants like Facebook, Twitter etc. Data is growing at an alarming rate and 90 % of the data available in the world was collect in the previous 2 years and 80 % of that data comes from unstructured sources such as social media [39].

The main advantage of harvesting social media big data is the ready availability of bulk data and continuous monitoring which reduces the response time to a minimum. Another advantage is the empowerment of new marketing strategies and customized algorithms which help companies analyse and make effective marketing efforts. It enables the marketers to look into the future with increased clarity to gauge the likely effectiveness of as strategy, rather than just relying on past experiences.

Despite the various recent developments in data mining and analytic tools, there are various challenges in that remain in capturing, analysing and interpreting the big health data and converting it into actionable public health solutions. Some of these issues include offline-user behaviour and privacy issues over the acquired data usage [39, 40].

9 Three P's of Successful Social Media in Healthcare

The 3 P's of social media include Personalization, Presentation and Participation. We know that that social media has started to gain acceptance in Healthcare community which means that patients are now communicating with other patients and Physicians and relying on the social media platform, which provide credible, evidence-based health information. One of the major challenges for social media platforms is protection of patient information and other ethical issues [6].

Especially for Physicians and medical organizations the three P's of social media can be highly effective as it is possible to leverage this emerging communication technology for medical practices. Social media can be used to target new patients, communication of transparent exchange of credible information and reinforcing advice.

Personalization: Timely and unbiased information should be focused upon and should be scientifically accurate, and patients and users should be allowed to personalize the media application according to one's need [6].

Presentation: This is most important of the three as physicians and other medical organizations can attract more customers and other properties such as, participation and personalization depends on it. Presentation depends upon the user interface and usage of other multimedia experience that attracts more customers and allows better personalization; and enhances participation of customers henceforth differentiating organization from the competition [6].

Participation: Any communication medium is useless without the availability of human resource hence actively communicating clients base is required to leverage the power of social media. Human resource is required that engage with campaigns and participate in healthcare promotions using social media and other means. Some other functionalities of client base include communication during epidemic or crisis, unbiased medical information sharing among the peers. Active participation by the clients also depends upon the presentation of content as explained above [6].

10 Recent Trends in Social Media

Social media continues to evolve at a rapid pace. Live Video Streaming is considered to be the next big development in social media. Periscope, Blab, Facebook Live and YouTube have been rising rapidly. As of 2016, people now watch an average of 5 h 31 min of video every day. Another recent trend that could be easily observed is the importance of Mobile Phones over other devices. Mobile devices especially smartphones, tablets and smartwatches should be the main focus of any social media analyst. Social commerce has also been booming. Social media plays a crucial role in influencing customer decisions. Therefore, keeping up with social media trends is a must and it's time to adapt to the recent trends and embrace these trends [42, 43].

11 Risks Involved in Using Social Media for Healthcare

There are various risks involved in social media that need to be carefully understood by patients and healthcare professionals. Most common risk is breaching of patient privacy. Many sensitive information including PHI is usually posted unencrypted and can be read by anyone. Protected Health Information generally includes information relating to health status or payment of health care that can be related to a specific individual. Information such as Phone numbers, Account numbers, Social security numbers and so on come under this category and they must be treated with special care. Some information can also be disclosed by third party and put harm the patient's reputation.

Another significant threat is the spread of unprofessional material that can harm the organization. There have been various cases of using discriminatory language, images of sexual suggestiveness or intoxication, abysmal comments on a firm, etc. Such events have actually been recorded where doctors have posted images with alcohol or have taken selfies in the middle of a surgery. Healthcare Professionals should continuously monitor their profile online to ensure that their social media presence projects a professionality image [31].

Lack of proper social media use plan can have negative effects. Some healthcare organizations enter into social media just to be in par with their competitors. An efficient social media policy and related procedures should be developed as part of the social media usage plan. Proper training of workforce is also a must because they are more likely to misuse social media. If they are aware of what has to be posted and what has to be kept concealed, they could inadvertently post sensitive information ultimately damaging the entire organization's reputation. In the United States, Health Insurance Portability and Accountability Act (HIPAA) is the governing legislation for data privacy and security measures relating to medical information. They have laid down some strict rules to be followed while communicating in the medical social media. According to the Health and Human Resources (HHS) of the United States, the most common violations occurring in medial social media are:

- Misusing and Disclosing PHI
- Unprotected Health Information
- Patients unable to access their own health information
- Disclosing more than the minimum necessary health information that is protected.

Let us look at an incident understand how important data privacy is in medical social media [32]. In 2011, about 4.9 million people very victims of health information breaching when data was stolen from the TRICARE healthcare program [33]. The TRICARE health program is by the United States defense department that serves active military troops and their dependents as well as military retirees. The data tapes were stolen from a car which was being used to transport the data tapes between federal facilities. What's even worse is that most of the data was not encrypted and the encrypted data part was not in accordance with the compliant with the federal standards. Information present in the tapes included Social Security numbers, Names, Contact Information and also personal health data such as lab tests, clinical notes and prescriptions. All the people affected were quickly identified to warn them. They were asked to place a fraud alert in case any of their personal or financial information had been leaked.

12 Conclusions

Social media networks when combined with Big Data applications is a growing domain which has the potential to provide us with key insights in healthcare. Despite providing patients with moral support it helps in raising funds for impecunious patients. Social media is not being fully utilized by healthcare agencies. Out of the 50 largest drug makers only half of them even dabble in social media and hardy 10 uses Facebook, Twitter and YouTube. The main reason being fear especially fear of adverse effects reporting which can prove very detrimental to an organization. Doctors should also use social media strategically. There is always a constant need for an organization to be above its competitors. After all, no one visits the 5th or the 6th pages of google searches. The main reason why social media is sought after is its capability of support and interaction. It is this interaction and support that differentiates a social media from Web 2.0 which provides the tools for interaction rather than providing the true interaction itself. Social media has also been very beneficial in promoting fitness awareness among users by allowing health clubs to share motivational videos and messages. Technology is ever improving and with the recent launch of 360 video capabilities in Facebook and YouTube doctors can almost have a real time experience with a patient. Google has already started implementing social contents available to their search engines. Companies like Facebook and Twitter have initiated deals with google and users are more likely to land up with tweets or Facebook content in their search results.

Acknowledgments Thank you for your cooperation and contribution.

References

1. Denecke, K.: Health Web Science. Springer International Publishing (2015)
2. Chretien, K.C., Kind, T.: Social media and clinical care ethical, professional, and social implications. Circulation **127**(13), 1413–1421 (2013)
3. Taylor, K.: Deliotte Solutions.How digital technology is Transforming Health and Social Care (2015)
4. Raghupathi, W., Raghupathi, V.: Big data analytics in healthcare: promise and potential. Health Inform. Sci. Syst. **2**(1), 1 (2014)
5. Raghupathi, W., Raghupathi, V.: An overview of health analytics. J. Health Med. Informat. **4**, 132 (2013). doi:10.4172/2157-7420.1000132
6. Fan, Weiguo, Gordon, Michael D.: The power of social media analytics. Commun. ACM **57** (6), 74–81 (2014)
7. Cottle, M., Hoover, W., Kanwal, S., Kohn, M., Strome, T., Treister, N.: Transforming health care through big data strategies for Leveraging Big Data in the Health Care Industry. Institute for Health Technology Transformation. http://ihealthtran.com/big-data-in-healthcare (2013)
8. Raghupathi, W., Kesh, S.: Interoperable electronic health records design: towards a service-oriented architecture. E-Serv. J. **5**(3), 39–57 (2007)
9. Borkar, V.R., Carey, M.J., Li, C.: Big data platforms: what's next?. XRDS: crossroads. ACM Mag. Stud. **19**(1), 44–49 (2012)
10. Ohlhorst, F. J.: Big Data Analytics: Turning Big Data into Big Money. John Wiley (2012)
11. Zikopoulos, P., Parasuraman, K., Deutsch, T., Giles, J., Corrigan, D.: Harness the Power of Big Data. The IBM Big Data Platform. McGraw Hill Professional (2012)
12. Zikopoulos, P., Eaton. C.: Understanding Big Data: Analytics for Enterprise Class Hadoop and Streaming Data. McGraw-Hill Osborne Media (2011)
13. Wiggin. D, Teradata.: Optimizing Social Media Analytics in Healthcare (2013)
14. Honigman, B.: 24 Outstanding Statistics and Figures on How Social Media has Impacted the Health Care Industry (2015)
15. Weeks, W.: 8 Exceptional Examples of Social Media Marketing in Healthcare (2015)
16. Adedoyin-Olowe, M: A Survey of Data Mining Techniques for Social Network Analysis (2013)
17. Marianne, K.M: Social Media: Teach Patients the Risks (2014)
18. HIMSS Privacy and Security Committee: Social Media in Healthcare: Privacy and Security Considerations (2013)
19. Nandi, S., et al.: Cellular Automata Based Encrypted ECG-hash Code Generation: An Application in Inter Human Biometric Authentication System (2014)
20. Biswas, S., Roy, A.B., Ghosh, K., Dey, N.: A biometric authentication based secured ATM banking system. Int. J. Adv. Res. Comput. Sci. Softw. Eng., 128X, **2** (4),2012
21. Bose, S., et al.: Effect of Watermarking in Vector Quantization based Image Compression (2014)
22. Suri, J.S., et al.: Effect of Watermarking on Diagnostic Preservation of Atherosclerotic Ultrasound Video in Stroke Telemedicine (2016)
23. Pal, A.K., Dey, N., Samanta, S., Das, A., Chaudhuri, S.S.: A hybrid reversible watermarking technique for color biomedical images. In: IEEE International Conference on Computational Intelligence and Computing Research (ICCIC) (2013)
24. Acharjee, S., et al.: Watermarking in Motion Vector for Security Enhancement of Medical Videos (2014)
25. Islam, S.R., et al.: The Internet of Things for Healthcare: A Comprehensive Survey (2015)
26. Atzori. L., et al.: SIoT: The Social Internet of Things (2011)
27. Cruse, D.: 5 Essential and Easy Social Media Metrics You Should be Using Right Now (2012)
28. Demographic Pro [website] www.demographicspro.com
29. Dunlop, D.: Demographic Analysis of Your Hospital's Twitter Followers (2014)

30. American Medical Association-Principle of Medical Ethics.: http://www.ama-assn.org/ama/pub/physician-resources/medical-ethics/code-medical-ethics/principles-medical-ethics.page (2001)
31. Ventola, C.L.: Social Media and Healthcare Professionals: Benefits, Risks and Best Practices (2014)
32. TRICARE Health Program www.tricare.mil
33. Anderson, H.: TRICARE Breach Affects 4.9 Million (2011)
34. Friedel, S.L.: Pharma Challenges: Adverse Event Reporting And Social Media (2012)
35. Lee,. K.: Know What's Working on Social Media: 19 Free Social Media Analytics Tools (2014)
36. Gilpin, L.: How an Algorithm Detected the Ebola Outbreak a Week Early, and What it could do Next (2014)
37. PubMed: Finding Systematic Reviews at PubMed Health www.ncbi.nlm.nih.gov/pubmedhealth/finding-systematic-reviews (2016)
38. Alan, R.: MetaMap Variant Generation (2001)
39. Hung, D.: The Impact of Big Data on Social Media Marketing Strategies (2016)
40. Alkay, A., et al: Mining Social Media Big Data for Health (2015)
41. McKenna, M.: Polio Eradication: Is 2016 the Year? (2016)
42. Radice, R.: Top Social Media Trends That'll Change Your Business in 2016
43. Beese, J.: 6 Social Media Trends That Will Take Over 2016

A Decision Support System in Brain Tumor Detection and Localization in Nominated Areas in MR Images

Omid Mahdi Ebadati E. and Mohammad Mortazavi T.

Abstract Manual brain tumor detection is time-consuming and bestows ambiguous classification. Hence, there is a needed for automated classification of brain tumor. With brain segmentation, the pixels within an image can be divided into sub regions or areas that they have similar features or characteristics for identification and detection of different objects. Segmentation of magnetic resonance (MR) image of human brain has got significant focus in the field of biomedical image processing. MR image segmentation has a wide application in medicine. This act can increase accuracy, and it helps doctors to minimize the errors. Tumor detection system can be used as a decision and diagnosis support system by doctors, nurses and who is working in this area. The proposed method for tumor segmentation is implemented in three stages by using image processing and machine learning approaches: extract histogram and train SVM, remove skull bone and *k*-mean clustering. The experimental results shown a high accurate detection of the tumor.

Keywords Tumor detection · Magnetic resonance imaging · Decision support system · Image processing · Machine learning

1 Introduction

62,930 new cases of human brain tumors estimated by The American Brain Tumor Association (ABTA) would be diagnosed in 2010. In addition, The National Cancer Institute (NCI) estimated that 22,070 new cases of human cancers would be

O.M. Ebadati E. (✉)
Department of Mathematics and Computer Science, Kharazmi University,
#242, Somayeh Street, Between Qarani & Vila, Tehran, Iran
e-mail: omidit@gmail.com

M. Mortazavi T.
Department of Knowledge Engineering and Decision Science,
Kharazmi University, #242, Somayeh Street, Between Qarani & Vila, Tehran, Iran
e-mail: Mortazavie@outlook.com

C. Bhatt et al. (eds.), *Internet of Things and Big Data Technologies for Next Generation Healthcare*, Studies in Big Data 23,
DOI 10.1007/978-3-319-49736-5_14

diagnosed in the United States of America in 2009 [1]. This statistic shows that tumor and white matter detection in the brain is an important issue in health care area. One of the useful tools for this work is medical imaging. Medical imaging can be more helpful in healthcare area with use of computer science. The blood vessels' segmentation [2], brain tumor detection [3], breast density classification [4] and etc. are many applicable and useful tools in medical imaging and healthcare.

Image processing has a wide usage like object detection, segmentation, hand writing recognition and others. It can also be used in industrial, medical, martial, etc. In medical usage, magnetic resonance imaging (MRI) is a type of imaging method that is used in radiology to visualize the structure of the body. This imaging method provides detailed images of the different body parts in any plane. In neurological imaging, MRI makes the much greater contrast between the different of tissues of the different parts of a body than does computer tomography (CT). The MR imaging has many advantages over other diagnostic medical imaging methods. One of the great difference in this area is high spatial resolution and great discrimination of soft tissues like skin, muscle, vessel and others. MRI is more useful in brain imaging also [5].

The MRI tumor brain detection is one of the useful applications of the image processing in medicine. Nowadays, there are several methodologies for tumor detection in MR images. There are many researches on tumor detection that uses a different method to do this work.

An approach based on probabilistic neural network (PNN) and other method named learning vector quantization (LVQ) are proposed to do a brain tumor detection and classification using MRI scans automatically. In this model with use of LVQ-based PNN system decreases the processing time, and it increases accuracy. This method runs in three steps: Image acquisition, Image segmentation and Edge detection [1, 6].

In another research work, a model proposed to use knowledge based (KB) system. In this method, an unsupervised clustering isused for initial segmentation and then multispectral histogram analysis separates a suspected tumor from the rest of the intracranial part, with region analysis used in performing the final tumor labelling. The proposed method is experienced on three different datasets, and it is tested on thirteen new and unseen volume datasets [7].

In a research from [8], they used genetic algorithm (GA) for image segmentation in tumor detection. GAs are the heuristic methods of search algorithms based on the evolutionary ideas of natural selection and genetics. This heuristic algorithm uses a method that is named random search for solving many optimization issues and problems [9, 10]. GA is a heuristic algorithm that it has done in several steps. Initial population step is first step that it determines the number of population, size of the chromosome and etc. fitness function in GA calculates the fitness of each individual and improves the answer. Cross over and mutations are two operators in GA that create new population based on the past population for next-generation [9, 11].

Another research by [12–14] worked on tumor classification and segmentation for brain computed from tomography image data. They proposed an algorithm with using of watershed and threshold. It is a tumor detection algorithm that works based on segmentation and morphological operators. They used 30 male and 30 female patients, who have ages ranging between 20–60 years old. In pre-processing stage, they used noise removal and image sharping. The processing stage contains segmentation and at last stage watershed segmentation, and morphological operator was done [6].

In another study [15], proposed an edge detection technique for segmentation of human brain tumor. It is based on Sobel's approach for edge detection. In this method, detecting edges are based on local changes in the brightness value of the image pixels. This method works with acombinatory approach like Sobel and dependent threshold approach, and it finds different regions using a closed contour algorithm. At last, tumors' regions and white matters are extracted from the MR image using intensity and brightness information within the closed contours.

Another research [16, 17] proposed a method, which studies estimating the efficacy of statistical features over Gabor wavelet features using numerous classifiers for tumor of brain detection and segmentation. Statistical feature stage consists mean, average contrast, median, energy, entropy and many others as useful first-order statistical features. The second stage in statistical features is grey level co-occurrence matrix features that are related to second-order statistics. The third level calculated grey level to run length method (GLRLM) features, and the fourth level calculated histogram of oriented gradient (HOG) features. At the final level linear binary pattern (LBP) features is calculated. HOG is a feature descriptor algorithm that it is similar to geometric and photometric transformations, but it is variant for object orientation. After applying a derivative mask on image in two direction axis, each image has been divided to several sub regions and each pixel in the cell based on the values that is found in the gradient calculation casts a weighted vote for an orientation-based histogram channel [18–20].

Furthermore, in other research support vector machine (SVM) is used fordetection of human brain tumor. This approach contains of three levels: the first step is automatically training the SVM; the second step is to classify the tumor tissues, and the last step is to increase the classification results [21]. SVMs are useful tools for classification, and its applications cover a wide area in research, ranging from pattern recognition, text categorization and biomedicine [21–24]. Additionally, for classification, there are many other algorithms.

In this area, an approach in three stages based on SVM is Proposed [25]. Firstly, they used a paired support vector kernel machine by using metabolic data from affected and normal voxels. Secondly, they quantify the performance of an optimal reduced feature set and at last stage, expanded their past formulation to full multiclass classification.

Another tool for tumor detection and image of brain segmentation is clustering that is an unsupervised method. There is a research from [26, 27] that proposed an approach that contains several methods for detecting the brain tumor. This method presents an image segmentation method utilizing *k*-means [28] and fuzzy c-means (FCM) [2, 29–31]. Clustering has a wide application in this issue, and it can partition brain into several segments. In clustering, dataset is divided to several groups that have no intersection, and the union of these clusters is empty [32].

Unsupervised classification methods can work without utilizing any past information and data [33, 34]. Another study [35] used both unsupervised clustering and supervised classification technique. For clustering, proposed method uses brightness levels of the brain human pixel points as the main features. Three cluster validity indices are used that cluster one and two validity indices are symmetry distance. Cluster three is a supervised information-based cluster validity index.

In another research [36], they start this model with data samples that generated from past tissue probability maps. The method at first stage, reduces the fraction of incorrectly labeled instances in this set by using a minimum spanning tree (MST). After that, the set of data samples that is corrected is used by a supervised k-nearest neighbor (k-NN) classifier for classifying the entire 3D image.

Furthermore, there are many methods for brain tumor image classification, segmentation and detection. Like fuzzy c-means [29, 37], multi-layer perceptron (MLP), artificial neural network (ANN) [23, 38], decision tree (DT) [24, 39], radial basis function (RBF) [40, 41] and many more [42]. Based on research from [3], ANN classifier can classify big datasets with good classification results. From the other side back propagation neural network (BPNN) [43] can obtain an accurate classification.

Another research proposed a method for detection and localization tumor in MR images [44]. This method has five levels: at first level, image acquisition is done. In this level, 50 neuro images are used. The resolution of all images is 256×256 in grey scale. At second level for pre-processing, removing noise, sharping image and improving image quality are done. At next level, edge detection to specify the boundaries of the matter in MR images is used. For this work, canny filter is applied to images. In fourth level, histogram clustering is used to clustering similar neighbored bins and grouped together. At last level, morphological operator dilation and erosion are used. This system error rate is only 8 %.

In another study [45], they used k-NN for lung cancer detection and classification. In this method, the dataset includes more than 300 MR images with different sizes. The region of 256×256 were extracted from the different size MR images. This method contains two steps: preprocessing and KNN. In preprocessing step, they used dilation and erosion process on the images. In KNN step, the distance between new sample and instances that exist in dataset is calculated, and it is classified according to the nearest k sample based on the training data. In this method, distance function is Euclidean distance. The result shows classification accuracy of this model is 97 % and misclassification rate is 3 %.

Kriti et al. [4] proposed a research for comparing performance of two methods for classification breast tissue density. They used Mammographic Image Analysis Society (MIAS) that contains 322 images. Five features like mean, entropy, kurtosis, skewness and standard deviation in lengths of 5, 7 and 9 are used. After extracting these features, SVM and PNN classifier can classify the ROI in 3 classes as fatty, fatty-glandular and dense-glandular.

In continue of this chapter, the proposed method is introduced a different approach, which can detect tumor brain in MR images. In section two, the proposed method is described. In section three, the experimental work of the proposed method is implemented on several examples; and conclusion of the model is brought in section four.

2 Methodology

2.1 Support Vector Machine

In machine learning and pattern recognition, SVM is a supervised method for regression and classification. SVM tries to maximize predictive accuracy with use of machine learning theory. It can classify the input data into two groups. The accuracy of SVM is comparable to neural networks [46].

The dataset includes a set of input examples $\{(x_i, y_i)\}_{i=1,\ldots,m}$, where $x_i \in \mathbb{R}^n$ are the inputs and $y_i \in \{0, 1\}$ are the outputs. The regularization term is $\frac{1}{2}\|w\|^2$ and error variables are $\xi = (\xi_1, \ldots, \xi_m)^t$. Optimization problem is shown in Formula 1.

$$\min_{w,e} \frac{1}{2} w^t w + Ce^t \xi \tag{1}$$

$$\mathrm{s.t.}\, \mathrm{y_i}(\mathrm{w^t}\phi(\mathrm{x_i}) + \mathrm{b}) \geq 1 - \xi_\mathrm{i}$$

$$\xi_i \geq 0 \quad \forall i = 1, \ldots, m$$

Where $C > 0$ is the regularization parameter, $\phi(\cdot)$ is for transform function and b is for bias. For primal problem, SVM solves by its Lagrangian dual problem, which presents in Formula 2.

$$\min_{\alpha} \frac{1}{2} \sum_{i=1}^{m} \sum_{j=1}^{m} \alpha_i \alpha_j y_i y_j K(x_i, x_j) - \sum_{i=1}^{m} \alpha_i \tag{2}$$

$$\mathrm{s.t.} \sum_{\mathrm{i}=1}^{\mathrm{m}} \mathrm{y_i} \alpha_\mathrm{i} > 0$$

$$0 < \alpha_i < C$$

Where $K(.,.)$ is the linear kernel function, which linear function is $K(x, x_i) = x^T x_i$ [22, 47].

2.2 K-Means

In pattern recognition area, k-mean clustering algorithm is widely used. Organizing data into several groups is one of the useful methods for understanding and learning. k-mean algorithm is an unsupervised method that clusters data into k groups without any intersection. Each similar data has a same group, and the usual similarity function is Euclidean distant [32]. k-means algorithm is used for clustering, which it can cluster the new unseen data $x = \{x_1, x_2, ..., x_k\}$, and the clustering method tries to minimize sum square error (SSE). At first, the number of clusters is set as $(k = 3)$ cluster that are exclusive $S = \{S_1, S_2, S_3, ..., S_k\}$, $\bigcup_{k=1}^{K} S_k = S, S_i \bigcap S_j = \emptyset, where\ 1 \leq i \neq j \leq k$ by minimizing the SSE. Formula 4 shows this method.

$$SSE = \sum_{k=1}^{K} \sum_{x_i \in S_k} \|x_i - C_k\|_2^2 \tag{4}$$

Where $\|.\|_2$ is a Euclidean normand C_k is the value of center of each cluster. For calculating the Euclidean distance between two points $x = \{x_1, x_2, ..., x_n\}$ and $y = \{y_1, y_2, ..., y_n\}$, Formula 5 is used [48].

$$d = \sqrt[2]{\sum_{i=1}^{n} (x_i - y_i)^2} \tag{5}$$

k-means clustering algorithm has two steps:

1. Assignment step: each input values of data assigns to the nearest cluster,

$$S_i^{(t)} = \left\{ x_p : \left\| x_p - m_i^{(t)} \right\|^2 \leq \left\| x_p - m_j^{(t)} \right\|^2 \ \forall j, 1 \leq j \leq k \right\} \tag{6}$$

2. Update step: in every cluster, the means of each point is calculated and then the values of centers are updated,

$$m_i^{(t+1)} = \frac{1}{\left| S_i^{(t)} \right|} \sum_{x_j \in S_i^{(t)}} x_j \tag{7}$$

Where $m_1, m_2, ..., m_i$ are initial values of centers of each cluster.

3 Proposed Work

One of the important issues with brain tumor is detecting and finding a tumor or an unusual part in MR images manually. In this work, T1-weighted experimented images, are taken from the Internet. This type of image weighting is helpful for detecting the cerebral cortex, detecting the fatty tissue, identifyingan unusual area, characterizing focal liver lesions and in general for obtaining morphological information, as good as for post-contrastimaging. In Fig. 1 the workflow of the presented method is shown.

The workflow contains several steps that are described in continue.

1. Read Data: in this step, 100 MR images are loaded. Each image is converted to grey scale.
2. Extract Histogram: for each image, histogram is calculated. The intensity values of the pixels in grey scale images have a wide range from 0 to 255 [49].
3. Train SVM: a SVM is trained with the data of histograms.
4. Decision Section: in this step, SVM is applied on both sides of MR image and if each side that has a tumor is detected.
5. Remove Skull: with use of morphological operators, the skull bone is removed.
6. k-means: brain is segmented to three clusters ($K = 3$).
7. Show Segmented Image: the brightest area that is segmented is shown as tumor.

In first stage, 100 MR images are used from the Internet that half of them are healthy brain and half of them have a tumor. MR images are grey scale and tumors in these images have bright pixels. A grey scale 8 bit image is a digital image that each pixel has an intensity between [0, 255], which 0 is for black and 255 is for white with any different values in this between. Pixels in grayscale images are the result of measuring the intensity value of light in a single band at each pixel.

A histogram is a graphical representation. It used a graph to display the distribution of numerical data, and count the number of values that fall into each range.

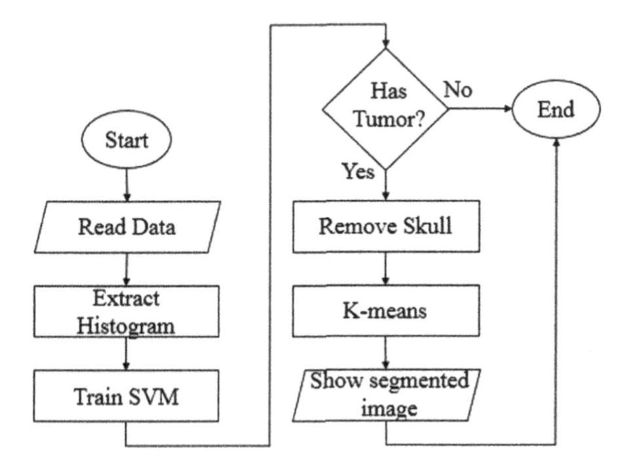

Fig. 1 A view of the proposed method workflow

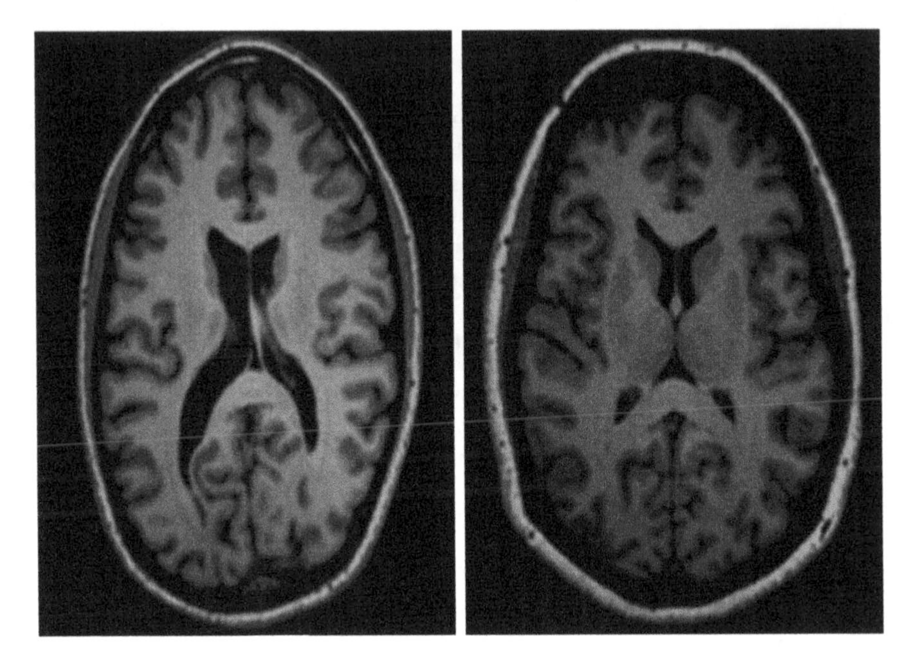

Fig. 2 A view of a healthy brain

The histogram with $bin = 35$ is used to divide the entire range of values into a series of intervals. These values should be tested for several images in dataset to identify the closest threshold value. This work is an experimental work, and it is tested for different values. A T1-weighted MR image with tumor has more white pixels. On the other hand, left side of the brain is more similar to the right side of the human brain. In Fig. 2, there are two healthy brain.

The difference between these histograms is low (Fig.3). These sides have almost same intensity and same distribution. Figure 4 presents this difference.

However, these histograms are different in a brain with and without tumor. The side of a brain that has a tumor has more brightness pixels. These pixels can help to detect which side of a brain has tumor and, which hasn't a tumor. The difference between the left and right side of a brain crate a difference in histograms of two sides. In Fig. 5, the difference for a MR of the brain with tumor is shown.

Therefore, each side of the brain for a classifier can be used. This difference in histograms is an advantage point for tumor detection. In continue, a linear SVM on dataset for classification will be trained. After detecting the tumor in one or two sides of the brain with SVM, with use of the morphological operators, the skull from the image can be removed. For this work at first, the image should be normalized in [0, 1] range. In next step for each pixel, formula 3 is calculated.

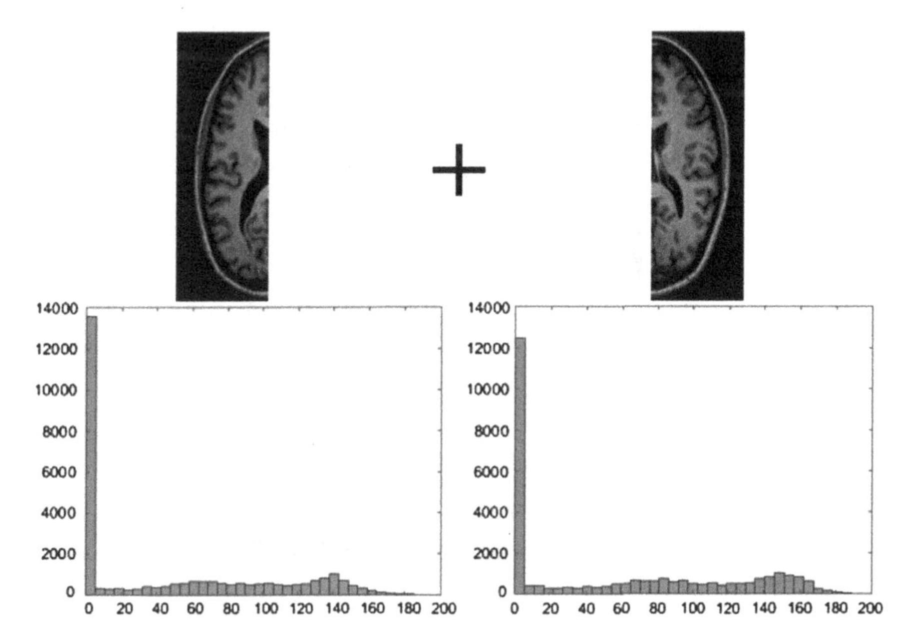

Fig. 3 A view of the histogram of two sides

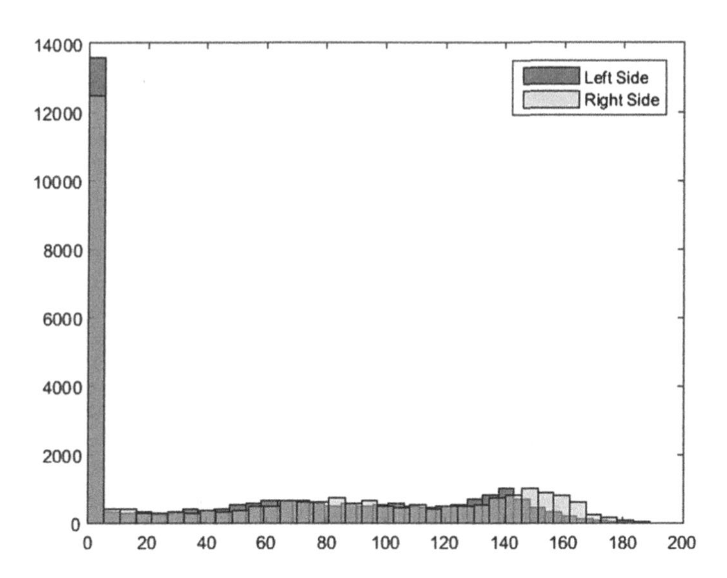

Fig. 4 A view of different between two histograms

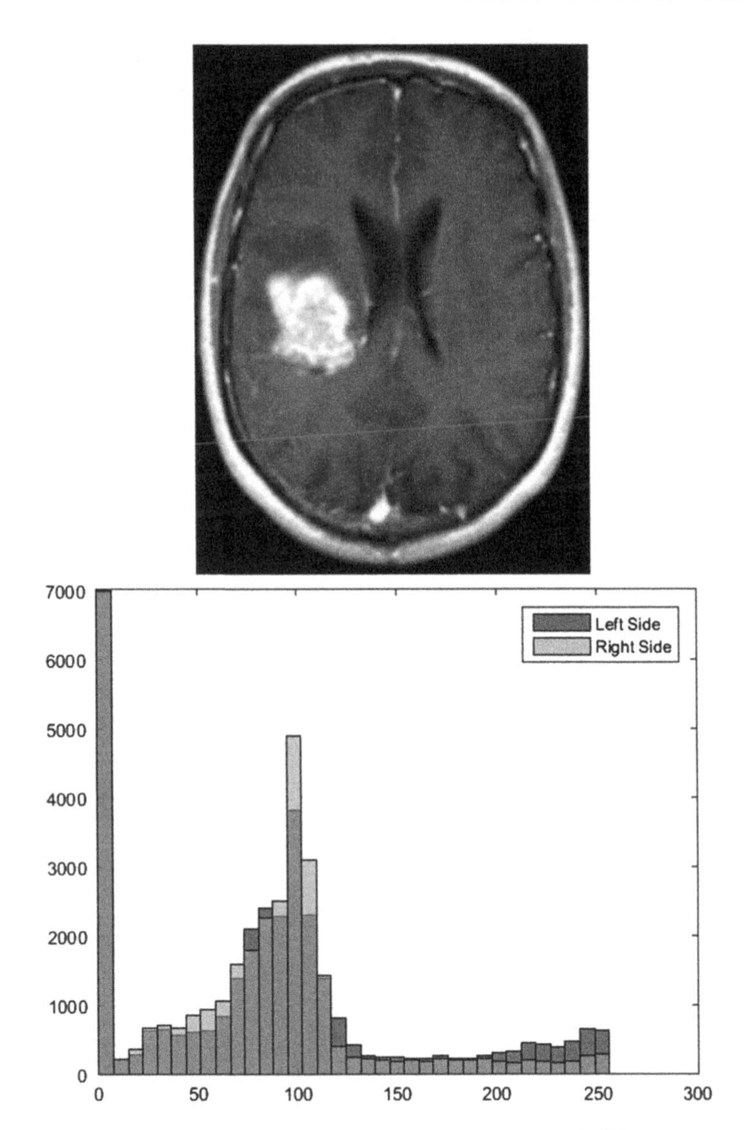

Fig. 5 *(Up image)* a brain with tumor, *(down image)* A view of difference between two histograms of a brain with tumor

$$pixel(x, y) = \begin{cases} 1, & x \geq 0.5 \\ 0, & x < 0.5 \end{cases} \quad (3)$$

Now, the gray image is converted to a binary image. Each pixel in a binary image has 0 or 1 value. In Fig. 6, this operation is shown.

In next stage, the determination of the connected components and count the pixels in each component is made. With this work, the area of each component is

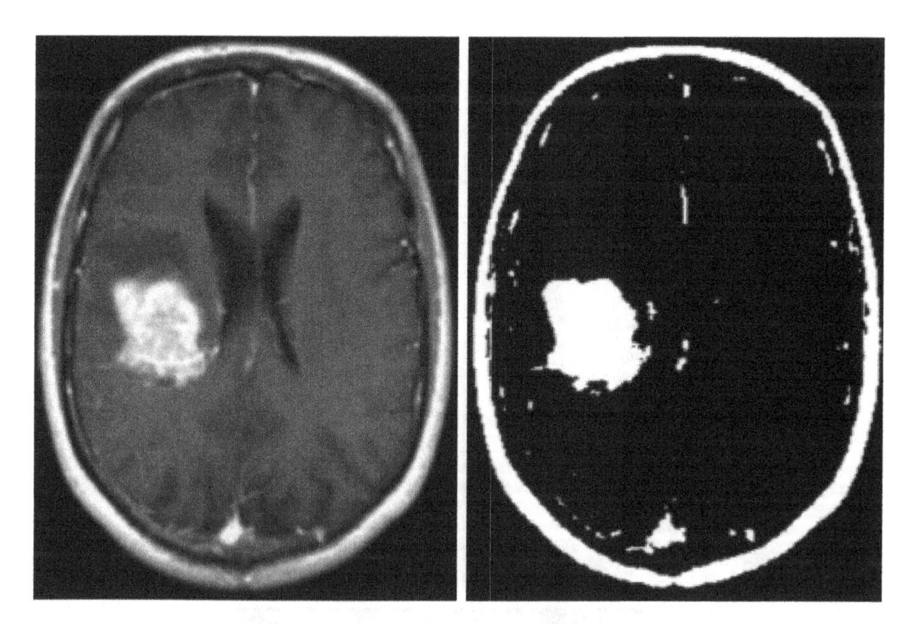

Fig. 6 (*Left image*) the original image, (*right image*) binaries image

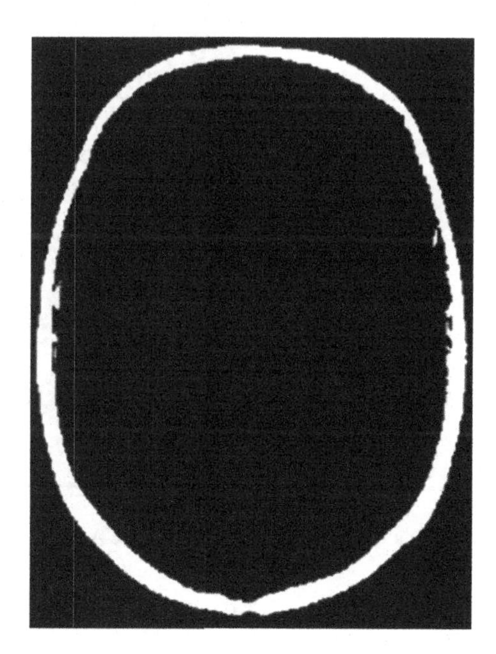

Fig. 7 Binary image mask of skull bone

computed. Now, the small regions can be removed from the binary image. For removing all the small regions, a big area value is selected that each region is smaller than this value is removed. Figure 7 is shown the result of this work.

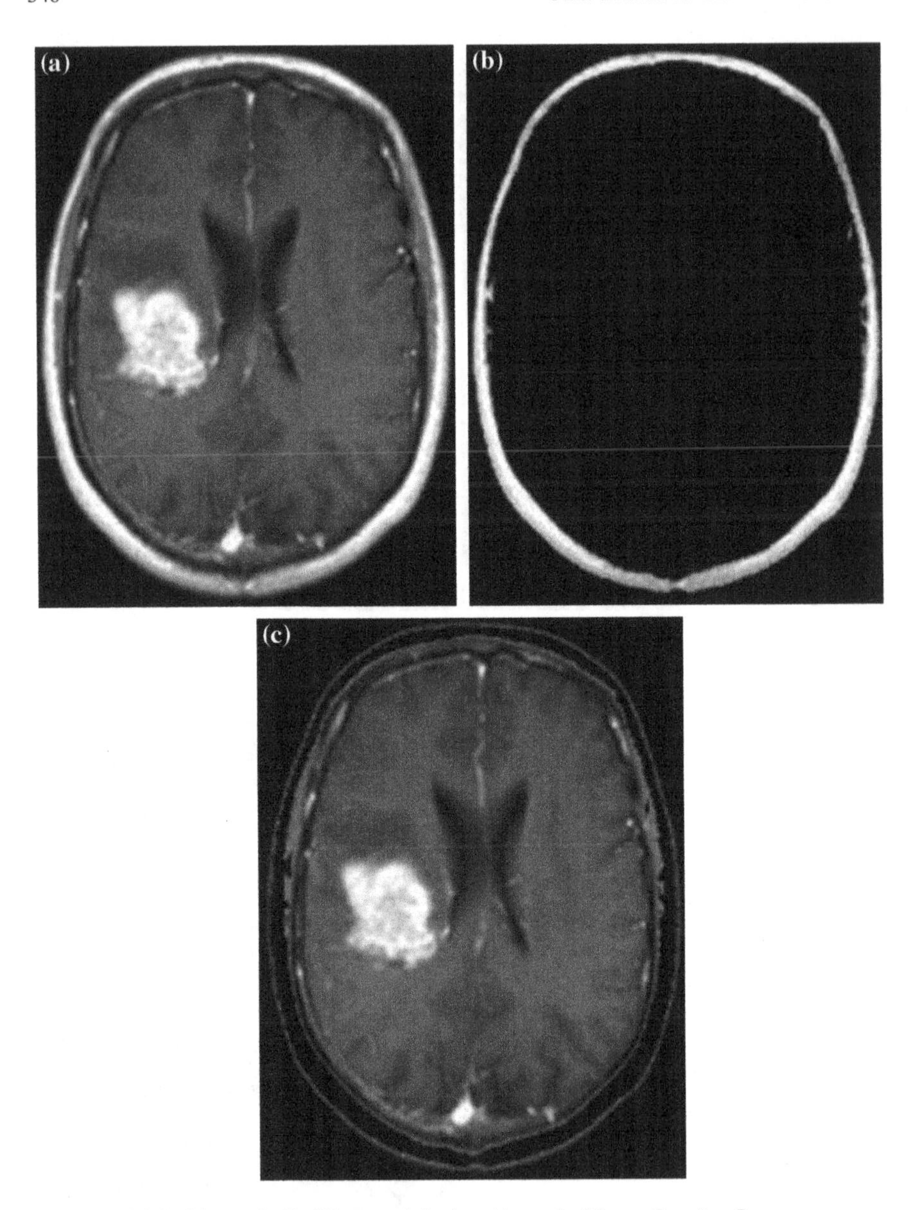

Fig. 8 **a** Original image **b** Skull bone **c** A brain without skull bone $C = A - B$

The calculated mask can be applied to the original image and the area, which contains skull bone can be subtracted from the primal MR image. The result is shown in Fig. 8.

Now, the classifier can classify the two sides of the brain image as positive or negative. If one side of the brain image has tumor, then classifier can detect it.

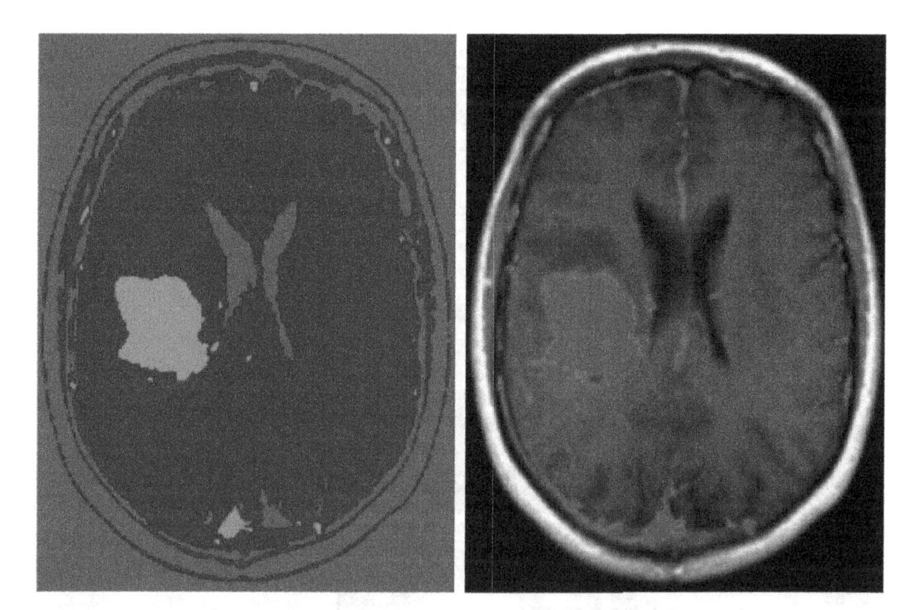

Fig. 9 (*Left image*) clustered image to 3 sections, (*right image*) bright pixel is detected and is localized on original image

At last step, each side that has tumor clusters into 3 sections (tumor, tissue, background). k-mean algorithm is used in this step. k-mean clustering is used for image segmentation because for detecting white area it is needed to know the values of centers. Then in this step, other segmentation methods are useless. K-mean method returns the clusters with center values, and each center which has the brightest value is white matter and tumor area.

After clustering, the segmentation of the sections of different parts of the brain should be done. Figure 9 presents a brain with tumor that is segmented. At the last step, the result of k-mean is applied on original image and extracted the unusual area. Red part in Fig. 9 is shown the unusual area.

The processed MR image can help doctors and others in this area for an accurate diagnosis. This process on MR images can decrease errors by highlighting the unusual area.

4 Results and Discussion

In present method, one hundred T1-weighted MR images are used from the Internet and Neuroimaging Informatics Tools and Resources Clearinghouse (NITRC) [50]. Half of these images have tumor and half of them are healthy. All of these images have the resolution of 346×587. Figure 10 shows a short view of them.

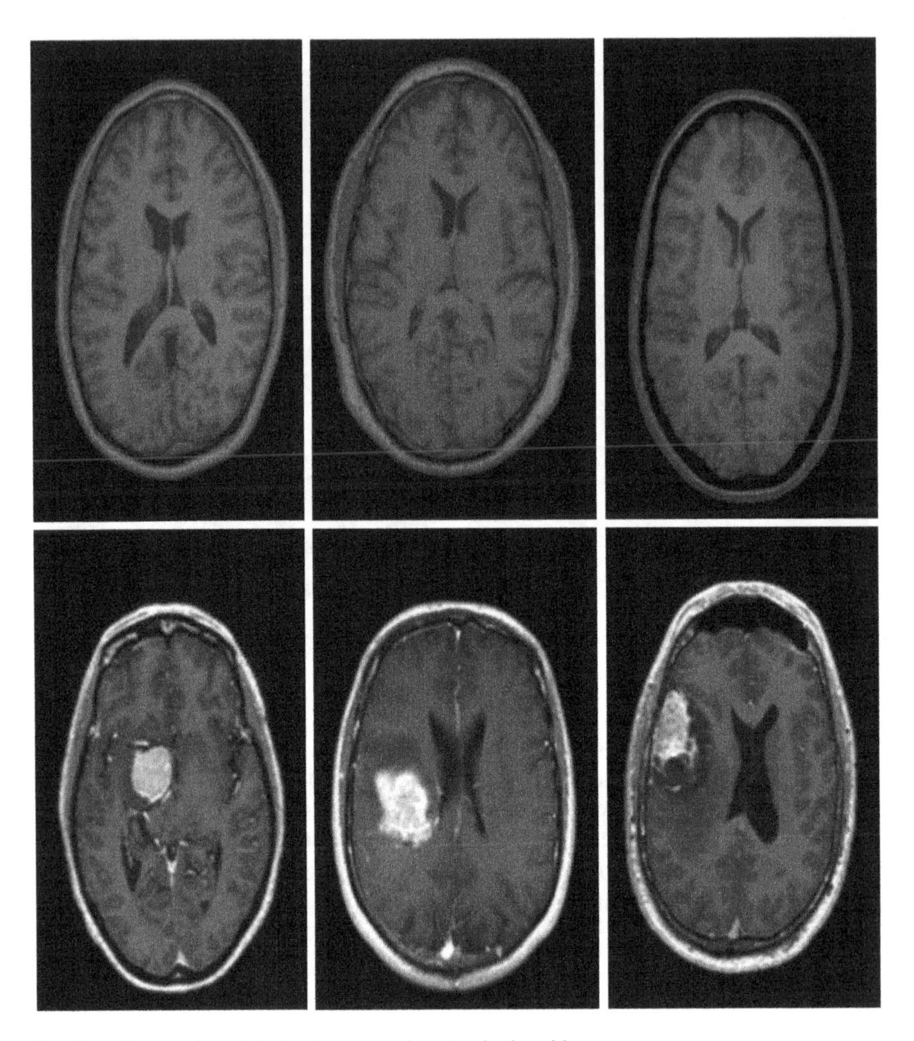

Fig. 10 (*First row*) healthy brain, (*second row*) a brain with tumor

A dataset from the histograms of these images is created with a supervised column $y = \{0, 1\}$ for healthy and tumor brains.

A SVM is trained on the dataset to detect what side of a brain has the tumor. It does this work with help of the histogram features. Skull bone is removed after the detection on brain, and the last step is segmentation with the k-means. For removing skull from the MR image, the skull image is subtracted from the original image.

Each image if hasn't the tumor the result is only "No" and if it has the tumor in each side or both sides the results determine the side of tumor and segment the brain image to three clusters. One of these clusters have the brightest center. A cluster with the brightest center contains tumor or some white matters. In Table 1, some example of this work is shown.

Table 1 Some experimental results

Ex.	Original image (A)	SVM side detected	Skull bone (B)	Skull removed (C = A − B)	Final result
1		Right			
2		Right			

(continued)

Table 1 (continued)

Ex.	Original image (A)	SVM side detected	Skull bone (B)	Skull removed (C = A − B)	Final result
3		Left			
4		Right			

(continued)

Table 1 (continued)

Ex.	Original image (A)	SVM side detected	Skull bone (B)	Skull removed (C = A − B)	Final result
5	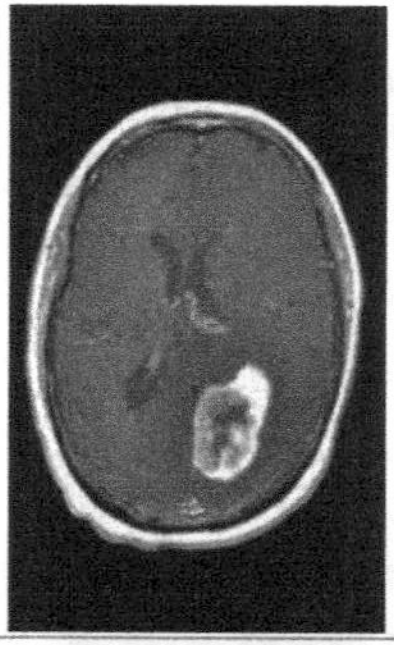	Right	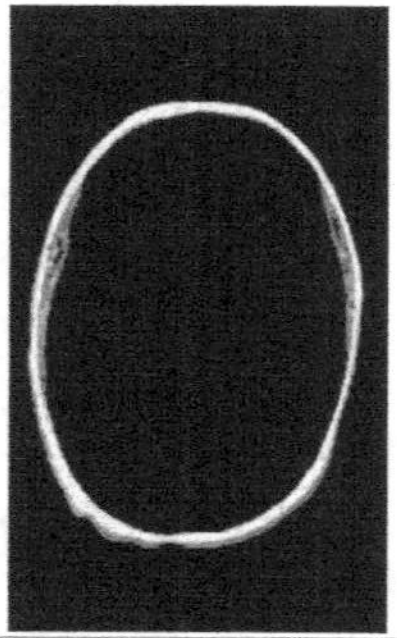	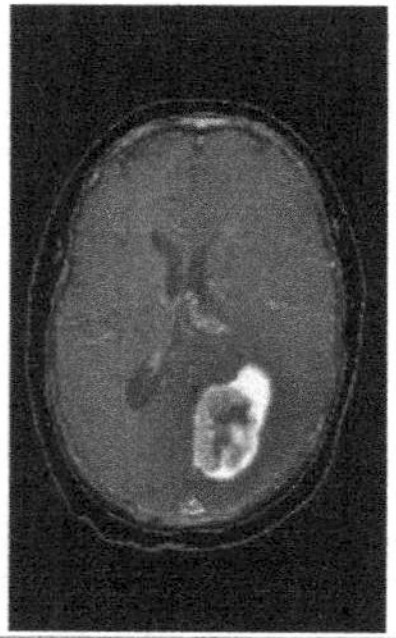	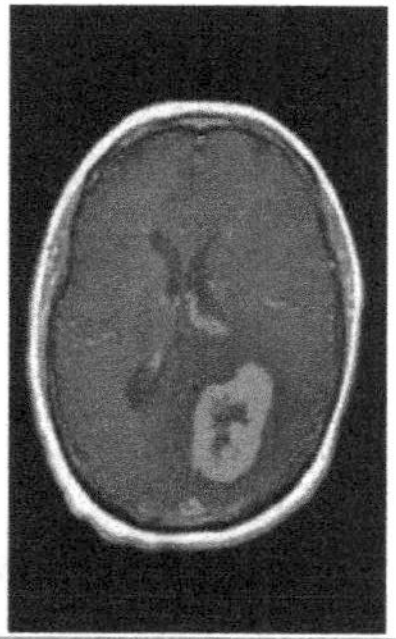
6	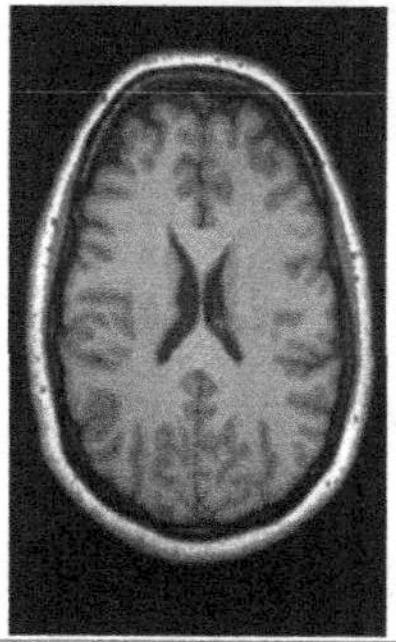	No	–	–	–

Table 2 *k*-mean segmented and center values

Ex.	Original	*k*-mean segmented	Clusters	Values of centers
1	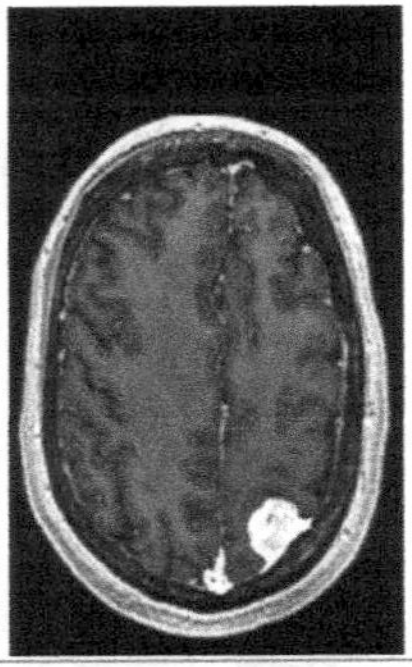	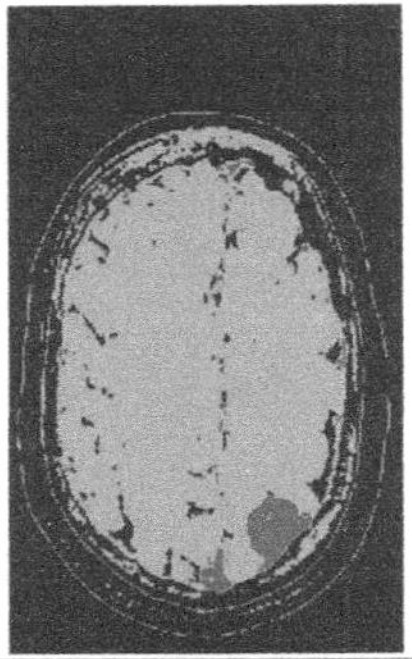	Red	0.506672
			Green	0.029269
			Blue	0.315362
2	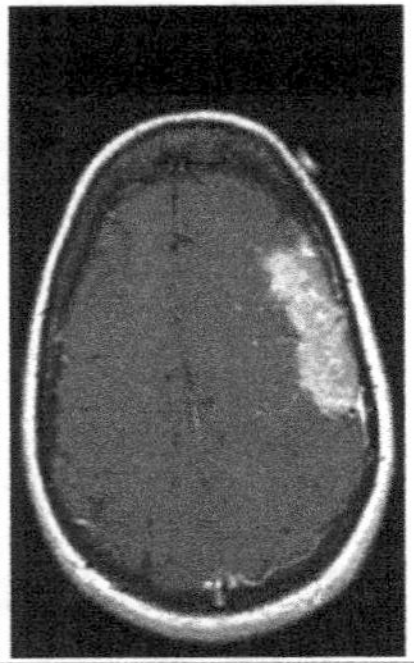	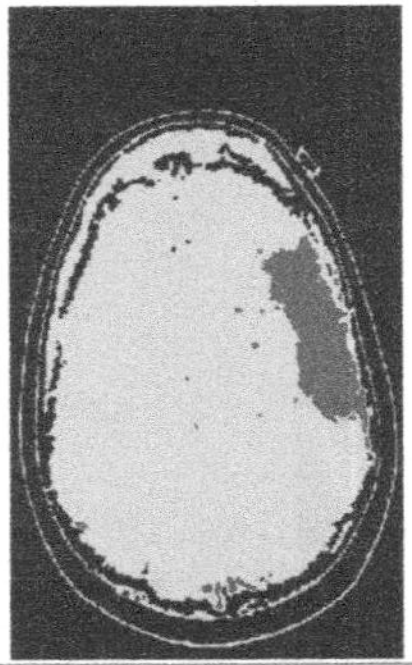	Red	0.785960
			Green	0.417679
			Blue	0.058261

(continued)

Table 2 (continued)

Ex.	Original	*k*-mean segmented	Clusters	Values of centers
3	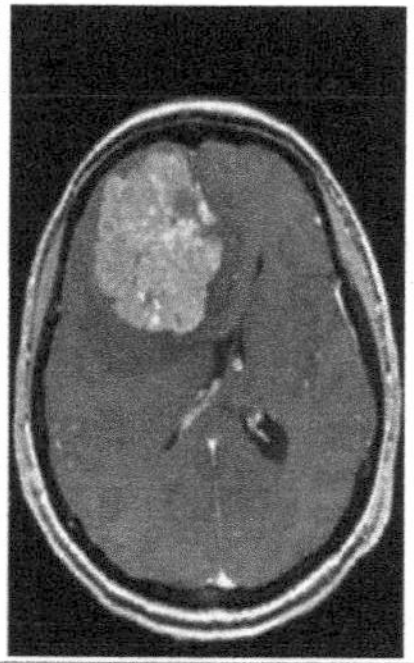	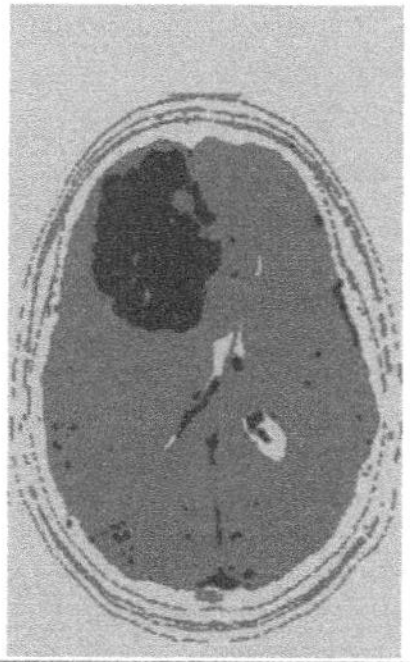	Red	0.435722
			Green	0.019039
			Blue	0.698160
4	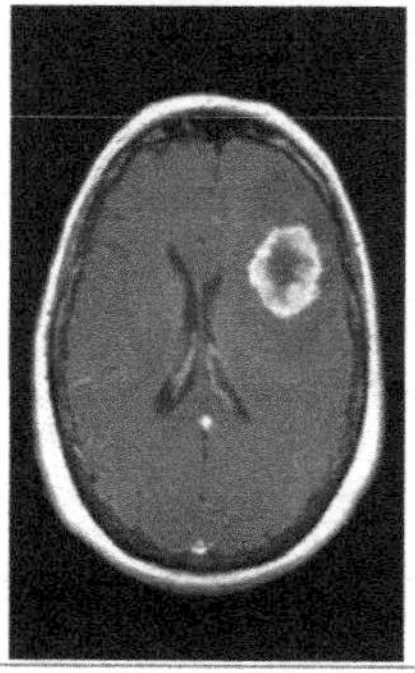	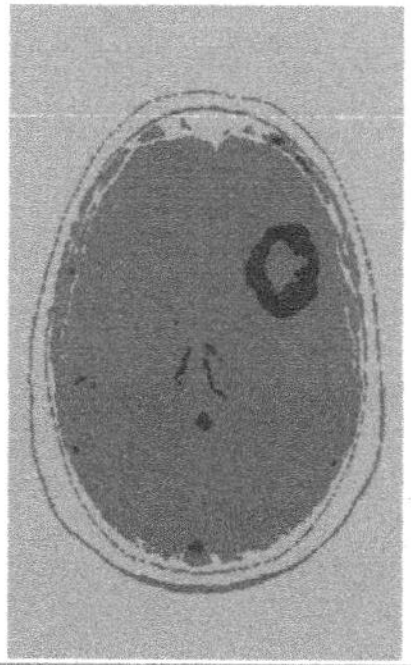	Red	0.448078
			Green	0.013211
			Blue	0.816942

(continued)

Table 2 (continued)

Ex.	Original	k-mean segmented	Clusters	Values of centers
5			Red	0.007242
			Green	0.399890
			Blue	0.764941

Table 3 Contingency table

Classification outcome	Goal	
	Tumor (Positive)	Non-tumor (Negative)
Tumor (Positive)	TP = 45	FP = 5
Non-tumor (Negative)	FN = 4	TN = 46

In Table 2, there are four examples of Table 1 that are segmented with values of each center. Tumor and white matters' cluster have brightest centers of others. Then great number value of each center belongs to a cluster with tumor and white area pixels.

A contingency table can describe all the different situation of combinations of correct and incorrect classification. In Table 3, detail is shown. True positive (TP) is a value for brain tumor that is detected correctly; false positive (FP) is a value for brain with no tumor that detected incorrectly; false negative (FN) is a value for brain tumors that is not detected, and true negative (TN) is a value for non-tumor brain that detected correctly as non-tumor.

With this data, the proposed method have 91 % ($\frac{TP}{FN+TP} = \frac{45}{49}$) sensitivity and 90 % ($\frac{TN}{FP+TN} = \frac{46}{51}$) specificity. That is a high accuracy for tumor detection and it can classify tumor brain with the best performance. The accuracy of this model is 91 % ($\frac{TP+TN}{TP+FP+FN+TN} = \frac{91}{100}$). The proposed approach is implemented on a system with 8 GB RAM and Intel Core i5 M460 2.53 GHz CPU with MATLAB 2015a.

5 Conclusion

MR images have wide usage in medicine and health care. These gray scale images contain important information of the brain. This chapter presents an automated recognition system for the MR image by using the morphological operator, histogram, SVM and *k*-mean. In this method, SVM is trained with histograms that extracted from the MR images. All input images are classified as with tumor and without tumor segments. The skull bone of the images that have tumor removed in the next stage, and they become ready for clustering. These images are segmented into 3 clusters as tumor, tissue and background. The area that contains the tumor has brighter pixels than others. In Sect. 3, the results show a suitable segmentation on MR images. Further more, the result of contingency table shows 91 % sensitivity, 90 % specificity and 91 % accuracy for SVM classification on dataset.

Focusing on medical imaging has been various beneficent in healthcare area. Medical imaging has been meaning when a good process done on it, and different features and results extracted. One the main limitation on this area is accessing to patients' data.

For the future work in this area, using of meta-heuristic algorithms like memtic or genetic to increase the accuracy of the clustering part and for feature extracting from MR images, edge detection algorithms can be added to this method.

References

1. Dahab, D.A., Ghoniemy, S.S., Selim, G.M.: Automated brain tumor detection and identification using image processing and probabilistic neural network techniques. Int. J. Image. Proc. Vis. Commun. **1**(2), 1–8 (2012)
2. Dey, N., et al.: FCM based blood vessel segmentation method for retinal images. arXiv preprint arXiv:1209.1181 (2012)
3. Khan, P., Singh, A., Maheshwari, S.: Automated brain tumor detection in medical brain images and clinical parameters using data mining techniques: a review. Int. J. Comput. Appl. **98**(21) (2014)
4. Virmani, J., Dey, N., Kumar, V.: PCA-PNN and PCA-SVM based CAD systems for breast density classification. In: Applications of Intelligent Optimization in Biology and Medicine, pp. 159–180. Springer (2016)
5. Kekre, H., Sarode, T.K., Gharge, S.M.: Detection and demarcation of tumor using vector quantization in MRI images. arXiv preprint arXiv:1001.4189 (2010)
6. Hasan, S.A., Ko, K.: Depth edge detection by image-based smoothing and morphological operations. J. Comput. Des. Eng. (2016)
7. Clark, M.C., et al.: Automatic tumor segmentation using knowledge-based techniques. IEEE Trans. Med. Imaging **17**(2), 187–201 (1998)
8. Chandra, G.R., Rao, K.R.H.: Tumor detection in brain using genetic algorithm. Procedia. Comput. Sci. **79**, 449–457 (2016)
9. Razavi, S., et al.: An efficient grouping genetic algorithm for data clustering and big data analysis. In: Acharjya, D.P., Dehuri, S., Sanyal, S. (eds.) Computational Intelligence for Big Data Analysis, pp. 119–142. Springer International Publishing (2015)
10. Kaushik, K., Arora, V.: A hybrid data clustering using firefly algorithm based improved genetic algorithm. Procedia. Comput. Sci. **58**, 249–256 (2015)
11. Chatterjee, S., et al.: Forest Type Classification: A hybrid NN-GA model based approach. In: Information Systems Design and Intelligent Applications, pp. 227–236. Springer (2016)
12. Mustaqeem, A., Javed, A., Fatima, T.: An efficient brain tumor detection algorithm using watershed and thresholding based segmentation. Int. J. Image, Graphics. Signal. Process. **4** (10), 34 (2012)
13. Bhattacherjee, A., et al.: Classification Approach for Breast Cancer Detection Using Back Propagation Neural Network: A Study. Biomedical Image Analysis and Mining Techniques for Improved Health Outcomes, 2015: p. 210
14. Cheriguene, S., et al.: Optimized tumor breast cancer classification using combining random subspace and static classifiers selection paradigms. In: Applications of Intelligent Optimization in Biology and Medicine, pp. 289–307. Springer (2016)
15. Aslam, A., Khan, E., Beg, M.S.: Improved edge detection algorithm for brain tumor segmentation. Procedia. Comput. Sci. **58**, 430–437 (2015)
16. Nabizadeh, N., Kubat, M.: Brain tumors detection and segmentation in MR images: Gabor wavelet vs. statistical features. Comput. Electr. Eng. **45**, 286–301 (2015)
17. Saba, L., et al.: Automated stratification of liver disease in ultrasound: An online accurate feature classification paradigm. Comput. Methods. Programs. Biomed. **130**, 118–134 (2016)
18. Liu, S.-L., et al.: Gabor filter-based edge detection: a note. Opt-Int. J. Light. Electron. Opt. **125**(15), 4120–4123 (2014)

19. Liang, C.-W., Juang, C.-F.: Moving object classification using local shape and HOG features in wavelet-transformed space with hierarchical SVM classifiers. Appl. Soft. Comput. **28**, 483–497 (2015)
20. Pang, Y., et al.: Efficient HOG human detection. Sig. Process. **91**(4), 773–781 (2011)
21. Zhang, N., et al.: SVM based follow-up system for brain tumor evolution from magnetic resonance images. In: Modeling and Control in Biomedical Systems, (2009)
22. Tanveer, M.: Robust and sparse linear programming twin support vector machines. Cognitive. Comput. **7**(1), 137–149 (2015)
23. Wong, W.-T., Hsu, S.-H.: Application of SVM and ANN for image retrieval. Eur. J. Oper. Res. **173**(3), 938–950 (2006)
24. Cervantes, J., et al.: Data selection based on decision tree for SVM classification on large data sets. Appl. Soft. Comput. **37**, 787–798 (2015)
25. Dimou, I., et al.: Brain lesion classification using 3T MRS spectra and paired SVM kernels. Biomed. Signal. Process. Control. **6**(3), 314–320 (2011)
26. Abdel-Maksoud, E., Elmogy, M., Al-Awadi, R.: Brain tumor segmentation based on a hybrid clustering technique. Egypt. Inform. J. **16**(1), 71–81 (2015)
27. Azween, A., Kausar, N., Dey, N.: Ensemble clustering algorithm with supervised classification of clinical data for early diagnosis of coronary artery disease. J. Med. Imaging Health Inf. pp. 226–239 (2014)
28. Arora, P., Varshney, S.: Analysis of K-Means and K-Medoids algorithm for big data. Procedia. Comput. Sci. **78**, 507–512 (2016)
29. Wikaisuksakul, S.: A multi-objective genetic algorithm with fuzzy c-means for automatic data clustering. Appl. Soft. Comput. **24**, 679–691 (2014)
30. Roy, P., et al.: Image segmentation using rough set theory: a review. Int. J. Rough. Sets. Data Anal. (IJRSDA). **1**(2), 62–74 (2014)
31. Pal, G., et al.: Video segmentation using minimum ratio similarity measurement. Int. J. Image. Min. **1**(1), 87–110 (2015)
32. Jain, A.K.: Data clustering: 50 years beyond K-means. Pattern. Recogn. Lett. **31**(8), 651–666 (2010)
33. Dhanachandra, N., Manglem, K., Chanu, Y.J.: Image segmentation using K-means clustering algorithm and subtractive clustering algorithm. Procedia. Comput. Sci. **54**, 764–771 (2015)
34. Barbakh, W.A., Wu, Y., Fyfe, C.: Review of clustering algorithms, Springer (2009)
35. Saha, S., Alok, A.K., Ekbal, A.: Brain image segmentation using semi-supervised clustering. Expert. Syst. Appl (2016)
36. Cocosco, C.A., Zijdenbos, A.P., Evans, A.C.: A fully automatic and robust brain MRI tissue classification method. Med. Image. Anal. **7**(4), 513–527 (2003)
37. Yang, J.-F., Hao, S.-S., Chung, P.-C.: Color image segmentation using fuzzy C-means and eigenspace projections. Sig. Process. **82**(3), 461–472 (2002)
38. Hassanat, A.B., et al., Color-based object segmentation method using artificial neural network. Simul. Model. Pract. Theory (2016)
39. Xiaohu, W., Lele, W., Nianfeng, L.: An application of decision tree based on id3. Phys. Procedia. **25**, 1017–1021 (2012)
40. Li, S., Li, X.: Radial basis functions and level set method for image segmentation using partial differential equation. Appl. Math. Comput. **286**, 29–40 (2016)
41. Lin, S.: Linear and nonlinear approximation of spherical radial basis function networks. J. Complexity. **35**, 86–101 (2016)
42. AlShahrani, A.M., Al-Abadi, M.A., Al-Malki, A.S.: Automated system for crops recognition and classification. In: Handbook of Research on Applied Video Processing and Mining, IGI Global, (2016)
43. Wang, J.-Z., et al.: Forecasting stock indices with back propagation neural network. Expert. Syst. Appl. **38**(11), 14346–14355 (2011)
44. Azhari, E.-E.M., et al.: Brain tumor detection and localization in magnetic resonance imaging. Int. J. Inf. Technol. Convergence. Serv. **4**(1), 1 (2014)

45. Thamilselvan, P., Sathiaseelan, J.: An enhanced k nearest neighbor method to detecting and classifying MRI lung cancer images for large amount data. Int. J. Appl. Eng. Res. **11**(6), 4223–4229 (2016)
46. Jakkula, V.: Tutorial on support vector machine (svm). Washington State University, School of EECS (2006)
47. Fenghua, W., et al.: Stock price prediction based on SSA and SVM. Procedia. Comput. Sci. **31**, 625–631 (2014)
48. Ebadati, E.O.M., Tabrizi, M.M.: A hybrid clustering technique to improve big data accessibility based on machine learning approaches. In: Satapathy, C.S. et al.: (eds) Information Systems Design and Intelligent Applications: Proceedings of Third International Conference INDIA 2016, Vol. 1, pp. 413–423. Springer, India, New Delhi (2016)
49. Samantaa, S., et al.: Multilevel threshold based gray scale image segmentation using cuckoo search. arXiv preprint arXiv:1307.0277, 2013
50. Neuroimaging Informatics Tools and Resources Clearinghouse (NITRC). https://www.nitrc.org/ (2005)

Detecting Unusual Human Activities Using GPU-Enabled Neural Network and Kinect Sensors

Ricardo Brito, Simon Fong, Wei Song, Kyungeun Cho, Chintan Bhatt and Dmitry Korzun

Abstract Graphic Processing Units (GPU) and kinetic sensors are promising devices of Internet of Things (IoT) computing environments in various application domains, including mobile healthcare. In this chapter a novel training/testing process for building/testing a classification model for unusual human activities (UHA) using ensembles of Neural Networks running on NVIDIA GPUs is proposed. Traditionally, UHA is done by a classifier that learns what activities a person is doing by training with skeletal data obtained from a motion sensor such as Microsoft Kinect [1]. These skeletal data are the spatial coordinates (*x*, *y*, *z*) of different parts of the human body. The numeric information forms time series, temporal records of movement sequences that can be used for training an ensemble of Neural Networks. In addition to the spatial features that describe current positions in the skeletal data, new features called shadow features are used to improve

R. Brito (✉) · S. Fong
Department of Computer and Information Science, University of Macau,
Taipa, Macau SAR, China
e-mail: mb55405@umac.mo

S. Fong
e-mail: ccfong@umac.mo

W. Song
Department of Computer Science and Technology,
North China University of Technology, Beijing, China
e-mail: sw@ncut.edu.cn

K. Cho
Department of Multimedia Engineering, Dongguk University, Seoul, South Korea
e-mail: cke@dongguk.edu

C. Bhatt
Department of Computer Engineering, Charotar University of Science
and Technology (CHARUSAT), Changa 388421, Gujarat, India
e-mail: chintanbhatt.ce@charusat.ac.in

D. Korzun
Department of Computer Science, Petrozavodsk State University, Lenin Ave., 33,
Petrozavodsk, Republic of Karelia 185910, Russia
e-mail: dkorzun@cs.karelia.ru

C. Bhatt et al. (eds.), *Internet of Things and Big Data Technologies for Next Generation Healthcare*, Studies in Big Data 23,
DOI 10.1007/978-3-319-49736-5_15

the supervised learning efficiency of the ensemble of Neural Networks running on an NVIDIA GPU card. Shadow features are inferred from the dynamics of body movements, thereby modelling the underlying momentum of the performed activities. They provide extra dimensions of information for characterizing activities in the classification process and thus significantly improving the accuracy. We show that the accuracy of using a Neural Network as a classifier on a data set with shadow features can still be further increased when more than one Neural Network is used, forming an ensemble of networks. In order to accelerate the processing speed of an ensemble of Neural Networks, the model proposed is designed and optimized to run on NIVDIA GPUs with CUDA.

Keywords Unusual human activities · Neural network · Machine learning · GPU · Classification · Healthcare · Internet of Things

1 Introduction

1.1 Unusual Human Activities and Shadow Features

Unusual human activities (UHA) is a branch of human activity recognition [2–5] where some action sequences are very different from the normal activities. Computationally, machine learning techniques train up a classification model using historical activity records. When a classification model learned the underlying mapping relations between the input data attributes and the various categories of activities (both usual and unusual) sufficiently well, the model is able to differentiate unusual actions from the usual ones, when it is given some unseen activities. UHA has wide applications, ranging from abnormal behavior detection in security surveillance [6] and posture monitoring in tele-rehabilitation [7] for healthcare that includes sudden drop detection in old folks home and dangerous activities monitoring, to hand gesture recognition in augmented-reality [8] and virtual-reality systems [9].

One type of UHA is based on motion sensor data [10, 11] from which the UHA system tries to infer activity patterns for prediction and classification. The sensor data arrive in the form of continuous sequential values, similar to time series. Time series such as those collected from an accelerometer are usually multivariate, comprising tri-axial information, known in its simplest form as three features (x, y, z). These features plus the timestamp information represent the temporal-spatial displacement of a human body part in motion. More complicated time series may contain extra information, such as velocity, acceleration, rotational angle and relative distance to a reference point. In this chapter a new type of feature, which we call the shadow feature, is presented together with a training method that uses an ensemble of Neural Networks that is designed to fully run on a GPU [12].

In order to maximize the efficacy of applying neural network for UHA where the data are mainly characterized by streaming flows of time-series, a new dimension of information called shadow features are estimated from the existing features and they are added to the training dataset, that represent the longituational flows of the activities. The concept of shadow features is inspired by Etienne-Jules Marey (1880–1904) who instigated chronophotography or cinematographic movement recording [13] as a fundamental technique of capturing motion pictures. His lifetime passion to see the invisible motivated him towards a single goal: recording all existing movement produced by humans or anything else, on a recordable surface. In alignment with Etienne-Jules motivation, shadow features are derived from the dynamics of human body movements. The shadow feature values are subtly approximated by the underlying motion resulting from performing activities.

Unlike other feature transformation techniques that have been previously reported in the literature, the shadow features method does not transform and replace the original features; instead, it created a new set of motion dynamic data that augments the original spatial data. Hence the term shadow. Shadow features offer extra dimensions of information for characterizing activities in the UHA classification process. The extra feature information gives insight into the motion of the body in supervised learning. The classification algorithm tries to learn and induce relationship mapping between the input feature values and the target classes. It can better learn about and recognize the activities when provided with motion information in addition to spatial coordinate data. Extra maps between the motion information and the target activities can be built to complement the existing mapping based on spatial information.

The shadow features method is designed not only to improve classification accuracy; its advantage over the peer techniques is its incremental nature. Simple and lightweight in computation, this method can generate extra features on the fly, making it suitable for data mining time series data, such as sensor data used in the classification of UHA. This quality is important in the UHA environment, where the incoming data are fast-moving in nature and the sensing data can potentially amount to infinity. Shadow features can be incrementally extended such that the classification model learns incrementally as data streams in. In contrast, feature trans- formation techniques such as wavelet transformation [14] and statistical transformation techniques require all data to be available to calculate the new feature values. This includes heavy latency in UHA because the full dataset must be reloaded into the classification model to rebuild (instead of refreshing) the whole classifier all over again.

1.2 Neural Networks on the GPU

As it is known in the machine learning field, Neural Networks [15] are biologically inspired classifiers that are composed of layers, each layer does data processing at different levels of abstraction. The simplest forms of Neural Networks are the Feed

Forward Neural Networks [16, 17] which are usually composed of 3 or more layers. The most common and general ones usually only have 3 layers, which are the input layer, hidden layer and the output layer. In case there are more than 3 layers, it means that there are multiple hidden layers. The first layer is the input layer, which is where data is fed into. In the hidden layer, processing is done at a more abstract level and then it is forwarded to the output layer where the final classification is done. When the data is very large in the number of features or in the number of instances, then training is likely to be very slow, so from this low speed comes the need to use the GPU, because as we all know the GPU has multiple cores and therefore can process multiple nodes of a Neural Network at once. In the further sections we will provide the details on how data processing is done in the GPU for the neural networks.

Figure 1 shows a visual representation of a neural network. As we can see, the layers of the neural network are connected by lines, these lines actually are numeric weights. These weights are the variables that need to be updated when the neural network is being trained, so that the output can be more accurate. The number of input nodes depends on the number of features in the data and the number of output nodes depends on the number of classes we want to classify the data instance to and the number of hidden nodes can vary. For example, for a dataset with 63 features there would be 63 input nodes and if there were 6 outputs then there would be 6 output nodes and as we have already stated, the number of hidden nodes can vary.

The operations inside Neural Networks are basically matrix operations and this makes Neural Networks a good candidate to be implemented in the GPU, because the GPU can perform matrix operations in parallel. Basically when calculating the hidden and output layers, these are all matrix operations that can be implemented in

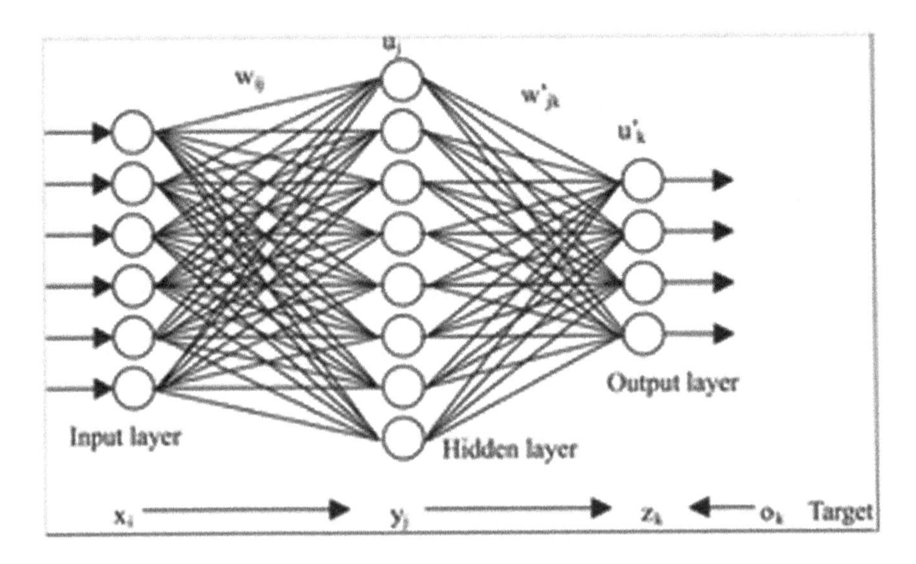

Fig. 1 A visual representation of a neural network

the GPU thus reducing a lot of processing time. Furthermore, when training a Neural Network there is also the need to back propagate the errors as feedbacks and update the weights, which again are basically matrix operations that can take advantage of the parallel architecture of the GPU.

Note that GPUs represent a growing class of IoT devices when, along with connectivity, richer graphics experiences appear in almost every application and every aspect of our lives. Such GPUs are able to perform smartphone-quality visuals even on wearable equipment. From this point of view, implementing neural networks with GPU opens a new opportunity for development of ambient intelligence applications and smart services in mobile healthcare.

2 Ensemble of Neural Networks

The idea for the ensemble of neural networks is that instead of having one neural network trying to predict 6 outputs, we can have N neural networks each specialized in two outputs: 1 if the instance of data represents a certain class and zero for all the others. The Kinect data that we use in our model is a time series, which has 6 classes for each activity it tries to predict. One approach for such a situation is to have a Neural Network which tries to predict 6 classes. But the idea with the ensemble of Neural Networks is to have e Neural Network specialized in each activity which means that each of the 6 neural networks will have 2 outputs (0 or 1) in case the instance of data corresponds to a certain activity. For example, Neural Network one will output 1 if a certain instance of data corresponds to activity 1 and 0 for all the other activities, Neural Network two will output 2 if a certain instance of data corresponds to activity 2 and 0 for all the other activities and so on for the remaining Neural Networks.

Figure 2 illustrates our idea of each activity is having a separate Neural Network for it. By using the GPU, we can greatly reduce the processing time for these Neural Networks. After training is complete the testing starts. For the testing phase, each Neural Network is used in each instance of the testing data. If the instance corresponds to the activity that a certain Neural Network was trained for, that Neural

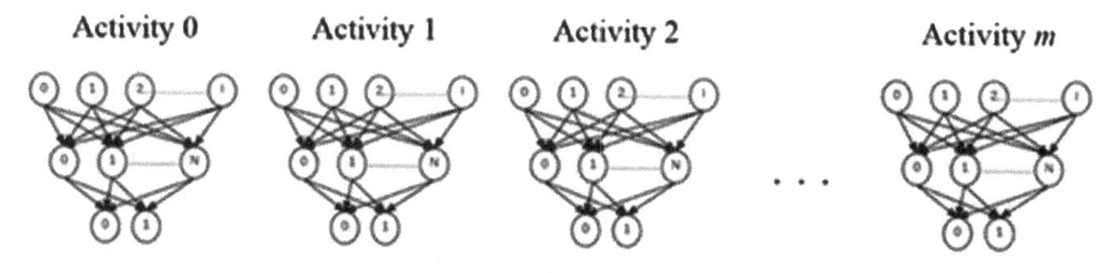

Fig. 2 Each of the neural network individually gets trained and recognizes its corresponding activity

Network outputs a 1 and all the others should output a 0. For example, for each instance of data, there should be the following output from the ensemble of networks:

0–0–0–0–1–0
0–0–0–0–1–0
0–0–0–0–1–0
0–0–0–0–1–0
0–0–0–0–1–0
0–0–0–0–1–0
0–0–0–1–0–0
0–0–0–1–0–0
0–0–0–1–0–0
0–0–0–1–0–0

This shows that for the first 6 instances of data the ensemble thinks that it should be activity 5 so only Neural Network 5 outputs a 1. But for the last 4 instances of data, the ensemble thinks it should be activity 4, so only the Neural Network 4 outputs 1. Of course, there may be exceptions in this procedure. Suppose we have the following output from the Ensemble of Neural Networks:

0–0–0–0–1–0
0–0–0–0–1–0
0–0–0–0–1–0
0–0–0–0–1–0
0–0–0–1–1–0
0–0–0–0–1–0
0–0–0–1–0–0
0–0–0–1–0–0
0–0–0–1–0–0
0–0–0–1–0–0

As we can see from above, in the fifth row of output, network 3 thinks the activity is activity 3 but network 4 thinks it is activity 4, so in this case we can check the history in order to know which network is correct and in this case it is network 4, because the data is a time series, so by checking that in the previous row of output the correct activity is activity 4 then the ensemble of networks can correct this situation by changing the output of Neural Network 3 to zero. This way the ensemble can predict the correct output when such exceptions happen.

3 Shadow Features Generation Method

In our proposed model, we generated the shadow features by attaching a new column to every feature column in the original data. This means that instead of having M columns of features like in the original data set, we will have $2 \times M$ columns of features after calculating the shadow features. The original features are not changed from the original data set, instead they have new Features that are appended to them.

For generating the shadow features, a column of new features is appended to every feature column, and the content of this column is calculated based on the column on its left side. To calculate the shadow features, we have to decide the Q size, and do the mean of $Q + 1$ elements in a column. This determines one data instance in the new features column, next we slide down by one in the original features column and take the average of the next $Q + 1$ elements until we have calculated all the new features—the shadow features. In the Fig. 3 we show a case where Q is equal to 1.

$$\text{Time} = t \quad \text{Time} = t+1 \quad \text{Time} = t+2$$

The left column represents the features from the original dataset while the right column represents the newly calculated shadow features. The first Q data elements in the second column are set to zero, and the next data elements are calculated by taking the mean of the previous $Q + 1$ elements in the original features column. The colors are just to show the progression in the calculation order, as each feature is generated. In the first colored pair of each picture the first instance is calculated, in the second colored pair the second instance is calculated, in the third color pair the third instance is calculated. The other instances of the shadow features are calculated in a similar fashion (Fig. 4).

$$\text{Time} = t \quad \text{Time} = t+1 \quad \text{Time} = t+2$$

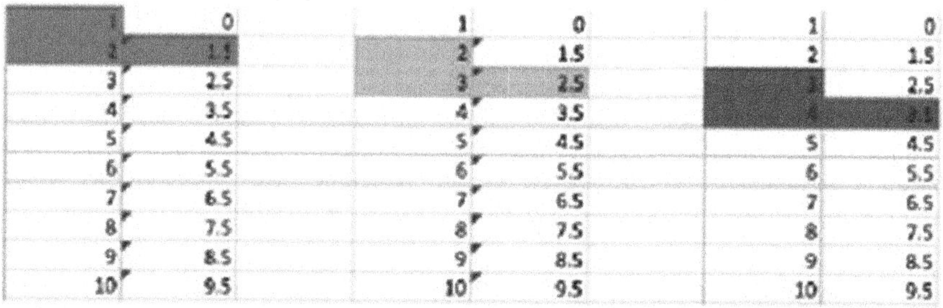

1	0	1	0	1	0
2	1.5	2	1.5	2	1.5
3	2.5	3	2.5	3	2.5
4	3.5	4	3.5	4	3.5
5	4.5	5	4.5	5	4.5
6	5.5	6	5.5	6	5.5
7	6.5	7	6.5	7	6.5
8	7.5	8	7.5	8	7.5
9	8.5	9	8.5	9	8.5
10	9.5	10	9.5	10	9.5

Fig. 3 Shadow features calculation with $Q = 1$

Time=t		Time=t+1		Time=t+2	
1	0	1	0	1	0
2	0	2	0	2	0
3	0	3	0	3	0
4	2.5	4	2.5	4	2.5
5	3.5	5	3.5	5	3.5
6	4.5	6	4.5	6	4.5
7	5.5	7	5.5	7	5.5
8	6.5	8	6.5	8	6.5
9	7.5	9	7.5	9	7.5
10	8.5	10	8.5	10	8.5

Fig. 4 Shadow features calculation with $Q = 3$

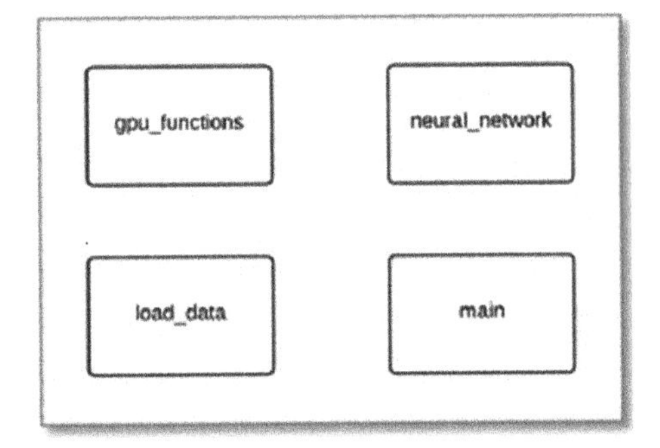

Fig. 5 Four major components of the GPU enabled neural network software program

4 GPU Neural Network Implementation

4.1 Overall Program Structure

The program is divided into different components so that each part has a specific function. In the following sections we describe each part in detail (Fig. 5).

4.2 Neural Network Class

In the Neural Network class, we have the hidden layers and the output layer definitions, the reason we don't have the input layer is because the input data will be the same for every neural network, so it would be a real waste of memory to include the input layer. Instead, the whole input data is read into the GPU once and every Neural Network accesses it. At first we had an input layer for every neural network but in cases when the input data is too large the program wouldn't even compile because it would exceed the memory limits, so instead, the data is copied only once to the GPU and then it is accessed by every Neural Network, which is more

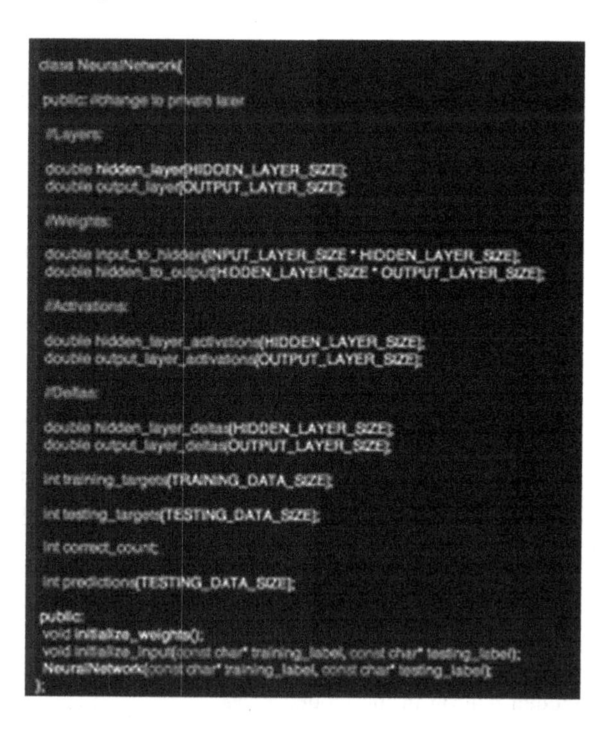

Fig. 6 Neural network class

efficient. Then we have other data definitions for the neural network like weights, deltas and activations which are all used in the training and testing process. We also have variables to count the number of correct predictions that the neural network has made (Fig. 6).

In the Neural Network class, we have the hidden layers and the output layer definitions, the reason we don't have the input layer is because the input data will be the same for every neural network, so it would be a real waste of memory to include the input layer. Instead, the whole input data is read into the GPU once and every Neural Network accesses it. At first we had an input layer for every neural network but in cases when the input data is too large the program wouldn't even compile because it would exceed the memory limits, so instead, the data is copied only once to the GPU and then it is accessed by every Neural Network, which is more efficient. Then we have other data definitions for the neural network like weights, deltas and activations which are all used in the training and testing process. We also have variables to count the number of correct predictions that the neural network has made.

4.3 GPU Functions

This subsection contains all the GPU functions used by our program. It contains the training and testing function definitions. In this section we will describe the most important GPU functions for the Neural Network in detail.

Feed Forward: This phase consists of two functions, one does the feed forward from the input layer to the hidden layer and the other does the feed forward from the hidden layer to the output layer (Fig. 7).

Feed Forward Input to Hidden: In this phase each input node is multiplied by the weight that connects that input node to a hidden node and the value is passed through a sigmoid function and stored in that hidden node. This is done for every hidden node in the hidden layer. Each hidden node is calculated in the following way.

X_0 to X_4 represents the input neurons, each input neuron is multiplied to the weight that connects it to the hidden node that is being calculated. For the case in the Fig. 8 we have one hidden neuron connected to 5 input nodes by 5 different weights, so the result of the activation is given by a dot product: $X_0 \times W_0 + X_1 \times W_{01} + X_2 \times W_{02} + X_3 \times W_{03} + X_4 \times W_{04}$, and then the result of this operation is passed through the sigmoid function (which we represent by σ) and then the result is stored in a hidden neuron. This operation is repeated for every hidden neuron in the hidden layer:

```
__global__ void feed_forward_input_hidden(NeuralNetwork *NN, double* training_data, int K){

 int j = blockIdx.x;
 int i = threadIdx.x;
 int size = blockDim.x;
 int weightIndex = i + size*j;
 int inputIndex = i + size*K;
 __shared__ double temp[INPUT_LAYER_SIZE];

 if(j == 0 && i == 0)
  NN->total_mse = 0;
 __syncthreads();

 temp[i] = training_data[inputIndex] * NN->input_to_hidden[weightIndex];

 __syncthreads();

 for(int stride = 1; stride < j; stride *=2){
  int index2 = 2 * stride * i;
  if(index2 < blockDim.x && index2 + stride < blockDim.x){
   temp[index2] += temp[index2 + stride];
  }

  __syncthreads();
 }

 if(i == 0){
  NN->hidden_layer_activations[j] = temp[0];
  NN->hidden_layer[j] = sigmoidal(NN->hidden_layer_activations[j]);
 }

}
```

Fig. 7 Feed forward input to hidden layer code

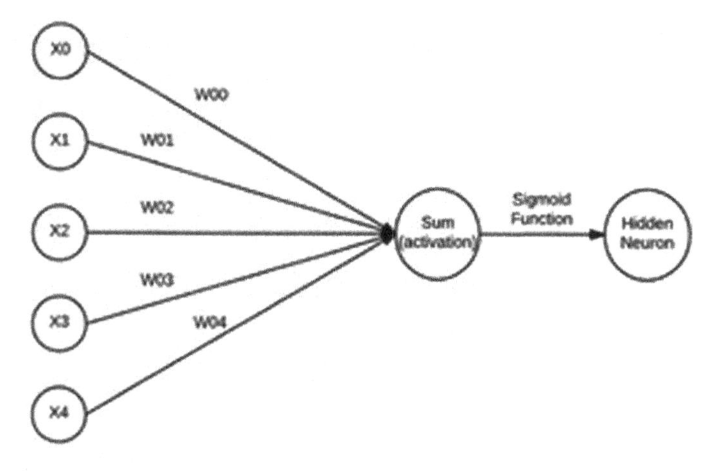

Fig. 8 Feed forward method

$$H_j = \sigma\left(\sum_{j=0}^{n} W_{ij} \times x_i\right),$$

where H_j is the hidden node j, W_{ij} is the weight matrix and x_i is the input node i.

To perform this computation on the GPU we take advantage of the fact that these operations are independent, and we perform them in parallel by using threads and blocks. The weights can be represented a matrix and all these operations are just matrix operations that can be done in parallel. The size of the weights matrix is *hiddenlayersize* × *inputlayersize*. So we can have each block calculating a hidden layer node and the operations inside each block represent the dot product such that each thread inside each block is multiplying one input node to one weight entry in the weight matrix, such that in every block we have *hiddenlayersize* × *inputlayersize* parallel operations. The result of this operation is stored inside the shared memory array (temporarily) that can be seen in the Fig. 7. Then memory is synchronized such that there is no risk of a thread reading inconsistent data. Next, parallel reduction is done to sum the results of the products and then the result is passed through the sigmoid function and stored in the hidden nodes.

Feed Forward Hidden to Output: This phase is really similar to the previous phase, instead it is from hidden layer to output layer, so the explanation given above can be used just by replacing the input nodes with the hidden nodes and the hidden nodes with the output nodes. The code for this operation is shown below (Fig. 9).

As we can see the code is very similar to the previous phase. The formula for this operation is

Fig. 9 Feed forward hidden to output layer code

```
__global__ void feed_forward_hidden_output(NeuralNetwork *NN){

int j = blockIdx.x;
int i = threadIdx.x;
int size = blockDim.x;
int weightindex = i + size*j;

__shared__ double temp[HIDDEN_LAYER_SIZE];

temp[i] = NN->hidden_layer[i] * NN->hidden_to_output[weightindex];

__syncthreads();

int m = blockDim.x/2;

while(m != 0) {
  if(threadIdx.x < m)
    temp[threadIdx.x] += temp[threadIdx.x + m];
  __syncthreads();
  m /= 2;
}

 if(threadIdx.x == 0){
  NN->output_layer_activations[j] = temp[0];
  NN->output_layer[j] = sigmoidal(NN->output_layer_activations[j]);
 }

}
```

```
__global__ void back_propagation(NeuralNetwork *NN, int k){

int index = threadIdx.x + blockIdx.x * blockDim.x;

if(index < OUTPUT_LAYER_SIZE){
 if(index != NN->training_targets[k]){
   NN->output_layer_deltas[index] = (NN->output_layer[index] - 0.0) * derSigmoidal(NN->output_layer_activations[index]);
   NN->rmse[index]+=((NN->output_layer[index] - 0.0) * (NN->output_layer[index] - 0.0));
 }
 else{
   NN->output_layer_deltas[index] = (NN->output_layer[index] - 1.0) * derSigmoidal(NN->output_layer_activations[index]);
   NN->rmse[index]+=((NN->output_layer[index] - 1.0) * (NN->output_layer[index] - 1.0));
 }
}

__syncthreads();

NN->hidden_layer_deltas[index] = 0.0;

for(int z = 0; z < OUTPUT_LAYER_SIZE; z++)
  NN->hidden_layer_deltas[index] += NN->output_layer_deltas[z] * NN->hidden_to_output[index + HIDDEN_LAYER_SIZE * z];
NN->hidden_layer_deltas[index] *= derSigmoidal(NN->hidden_layer_activations[index]);
}
```

Fig. 10 Back propagation code

$$O_j = \sigma\left(\sum_{j=0}^{n} W_{ij} \times H_i\right),$$

where O_j is the output node j, W_{ij} is the weight matrix and H_i is the hidden node i.

Back Propagation: In this phase, the errors from the output layer are calculated and then back propagated to the hidden layer where these are used to calculate the hidden layer errors (Fig. 10).

All this back propagation [18, 19] will be done inside one block where the output layer and hidden layer deltas (errors), will be calculated. First for every node in the output layer we calculate its error in the following way:

$$\Delta O_i = (O_i - T_i) \times \sigma'(a_i),$$

where ΔO_i is the delta for the output node O_i and T_i is the target for that node and σ' is the derivative of the sigmoid function, which is given by $\sigma \times (1 - \sigma)$ and a_i is the activation of the output node i, which is given by $\sum_0^n w_{ij} \times H_i$.

Each thread will calculate one entry in the output deltas array. Next for every node in the hidden layer we calculate its error in the following way:

$$\Delta H_i = \sum_{j=0}^{n} (\Delta O_i \times w_{i \times hidden_{layer_{size}} \times j}) \times \sigma'(a_i),$$

where ΔH_i is the delta for the Hidden node H_i and n is the number of output nodes, w is the matrix of weights that connects the hidden nodes to the output nodes and σ' is the derivative of the sigmoid function and a_i is the activation of the hidden node i.

Each thread will calculate one entry in the hidden deltas array.

Update input to hidden weights: After calculating the errors, the next step is to update the weight matrices. The code for this is shown below (Fig. 11).

This is done by using the deltas for the hidden layer that were calculated in the back propagation phase and multiplying them with a constant called the teaching step or learning rate, which controls the learning pace and also multiplying it to the input nodes $w_{ij} = w_{ij} - (TS \times \Delta H_i \times x_i)$, where w_{ij} is the weights matrix (which is updated in this step) that connects the input layer to the hidden layer, TS is the teaching step, ΔH_i is the hidden layer delta i and x_i is the input node i. Each thread updates exactly one weight entry of the weight matrix in parallel.

Update hidden to output weights: In this step the weights that connect the hidden nodes to the output nodes are updated. The code can be seen in the Fig. 12.

This is done by using the deltas of the output nodes which were obtained in the back propagation phase and multiplying them with the teaching step or learning rate and then the hidden layer $w_{ij} = w_{ij} - (TS \times \Delta O_i \times H_i)$.

```
__global__ void update_input_hidden_weights(NeuralNetwork *NN,double* training_data, int k){

  int j = blockIdx.x;
  int i = threadIdx.x;
  int size = blockDim.x;
  int inputIndex = i + k*size;
  int weightIndex = i + j*size;

  NN->input_to_hidden[weightIndex] -= TEACHING_STEP * NN->hidden_layer_deltas[j] * training_data[inputIndex];

}
```

Fig. 11 Input to hidden weights update code

```
__global__ void update_hidden_output_weights(NeuralNetwork *NN){

int j = blockIdx.x;
int i = threadIdx.x;
int size = blockDim.x;
int weightIndex = i + j*size;

NN->hidden_to_output[weightIndex] -= TEACHING_STEP * NN->output_layer_deltas[j] * NN->hidden_layer[i];

}
```

Fig. 12 Hidden to output weights update code

```
void train_network(NeuralNetwork *NN, double* training_data, int k){

feed_forward_input_hidden<<<HIDDEN_LAYER_SIZE, INPUT_LAYER_SIZE>>>(NN, training_data, k);
if ( cudaSuccess != cudaGetLastError() )
  printf( "Error!\n" );

feed_forward_hidden_output<<<OUTPUT_LAYER_SIZE, HIDDEN_LAYER_SIZE>>>(NN);
if ( cudaSuccess != cudaGetLastError() )
  printf( "Error!\n" );

back_propagation<<<1, HIDDEN_LAYER_SIZE>>>(NN, k);
if ( cudaSuccess != cudaGetLastError() )
  printf( "Error!\n" );

rmse_calculator<<<1,1>>>(NN);
if ( cudaSuccess != cudaGetLastError() )
  printf( "Error!\n" );

update_input_hidden_weights<<<HIDDEN_LAYER_SIZE, INPUT_LAYER_SIZE>>>(NN, training_data, k);
if ( cudaSuccess != cudaGetLastError() )
  printf( "Error!\n" );

update_hidden_output_weights<<<OUTPUT_LAYER_SIZE, HIDDEN_LAYER_SIZE>>>(NN);
if ( cudaSuccess != cudaGetLastError() )
  printf( "Error!\n" );

}
```

Fig. 13 Training the networks code

5 Training and Testing an Ensemble of Neural Networks

All the functions above are organized in a wrapper function for doing training. A snapshot is shown below about the wrapper function (Fig. 13).

It takes a series of step as follow:

Step 1. Feed Forward from input layer to hidden layer, called with the number of blocks equal to the number of nodes in the hidden layer (since each block calculates a hidden node entry) and the number of threads for each block is equal to the number of nodes in the input layer (since each thread performs one multiplication of an input node to a weight matrix entry).

Step 2. Feed Forward from hidden layer to output layer, called with the number of blocks equal to the number of nodes in the output layer (since each block calculates an output node entry) and the number of threads for each block is equal to the number of nodes in the hidden layer (since each thread performs one multiplication of a hidden node to a weight matrix entry).

Step 3. Back Propagation called with one block of threads equal to the number of nodes in the hidden layer, each thread calculates one entry for the delta matrices.

Step 4. Update the weights that connect the input layer to the hidden layer, called with the number of blocks equal to the number of hidden nodes and the number of threads equal to the number of input nodes, since the maximum size of that weight matrix is $inputlayersize \times hiddenlayersize$.

Step 5. Update the weights that connect the hidden layer to the output layer, called with the number of blocks equal to the number of output nodes and the number of threads equal to the number of hidden nodes, since the maximum size of that weight matrix is $hiddenlayersize \times outputlayersize$.

For the testing phase, after the networks have been trained, only the feed forward phase functions are used, because we are just trying to predict the output (Fig. 14).

To train the ensemble of Neural Networks in the GPU, first we initialize the Neural Networks on the CPU, then allocate memory for them in the GPU and then copy them to the GPU, train them, test them and copy them back to the CPU and evaluate the result on the CPU. The operation takes the following five steps:

```
void test_network(NeuralNetwork *NN, double* testing_data, int k){

 feed_forward_input_hidden_2<<<HIDDEN_LAYER_SIZE, INPUT_LAYER_SIZE>>>(NN, testing_data, k);
  feed_forward_hidden_output_2<<<OUTPUT_LAYER_SIZE, HIDDEN_LAYER_SIZE>>>(NN);
  check_result<<<1,1>>>(NN, k);
}
```

Fig. 14 Testing the networks code

```
//Initializing the Neural Networks

NeuralNetwork NN0(label_path_training0, label_path_testing);
NeuralNetwork NN1(label_path_training1, label_path_testing);
NeuralNetwork NN2(label_path_training2, label_path_testing);
NeuralNetwork NN3(label_path_training3, label_path_testing);
NeuralNetwork NN4(label_path_training4, label_path_testing);
NeuralNetwork NN5(label_path_training5, label_path_testing);

//Declaring the GPU Pointers

NeuralNetwork *GPU_NN0;
NeuralNetwork *GPU_NN1;
NeuralNetwork *GPU_NN2;
NeuralNetwork *GPU_NN3;
NeuralNetwork *GPU_NN4;
NeuralNetwork *GPU_NN5;
```

Fig. 15 Initializing the networks code

```
cudaMalloc((NeuralNetwork**)&GPU_NN0, sizeof(NeuralNetwork));
cudaMalloc((NeuralNetwork**)&GPU_NN1, sizeof(NeuralNetwork));
cudaMalloc((NeuralNetwork**)&GPU_NN2, sizeof(NeuralNetwork));
cudaMalloc((NeuralNetwork**)&GPU_NN3, sizeof(NeuralNetwork));
cudaMalloc((NeuralNetwork**)&GPU_NN4, sizeof(NeuralNetwork));
cudaMalloc((NeuralNetwork**)&GPU_NN5, sizeof(NeuralNetwork));

cudaMemcpy(GPU_NN0, &NN0, sizeof(NeuralNetwork), cudaMemcpyHostToDevice);
cudaMemcpy(GPU_NN1, &NN1, sizeof(NeuralNetwork), cudaMemcpyHostToDevice);
cudaMemcpy(GPU_NN2, &NN2, sizeof(NeuralNetwork), cudaMemcpyHostToDevice);
cudaMemcpy(GPU_NN3, &NN3, sizeof(NeuralNetwork), cudaMemcpyHostToDevice);
cudaMemcpy(GPU_NN4, &NN4, sizeof(NeuralNetwork), cudaMemcpyHostToDevice);
cudaMemcpy(GPU_NN5, &NN5, sizeof(NeuralNetwork), cudaMemcpyHostToDevice);
```

Fig. 16 Code for allocating the networks on the GPU

```
for(int epoch = 0; epoch < 300; epoch++)
 for(int k = 0; k < TRAINING_DATA_SIZE; k++){

  train_network(GPU_NN0, dev_training_data, k);
  train_network(GPU_NN1, dev_training_data, k);
  train_network(GPU_NN2, dev_training_data, k);
  train_network(GPU_NN3, dev_training_data, k);
  train_network(GPU_NN4, dev_training_data, k);
  train_network(GPU_NN5, dev_training_data, k);

 }
```

Fig. 17 Training the networks code—epoch is the number of training iterations

```
for(int k = 0; k < TESTING_DATA_SIZE; k++){

  test_network(GPU_NN1, dev_testing_data, k);
  test_network(GPU_NN2, dev_testing_data, k);
  test_network(GPU_NN3, dev_testing_data, k);
  test_network(GPU_NN4, dev_testing_data, k);
  test_network(GPU_NN5, dev_testing_data, k);

}
```

Fig. 18 Testing the networks code

Step 1. Initializing the Neural Networks (Fig. 15).

Step 2. Allocating memory for the Neural Networks on the GPU and copying the Neural Networks to the GPU. The ensemble of networks are coded and shown below (Fig. 16).

Step 3. Training the Neural Networks on the GPU (Fig. 17).

Step 4. Testing the Neural Networks on the GPU (Fig. 18).

Step 5. After all the above steps are complete, the neural networks are copied back to the CPU and the result is evaluated in the CPU.

6 Experiments

Five experiments were designed and conducted to verify the efficacy of the proposed Ensemble of Neural Networks for classification with shadow features. The dataset, "Kinect" data was collected from a Microsoft motion sensor, which is very sophisticated. In total experiments with 5 sets of Kinect sensors were set up and the Kinect sensors were laid out according to the configuration below. They represent different possible scenarios where the human activity data are captured from different angles of the camera—yet hopefully the classification model still can classify correctly well. A single participant in front of the Kinect sensors performed different activities, including the idle ones like standing still, and those active ones mimicking unusual human activities (Fig. 19).

The Kinect data is complex, with 63 attributes that describe six different human activities. The attribute data are spatial x-y-z information about various parts of the human body such as the head, shoulder, elbow, wrist, hand, spine, hip, knee, ankle and foot. The data was downloaded from the Data Repository of the D-lab of King Mongkut's University of technology Thonburi, Thailand. The volunteer performed in front of five Kinect sensors that placed at different positions. This arrangement represents that in real life scenario we do not always get perfect data which are always facing the subject directly. There may be different angles of views, fast moving subject, or even partial images being captured etc. The data of each position

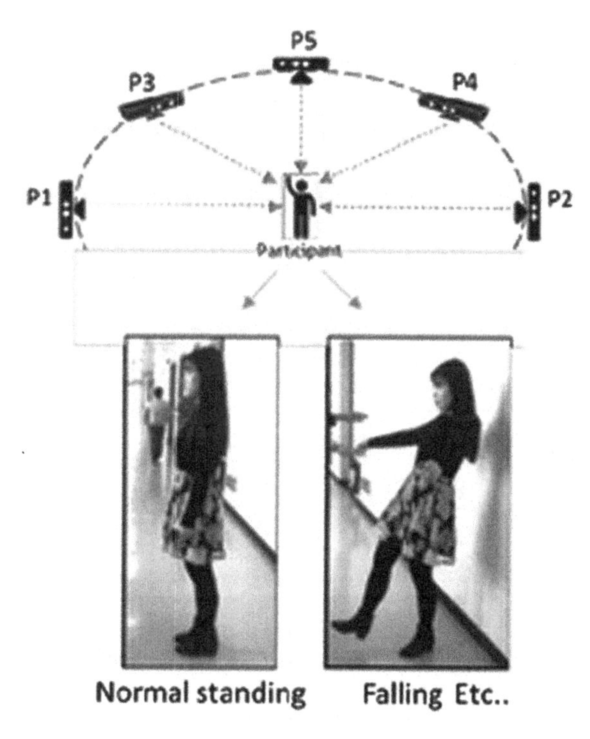

Fig. 19 Arrangement of Kinect sensors in the experiments

Table 1 Sample of Kinect sensor data

Head_xin3	Head_yin3	Head_zin3	Shoulder_center_xin3	Shoulder_center_yin3	Shoulder_center_zin3	Class
−0.8935909	0.9931934	2.708766	−0.860571	0.839574	2.758261	Stand
−0.8955113	0.9931067	2.706448	−0.8622427	0.8403043	2.75566	Stand
−0.8955278	0.994601	2.706552	−0.8627911	0.8415152	2.753539	Stand
−0.8953061	0.9966438	2.705594	−0.8627074	0.8426206	2.749703	Stand
−0.8978264	0.9957235	2.703982	−0.8631248	0.8417737	2.746142	Stand
−0.8985162	0.9953932	2.701781	−0.8660206	0.8414545	2.743067	Stand
−0.8992859	0.9950981	2.700636	−0.8679987	0.841422	2.742929	Stand
−0.863084	0.9990941	2.706844	−0.8695811	0.8413607	2.74163	Stand
−0.8650347	0.9933942	2.706177	−0.8720753	0.8391923	2.74159	Stand
−0.8643529	0.9910888	2.706824	−0.8732303	0.8373543	2.741842	Stand
−0.8321332	0.9922897	2.723943	−0.8738533	0.8369475	2.742155	Stand
−0.8300037	0.9919927	2.723763	−0.873325	0.8375872	2.74184	Stand
−0.8528603	0.9947926	2.715802	−0.8728629	0.8394547	2.741995	Stand
−0.8661485	0.9939991	2.712863	−0.8743425	0.8401586	2.745243	Stand
−0.8752261	0.9945456	2.711786	−0.8738497	0.8411217	2.746188	Stand
−0.8962126	0.9904791	2.708368	−0.8760409	0.8416366	2.749558	Stand
−0.9014133	0.9891821	2.707871	−0.8761206	0.8411717	2.749853	Stand
−0.8564351	1.009001	2.732582	−0.8763929	0.841782	2.751073	Stand
−0.8350045	0.9991518	2.732376	−0.8754745	0.8432102	2.752089	Stand
−0.8258742	1.008016	2.754112	−0.8742452	0.8429376	2.752358	Stand

(continued)

Table 1 (continued)

Head_xin3	Head_yin3	Head_zin3	Shoulder_center_xin3	Shoulder_center_yin3	Shoulder_center_zin3	Class
−0.8286709	1.008124	2.752595	−0.8723114	0.8434474	2.753454	Stand
−0.8303401	1.006768	2.750611	−0.8703818	0.8426715	2.754476	Stand
−0.8310919	1.007039	2.749743	−0.8695902	0.8420874	2.754701	Stand
−0.829497	1.009054	2.749041	−0.8659967	0.8436671	2.754232	Stand
−0.8321564	1.003287	2.738268	−0.8657405	0.8427323	2.754563	Stand
−0.8353055	1.00112	2.733313	−0.8656802	0.8418335	2.755323	Stand
−0.8352545	1.00067	2.731287	−0.865357	0.8417149	2.755033	Stand

was divided into training set and testing set. For these experiments, to show that the shadow features are really efficient, as well as the neural network that is designed to recognize between different activities, we train only with the data from the Kinect sensor placed at position 5 and test with all the remaining data from position 1 to position 5. So in our experiments training is only done with P5 but the results are tested with P1, P2, P3, P4 and P5 testing data and then we establish a comparison with a Neural Network without shadow features. A snapshot of the Kinect data which recorded the human activities in terms of the 64 attributes are shown in Table 1. However for simplicity only the first 6 out of 64 attributes are shown.

For the experiments the GPU card used was an NVIDIA GEFORCE GTX 980 Ti. The experiment is basically performed in the following order: For each Kinect sensor testing data located at position P (where P varies from 1 to 5).

1. Generate the shadow features on the P5 training set and P testing set (where P varies from 1 to 5).
2. After, generating the shadow features, the training and testing data have their features doubled, so instead of having 63 feature columns, the data set would have 126 feature columns.
3. Training is done with P5 training data.
4. Testing is done with P testing data (where P varies from 1 to 5).

7 Results

In this section we present the results in graph format so that it can be easy to visualize how the Q size for the shadow features has a big influence on the performance accuracy.

Our test data has about 16,000 instances and the data without shadow features has 63 features, whereas the data with shadow features has 126 features (which is 63×2). The testing was done with an ensemble of Neural Networks composed of 6 Neural Networks for each of the 6 outputs that we were trying to predict in the time series. As it can be seen from the graphs below, we can get great accuracy improvements when using shadow features, the graphs below help to describe patterns in order to figure out the best Q. Training with P5 training data and testing with P5 testing data (training data and testing data are disjoint) (Figs. 20, 21, and 22).

The next graph below shows results of testing the P5 testing data on a Neural Network trained on P5 training data without shadow features (Fig. 23).

Training with P5 and testing with P5: As it could be observed from the graphs above, the Shadow Features out-perform the non-shadow features networks in every case, with 60, 90 and 120 epochs. The highest accuracy obtained in each case for the ensemble of neural networks with shadow features outperforms the non-shadow features neural network.

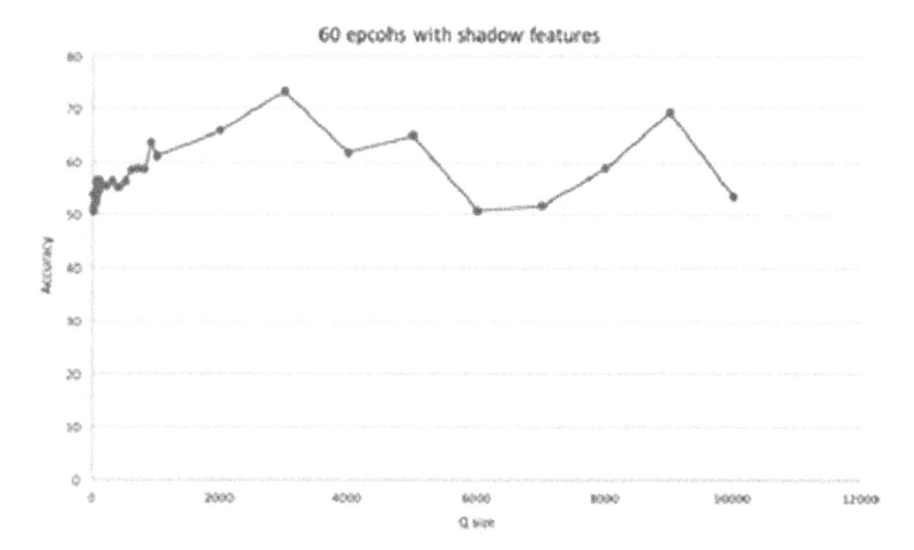

Fig. 20 Each neural network trained with 60 epochs

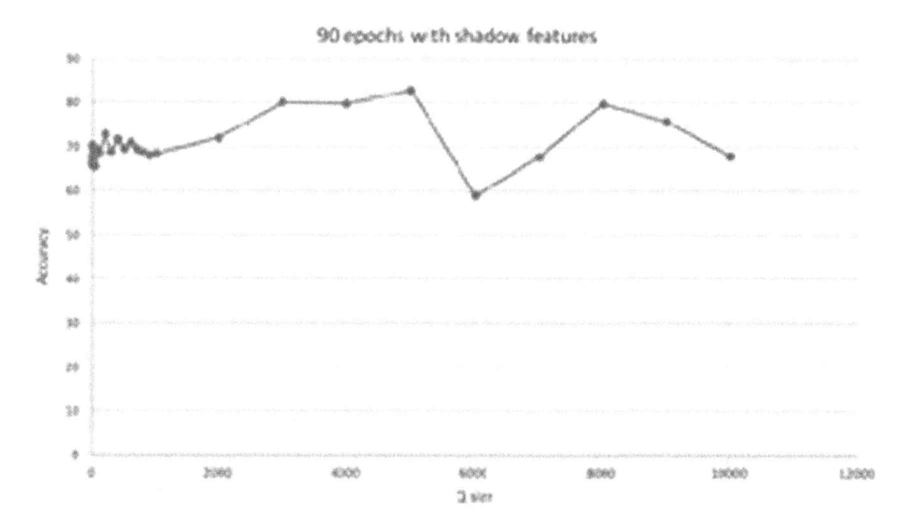

Fig. 21 Each neural network trained with 90 epochs

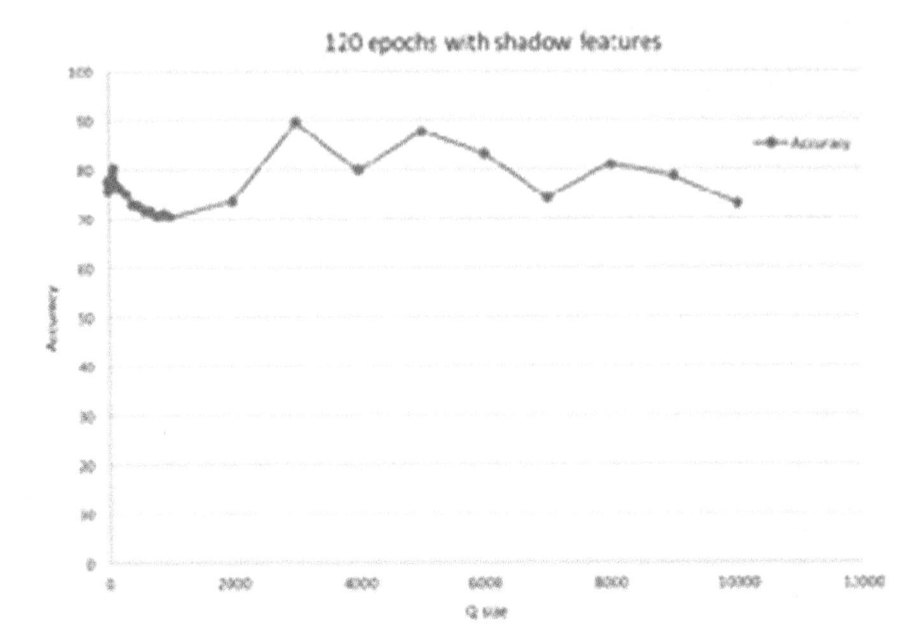

Fig. 22 Each neural network trained with 120 epochs

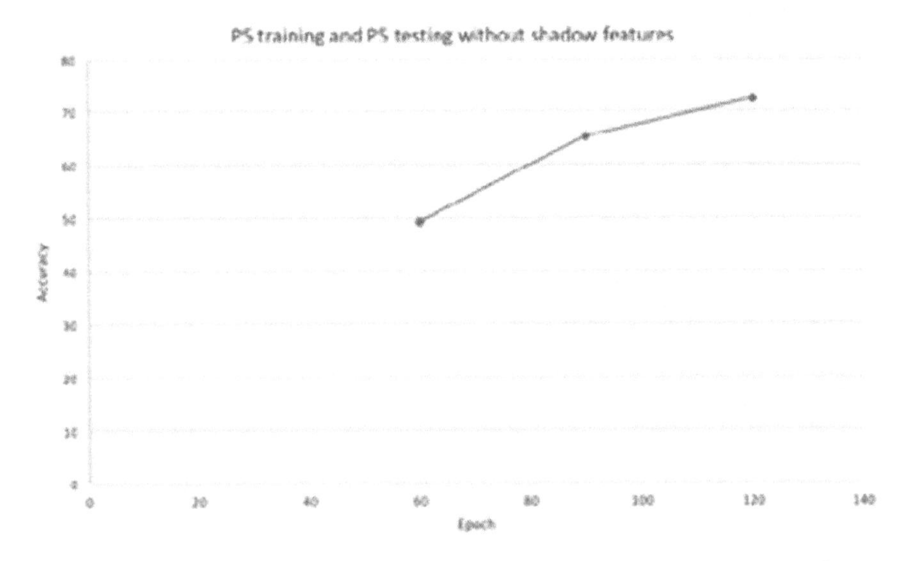

Fig. 23 P5 testing data on a neural network trained on P5 training data without shadow features

Here shows the results about shadow feature performance for P1–P5 datasets. Training with P5 training data and testing with P4 testing data (Figs. 24, 25 and 26).

The following scenario is the ensemble of neural network, training with P5 training data and testing with P3 testing data (Figs. 27, 28 and 29).

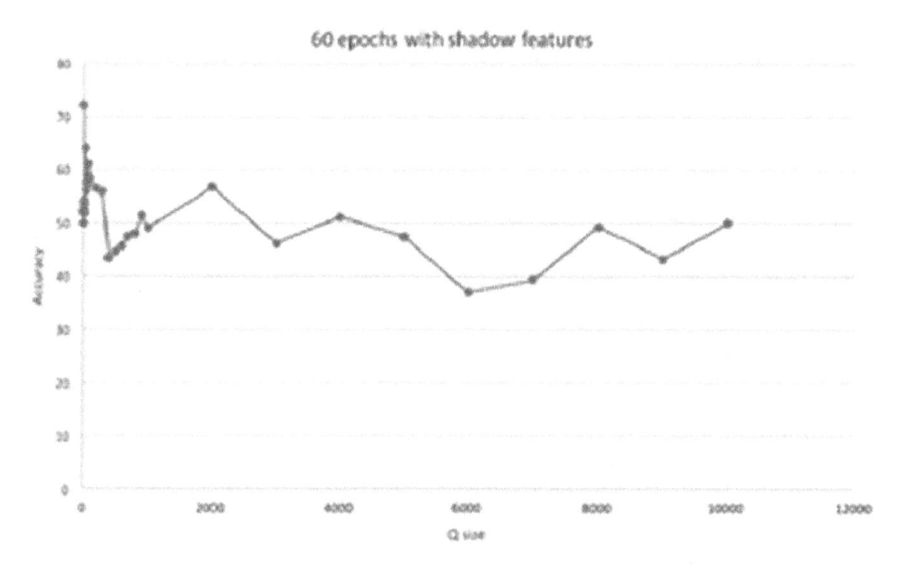

Fig. 24 Each neural network trained with 60 epochs

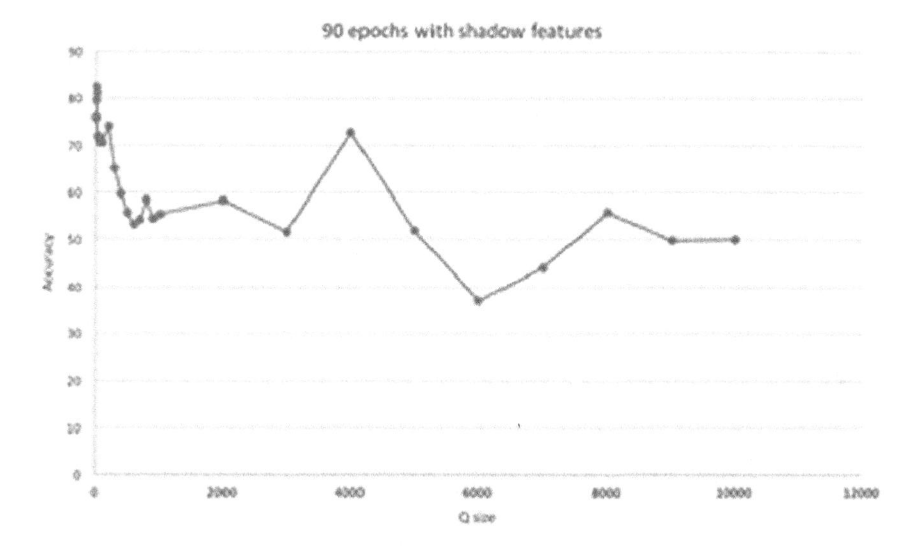

Fig. 25 Each neural network trained with 90 epochs

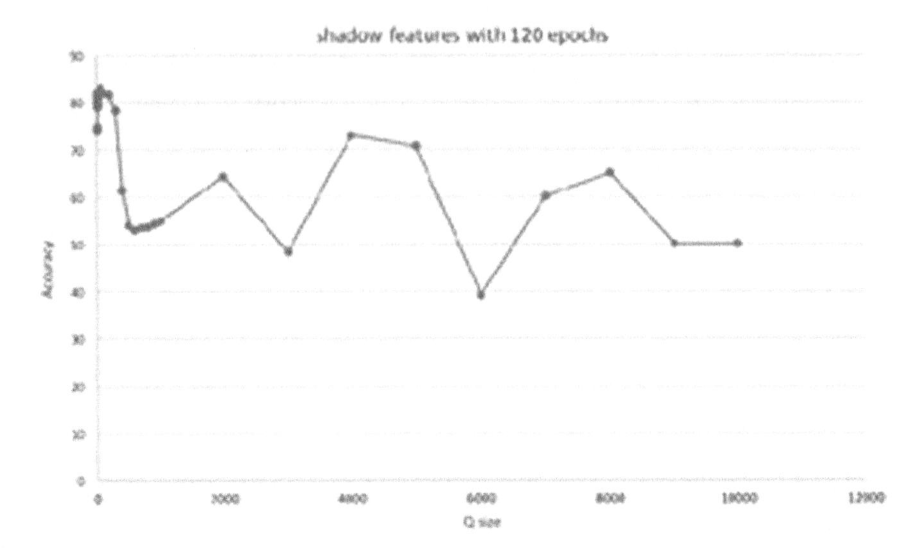

Fig. 26 Each neural network trained with 120 epochs

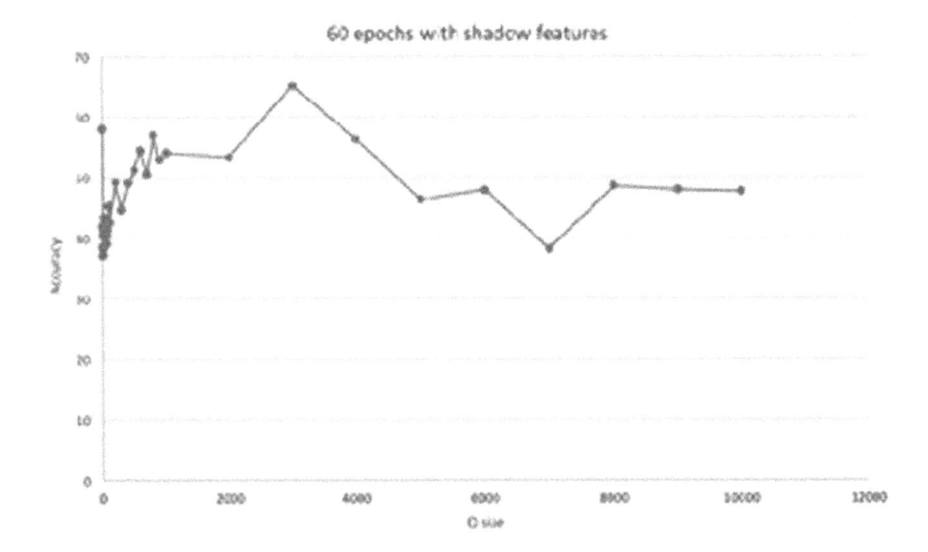

Fig. 27 Each neural network trained with 60 epochs

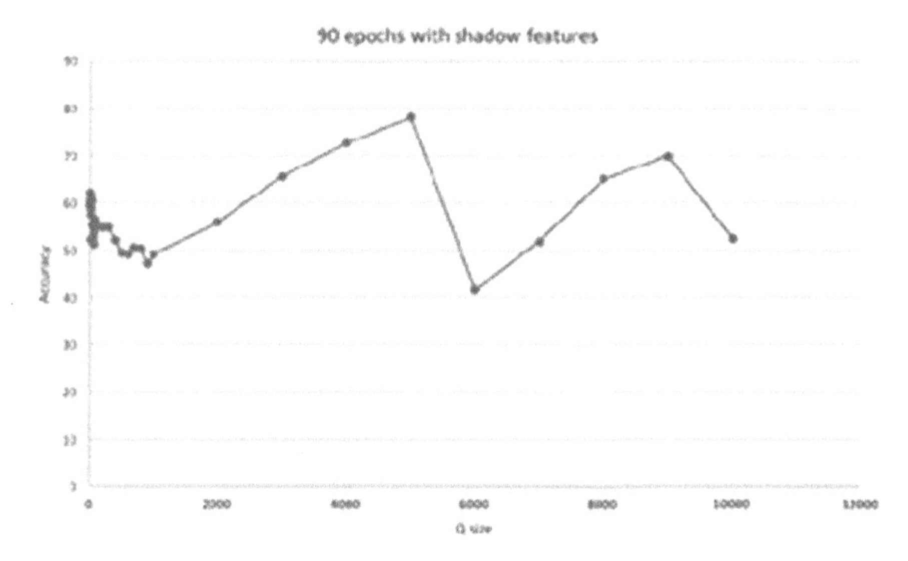

Fig. 28 Each neural network trained with 90 epochs

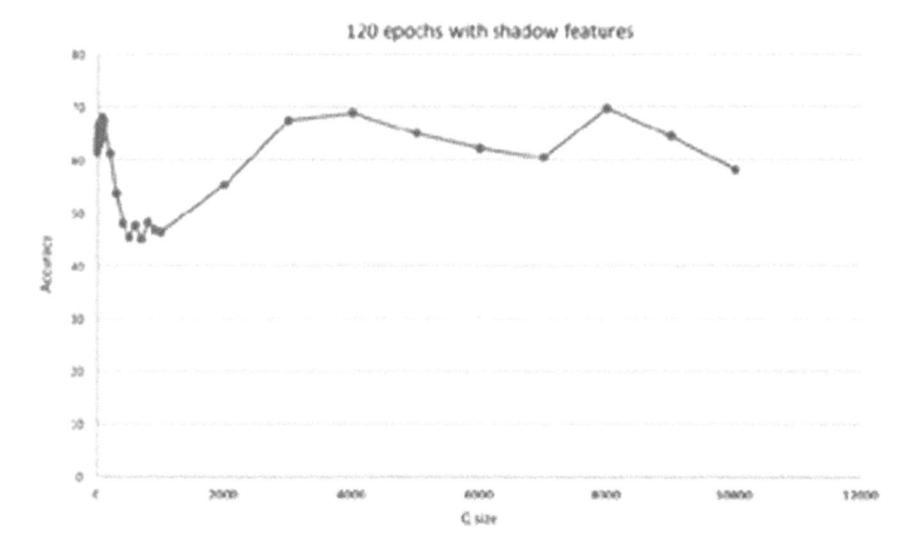

Fig. 29 Each neural network trained with 120 epochs

The following scenario is the ensemble of neural network, training with P5 training data and testing with P2 testing data (Figs. 30, 31 and 32).

The following scenario is the ensemble of neural network, training with P5 training data and testing with P1 testing data (Figs. 33, 34 and 35).

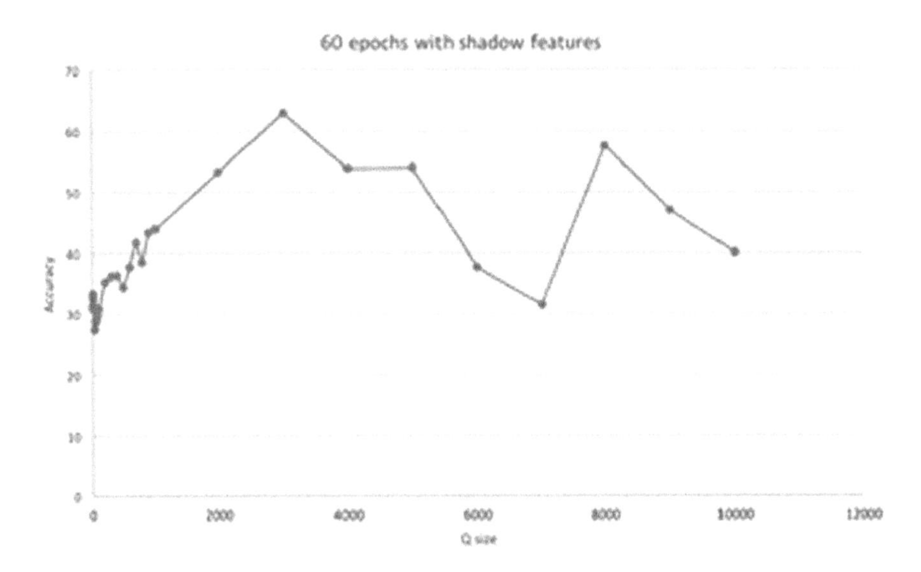

Fig. 30 Each neural network trained with 60 epochs

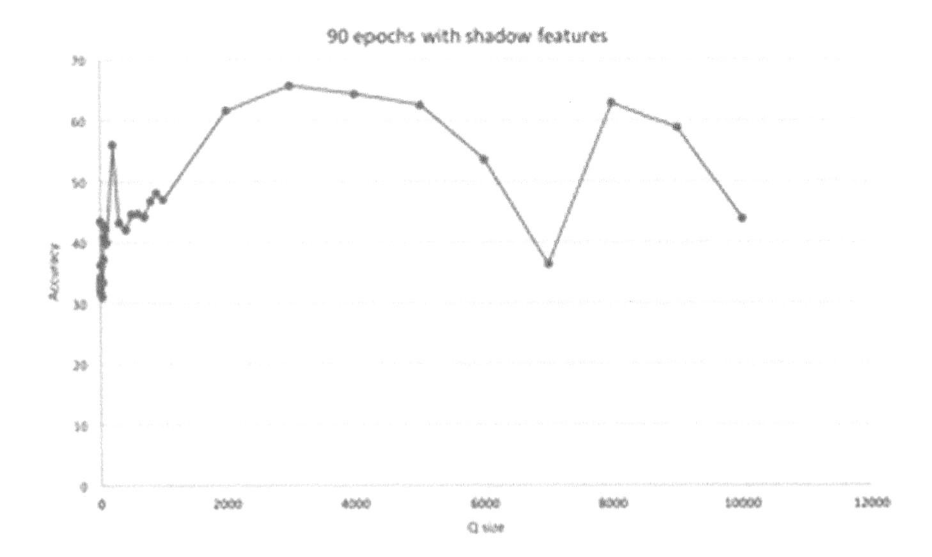

Fig. 31 Each neural network trained with 90 epochs

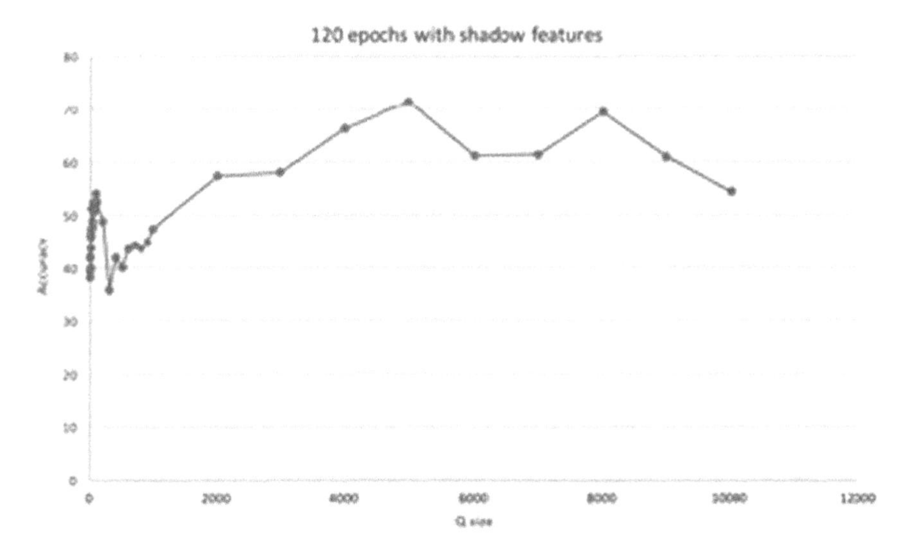

Fig. 32 Each neural network trained with 120 epochs

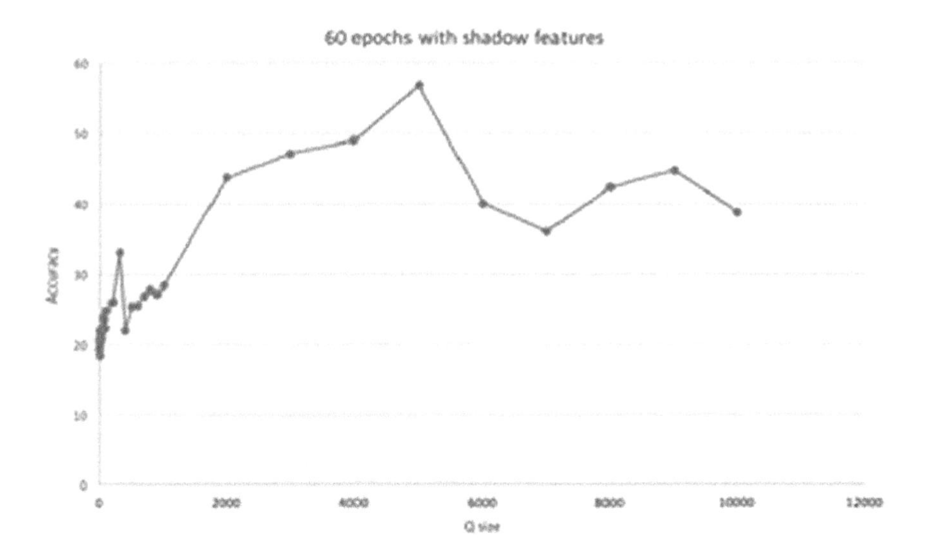

Fig. 33 Each neural network trained with 60 epochs

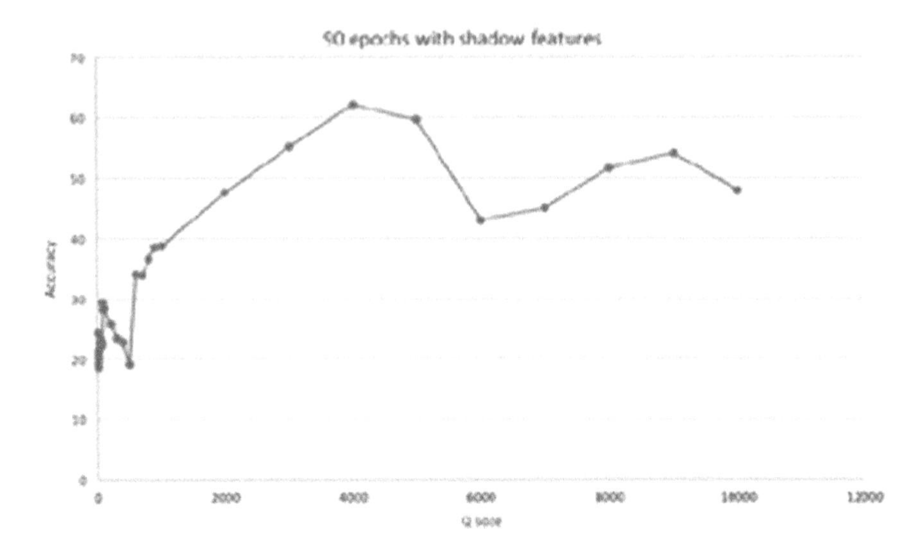

Fig. 34 Each neural network trained with 90 epochs

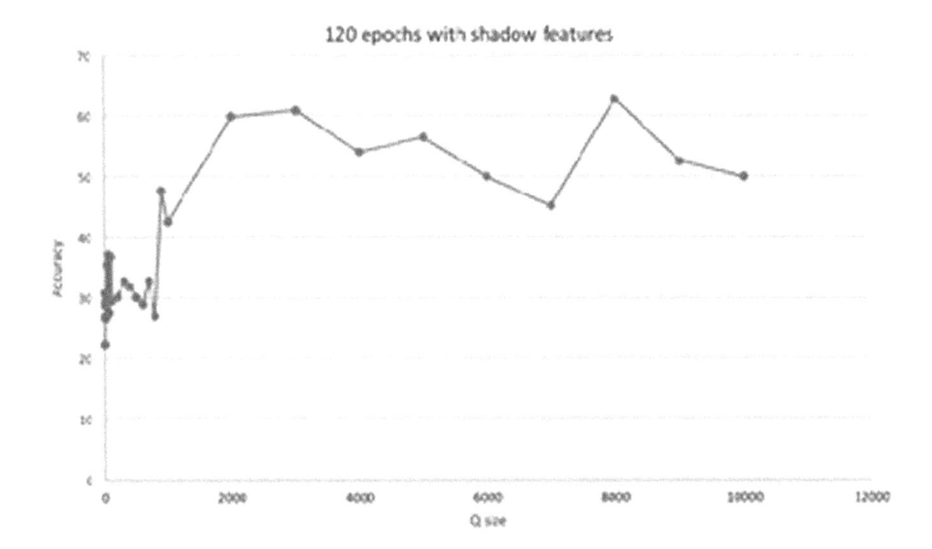

Fig. 35 Each neural network trained with 120 epochs

8 Conclusions

Unusual human activities (UHA) is a challenging machine learning problem, because of the dynamic and high speed sensing data that need to be processed quickly for inducing a prediction model. In this chapter, a novel pre-processing strategy called shadow features generation is proposed with the aim of improving the accuracy of the classifiers. The concept of shadow features is founded on the observations that bodily movements follow some flows of motions similar to the animation in chronophotography. in addition spatial information that are fed continuously to training a classification model, shadow features are inferred from them adding extra dimensions of information in terms of temporal sequence. In addition to the shadow feature strategy, we also proposed a new training model for Neural Networks which is ensemble of networks trained on the GPU. Instead of having one single Neural Networks trying to predict *M* classes of human activities, we can have *M* neural networks working together with each one focused on learning how to predict 1 out of *M* classes and when the *M* Neural Networks work together they can have a higher overall accuracy in predicting all the *M* classes. The computation costs incurred by using multiple neural networks are relieved by the parallel processing of GPU. The presented model showed good results. We also expect that implementing the machine learning computations on GPU opens a new IoT-enabled opportunity for development of ambient intelligence applications and smart services in mobile healthcare.

Acknowledgments The authors are thankful for the financial support from the Research Grant called “A scalable data stream mining methodology: stream-based holistic analytics and reasoning in parallel”, Grant no. FDCT-126/2014/A3, offered by the University of Macau, FST, RDAO and the FDCT of Macau SAR government. The work of D. Korzun is financially supported by Russian Fund for Basic Research (RFBR) according to research project # 16-07-01289.

References

1. Suvagiya, P.H., Bhatt, C.M., Patel, R.P.: Indian sign language translator using Kinect. In: Proceedings of International Conference on ICT for Sustainable Development, Vol. 2, February 2016, pp. 15–23 (2016)
2. Kim, E., Hetal, S., Cook, D.: Unusual human activities and pattern discovery. IEEE Pervasive Comput. **9**(1), 48–53 (2010)
3. Lara, O.D., Labrador, M.A.: A survey on human activity recognition using wearable sensors. IEEE Commun. Surv. Tutor. **15**(3), 1192–1209 (2011)
4. Tapia, E.M., Intille, S.S., Larson, K.: Activity recognition in the house using simple and ubiquitous sensors, LNCS. Pervasive Comput. **3001**, 158–175 (2002)
5. Max, A.B., Blanke, U., Schiele, B.: A tutorial on unusual human activities using body-worn inertial sensors. ACM Comput. Surv. **46**(3), Article No. 33 (2014)
6. Leo, M., D’Orazio, T., Spagnolo, P.: Human activity recognition for automatic visual surveillance of wide areas. Proceedings of the ACM 2nd International Workshop on Video Surveillance and Sensor Networks, pp. 124–130. ACM, New York, NY, USA (2004)

7. Chan, J.H., Visutarrom, T., Cho, S.-B., Engchuan, W., Mongolnam, P., Fong, S.: A hybrid approach to human posture classification during TV watching. J. Med. Imaging Health Inf. (American Scientific Publishers). ISSN: 2156-7018 (Accepted for publication) (2016)
8. Song, W., Lu, Z., Li, J., Li, J., Liao, J., Cho, K., Um, K.: Hand Gesture Detection and Tracking Methods Based on Background Subtraction, Future Information Technology. Lecture Notes in Electrical Engineering, Vol. 309, pp. 485–490 (2014)
9. Kim, Y., Sim, S., Cho, S., Lee, W., Jeong, Y.-S., Cho, K., Um, K.: Intuitive NUI for Controlling Virtual Objects Based on Hand Movements, Future Information Technology. Lecture Notes in Electrical Engineering, Vol. 309, pp. 457–461 (2014)
10. Mantyjarvi, J., Res, N., Center, F., Himberg, J., Seppanen, T.: Recognizing human motion with multiple acceleration sensors. IEEE Int. Conf. Syst. Man Cybernet. **2**(2001), 747–752 (2001)
11. Yang, J.: Towards physical activity diary: motion recognition using simple acceleration features with mobile phones. In: IMCE International Workshop on Interactive Multimedia for Consumer Electronics, pp. 1–10 (2009)
12. Brito, R., Fong, S., Cho, K., Song, W., Wong, R., Mohammed, S., Fiaidhi, J.: GPU-enabled back-propagation artificial neural network for digit recognition in parallel. J. Supercomput. 1–19 (2016)
13. The J. Paul Getty Museum: Photography: Discovery and Invention. ISBN 0-89236-177-8 (1990)
14. Vishwakarma, D.K., Rawat, P., Kapoor, R.: Unusual human activities using gabor wavelet transform and Ridgelet transform. In: 3rd International Conference on Recent Trends in Computing 2015 (ICRTC-2015), Vol. 57, pp. 630–636 (2015)
15. Hornik, K., Stinchcombe, M., White, H.: Multilayer feedforward networks are universal approximators. Neural Netw. **2**(5), 359–366 (1989)
16. Hornik, K.: Approximation capabilities of multilayer feedforward networks. Neural Netw. **4**(2), 251–257 (1991)
17. Svozil, D., Kvasnicka, V., Pospichal, J.: Introduction to multi-layer feed-forward neural networks. Chemometr. Intell. Lab. Syst. **39**(1), 43–62 (1997)
18. Jeng, J.J., Li, W.: Feedforward backpropagation artificial neural networks on reconfigurable meshes. Future Gen. Comput. Syst. **14**(5–6), 313–319 (1998)
19. Rudolph, G.L., Martinez, T.R.: A transformation strategy for implementing distributed, multi-layer feed-forward neural networks: backpropagation transformation. Future Gen. Comput. Syst. **12**(6), 547–564 (1997)

Printed in the United States
By Bookmasters